D1083137

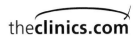

HEMATOLOGY/ ONCOLOGY CLINICS OF NORTH AMERICA

Multiple Myeloma

GUEST EDITOR
Kenneth C. Anderson, MD

December 2007 • Volume 21 • Number 6

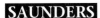

An Imprint of Elsevier, Inc.
PHILADELPHIA   LONDON   TORONTO   MONTREAL   SYDNEY   TOKYO

W.B. SAUNDERS COMPANY
A Division of Elsevier Inc.

Elsevier Inc. • 1600 John F. Kennedy Boulevard • Suite 1800 • Philadelphia, Pennsylvania 19103-2899

http://www.hemonc.theclinics.com

**HEMATOLOGY/ONCOLOGY CLINICS
OF NORTH AMERICA**
December 2007
Editor: Kerry Holland

Volume 21, Number 6
ISSN 0889-8588
ISBN-13: 978-1-4160-5082-7
ISBN-10: 1-4160-5082-5

Reprints: For copies of 100 or more, of articles in this publication, please contact the Commercial Reprints Department, Elsevier Inc., 360 Park Avenue South, New York, New York 10010-1710. Tel. (212) 633-3813; Fax: (212) 462-1935; e-mail: reprints@elsevier.com.

The ideas and opinions expressed in *Hematology/Oncology Clinics of North America* do not necessarily reflect those of the Publisher. The Publisher does not assume any responsibility for any injury and/or damage to persons or property arising out of or related to any use of the material contained in this periodical. The reader is advised to check the appropriate medical literature and the product information currently provided by the manufacturer of each drug to be administered to verify the dosage, the method and duration of administration, or contraindications. It is the responsibility of the treating physician or other health care professional, relying on independent experience and knowledge of the patient, to determine drug dosages and the best treatment of the patient. Mention of any product in this issue should not be construed as endorsement by the contributors, editors, or the Publisher of the product or manufacturers' claims.

Hematology/Oncology Clinics (ISSN 0889-8588) is published bimonthly by Elsevier Inc., 360 Park Avenue South, New York, NY 10010-1710. Months of issue are February, April, June, August, October, and December. Business and Editorial Offices: 1600 John F. Kennedy Blvd., Suite 1800, Philadelphia, PA 19103-2899. Customer Service Office: 6277 Sea Harbor Drive, Orlando, FL 32887-4800. Periodicals postage paid at New York, NY and additional mailing offices. Subscription prices are $262.00 per year (US individuals), $392.00 per year (US institutions), $131.00 per year (US students), $297.00 per year (Canadian individuals), $470.00 per year (Canadian institutions), $166.00 per year (Canadian students), $332.00 per year (international individuals), $470.00 per year (international institutions), $166.00 per year (international students). International air speed delivery is included in all *Clinics* subscription prices. All prices are subject to change without notice. **POSTMASTER:** Send address changes to *Hematology/Oncology Clinics of North America*, Elsevier Periodicals Customer Service, 6277 Sea Harbor Drive, Orlando, FL 32887-4800. Customer Service: 1-800-654-2452 (US). From outside of the US, call 1-407-345-4000.

Hematology/Oncology Clinics of North America is covered in *Index Medicus, EMBASE/Excerpta Medica*, and *BIOSIS.*

Printed in the United States of America.

ELSEVIER
SAUNDERS

HEMATOLOGY/ONCOLOGY CLINICS
OF NORTH AMERICA

Multiple Myeloma

GUEST EDITOR

KENNETH C. ANDERSON, MD, Chief, Division of Hematologic Neoplasia; and
Director, Jerome Lipper Multiple Myeloma Center; and Director, LeBow Institute
for Myeloma Therapeutics, Dana-Farber Cancer Institute; and Kraft Family
Professor of Medicine, Harvard Medical School, Boston, Massachusetts

CONTRIBUTORS

KENNETH C. ANDERSON, MD, Chief, Division of Hematologic Neoplasia; and
Director, Jerome Lipper Multiple Myeloma Center; and Director, LeBow Institute
for Myeloma Therapeutics, Dana-Farber Cancer Institute; and Kraft Family
Professor of Medicine, Harvard Medical School, Boston, Massachusetts

JOAN BLADÉ, MD, Senior Consultant, Institute of Hematology and Oncology,
Postgraduate School of Hematology, Farreras-Valentí, Institute d'Investigacions
Biomèdiques August Pi i Sunyer, Hospital Clínic, Barcelona, Spain

DANIEL R. CARRASCO, MD, PhD, Assistant Professor of Medicine, Department
of Medical Oncology, Dana-Farber Cancer Institute, Harvard Medical School,
Boston, Massachusetts

DHARMINDER CHAUHAN, PhD, Jerome Lipper Myeloma Center, Department
of Medical Oncology, Dana-Farber Cancer Institute, Harvard Medical School,
Boston, Massachusetts

MELETIOS A. DIMOPOULOS, MD, Department of Clinical Therapeutics, University
of Athens, School of Medicine, Athens, Greece

ANGELA DISPENZIERI, MD, Professor of Medicine, Division of Hematology,
Mayo Clinic, Rochester, Minnesota

LORI A. EHRLICH, MD, PhD, Research Associate, Division of Hematology/Oncology,
Veterans Administration Pittsburgh Healthcare System, Pittsburgh, Pennsylvania

RAFAEL FONSECA, MD, Professor of Hematology; and Consultant, Mayo Clinic
Arizona, Scottsdale, Arizona

JEAN-LUC HAROUSSEAU, MD, Professor of Hematology; and Head of Departments,
Centre Hospitalier Universitaire Hôtel-Dieu, Place Alexis Ricordeau,
Nantes Cedex, France

TERU HIDESHIMA, MD, PhD, Jerome Lipper Multiple Myeloma Center, Department of Medical Oncology, Dana-Farber Cancer Institute, Harvard Medical School, Boston, Massachusetts

EFSTATHIOS KASTRITIS, MD, Department of Clinical Therapeutics, University of Athens, School of Medicine, Athens, Greece

STEFFEN KLIPPEL, PhD, Jerome Lipper Myeloma Center, Department of Medical Oncology, Dana-Farber Cancer Institute, Harvard Medical School, Boston, Massachusetts

ROBERT A. KYLE, MD, Consultant, Division of Hematology, Mayo Clinic; and Professor of Medicine; and Professor of Laboratory Medicine, College of Medicine, Mayo Clinic, Rochester, Minnesota

SUZANNE LENTZSCH, MD, PhD, Assistant Professor of Medicine, Division of Hematology/Oncology, Department of Medicine, University of Pittsburgh, Pittsburgh, Pennsylvania

DOUGLAS W. McMILLIN, PhD, Jerome Lipper Myeloma Center, Department of Medical Oncology, Dana-Farber Cancer Institute, Harvard Medical School, Boston, Massachusetts

NIKHIL C. MUNSHI, MD, Associate Director, Jerome Lipper Multiple Myeloma Center, Dana-Farber Cancer Institute; Associate Professor, Department of Medicine, Harvard Medical School, Boston, Massachusetts

CONSTANTINE S. MITSIADES, MD, PhD, Instructor of Medicine, Jerome Lipper Multiple Myeloma Center, Department of Medical Oncology, Dana-Farber Cancer Institute, Harvard Medical School, Boston, Massachusetts

ANTONIO PALUMBO, MD, Associate Professor of Medicine, Division of Hematology, University of Turin, Azienda Ospedaliera S. Giovanni Battista, Ospedale Molinette, Turin, Italy

RAO H. PRABHALA, PhD, Instructor, Department of Medicine, Brigham and Women's Hospital/Dana Farber Cancer Institute; Research Health Scientist, Division of Hematology/Oncology, Veterans Administration Boston Healthcare System, West Roxbury, Massachusetts

S. VINCENT RAJKUMAR, MD, Consultant; and Professor of Medicine, Division of Hematology; and Professor of Medicine, College of Medicine, Mayo Clinic, Rochester, Minnesota

PAUL G. RICHARDSON, MD, Jerome Lipper Myeloma Center, Department of Medical Oncology, Dana-Farber Cancer Institute, Harvard Medical School, Boston, Massachusetts

LAURA ROSIÑOL, MD, PhD, Hematology Specialist, Institute of Hematology and Oncology, Postgraduate School of Hematology, Farreras-Valentí, Institute d'Investigacions Biomèdiques August Pi i Sunyer, Hospital Clínic, Barcelona, Spain

G. DAVID ROODMAN, MD, PhD, Professor of Medicine, Division of Hematology/Oncology; and Vice Chair for Research, Department of Medicine, University of Pittsburgh; Division of Hematology/Oncology, Veterans Administration Pittsburgh Healthcare System; Director, Center for Bone Biology, University of Pittsburgh Medical Center, Pittsburgh, Pennsylvania

JESUS SAN MIGUEL, MD, PhD, Hematology Department, University Hospital of Salamanca, Center for Cancer Research, Salamanca, Spain

GIOVANNI TONON, MD, PhD, Instructor in Medicine, Medical Oncology, Dana Farber Cancer Institute, Harvard Medical School, Boston, Massachusetts

ELSEVIER
SAUNDERS

HEMATOLOGY/ONCOLOGY CLINICS
OF NORTH AMERICA

Multiple Myeloma

CONTENTS

VOLUME 21 • NUMBER 6 • DECEMBER 2007

Several genetic mechanisms underlying the pathogenesis of multiple myeloma have been elucidated in the past decade. In particular, the presence of two distinct karyotypic patterns, that identify two patient groups and drive different pathogenetic and prognostic paths in the development of myeloma, have been identified, and the role of reciprocal chromosomal translocations and cyclin dysregulation have been identified. Despite this progress, several questions of critical importance remain to be addressed for the understanding of the pathogenesis of multiple myeloma. For example, little is known about the role of the primary events, including cyclin D overexpression and multiple myeloma set domain activity in the early pathogenesis of the disease. The additional lesions that promote the evolution of monoclonal gammopathy of undetermined significance to multiple myeloma (MM) and, within MM, the progression toward a more aggressive and proliferative disease is only starting to emerge. The heterotypic relationship between the stroma and the MM plasma cells also has not been fully explored. The understanding of the biology of MM cancer stem cells and of the pathways driving their maintenance, proliferation, and differentiation is still in its infancy. Recent and ongoing high-resolution genomic studies are leading the way toward a more refined and conclusive understanding of this disease.

Multiple myeloma (MM) is viewed as a prototypic disease state for the study of how neoplastic cells interact with their local bone marrow (BM) microenvironment. This interaction reflects not only the osteotropic clinical behavior of MM and the clinical impact of the lytic bone lesions caused by its tumor cells but also underlines the broadly accepted notion that nonneoplastic cells of the BM can attenuate the activity of cytotoxic chemotherapy and glucocorticoids. This article summarizes the recent progress in characterization, at the molecular and cellular levels, of how the BM milieu interacts with MM cells and modifies their biologic behavior.

Multiple myeloma is a plasma cell malignancy characterized by the frequent development of osteolytic bone lesions. The multiple myeloma–induced bone destruction is a result of the increased activity of osteoclasts that occurs adjacent to multiple myeloma cells. This activity is accompanied by suppressed osteoblast differentiation and activity, resulting in severely impaired bone formation and development of devastating osteolytic lesions. Recently the biologic mechanism involved in the imbalance between osteoclast activation and osteoblast inhibition induced by multiple myeloma cells has begun to be clarified. In this article, the pathophysiology underlying the imbalanced bone remodeling and potential new strategies for the treatment of bone disease in multiple myeloma are reviewed.

Multiple myeloma (MM) remains incurable despite high-dose chemotherapy with stem cell support. There is need, therefore, for continuous efforts directed toward the development of novel rational-based therapeutics for MM, which requires a detailed knowledge of the mutations driving this malignancy. In improving the success rate of effective drug development, it is equally imperative that biologic systems be developed to better validate these target genes. Here we review the recent developments in the generation of mouse models of MM and their impact as preclinical models for designing and assessing target-based therapeutic approaches.

The bone marrow (BM) milieu confers drug resistance in multiple myeloma (MM) cells to conventional therapies. Novel biologically based therapies are therefore needed. Preclinical studies have identified and validated molecular targeted therapeutics in MM. In particular, recognition of the biologic significance of the BM microenvironment in MM pathogenesis and as a potential target for novel therapeutics has already derived several promising approaches. Thalidomide, lenalidomide

(Revlimid), and bortezomib (Velcade) are directed not only at MM cells but also at the BM milieu and have moved rapidly from the bench to the bedside and United States Food and Drug Administration approval to treat MM.

In 1978, the term "monoclonal gammopathy of undetermined significance" (MGUS) was introduced. MGUS is defined as a serum monoclonal (M) protein less than 3.0 g/dL; less than 10% plasma cells in the bone marrow, if done; little or no M protein in the urine; and absence of lytic bone lesions, anemia, hypercalcemia or renal insufficiency. This article discusses the recognition, prevalence, natural history, and progression of MGUS. Management of the disease is discussed along with its association with other disorders. Information on smoldering multiple myeloma is included.

The field of multiple myeloma prognostication is replete with studies that have shown the value of independent predictors in determining clinical outcome. It is clear that host factors and factors intrinsic to the cells are the ultimate determinants of prognosis. In the immediate period after diagnosis, those factors related to the host are likely to be more relevant, whereas with passing time factors intrinsic to the cells predominate. At a minimum, we recommend that a comprehensive molecular cytogenetic assessment be performed at diagnosis, together with conventional evaluation, including β_2-microglobulin and albumin. In addition, information on proliferative activity of plasma cells may be of value. The introduction of novel methods of prognostication should be strongly considered in all clinical trials.

The treatment of multiple myeloma has changed dramatically in the last decade with the introduction of thalidomide, bortezomib, and lenalidomide. Patients eligible for autologous stem cell transplantation (ASCT) are treated with non-alkylating agent–containing regimens as initial therapy; typically thalidomide-dexamethasone or lenalidomide-dexamethasone. For patients not eligible for ASCT, the current standard of care is melphalan, prednisone, and thalidomide. Ongoing trials will soon assess if combinations including melphalan and prednisone plus bortezomib or MP plus lenalidomide may be considered an attractive option. Patients who have risk factors, such as deletion 13 or translation t(4;14) or t(14;16), are candidates for novel, more aggressive treatments.

Jean-Luc Harousseau

Hematopoietic stem cell transplantation (SCT) was introduced in the treatment of multiple myeloma in the 1980s. In the autologous setting, the use of peripheral blood stem cells instead of bone marrow has markedly improved feasibility. In fit patients who have normal renal function and are younger than 65 years of age, randomized studies have shown the superiority of autologous stem cell transplantation (ASCT) compared with conventional chemotherapy. ASCT is now considered the standard of care in this population of patients. It is currently challenged, however, by the introduction of novel agents, such as thalidomide, bortezomib, and lenalidomide. The role of allogenic SCT remains controversial, even with reduced intensity conditionings. Prospective studies still are needed to evaluate the impact of both autologous and allogeneic SCT in this new era.

Efstathios Kastritis, Constantine S. Mitsiades,
Meletios A. Dimopoulos, and Paul G. Richardson

Studies of bortezomib, thalidomide, and lenalidomide have shown promising clinical activity in relapsed/refractory multiple myeloma (MM). Bortezomib alone and in combination with other agents is associated with high response rates, consistently high rates of complete response, and a predictable and manageable profile of adverse events. Thalidomide-based regimens have also shown substantial clinical activity. The accumulating experience from ongoing trials of bortezomib/lenalidomide/dexamethasone combinations in patients who have relapsed/refractory or newly diagnosed MM will provide critical information that will determine the possible role of this combination as the basic backbone for combination regimens for management of advanced MM.

Rao H. Prabhala and Nikhil C. Munshi

Immune cells with specific functions and abilities are vital to cancer treatment prevention. Although there have been many accomplishments made in the areas of immunotherapy and immunobiology of myeloma, there are still many obstacles in the way of conceptualizing the interrelationships between immune cells and tumor cells. To provide better understanding of these concepts and to move toward improved therapies for myeloma, cell-based therapeutic approaches should be developed.

Multiple myeloma, also known as myeloma or plasma cell myeloma, is a progressive hematologic disease. Complications of multiple myeloma include renal insufficiency, hematologic complications (anemia, bone marrow failure, bleeding disorders), infections, bone complications (pathologic fractures, spinal cord compression, hyercalcemia), and neurologic complications (spinal cord and nerve root compression, intracranial plasmacytomas, leptomeningeal involvement, among others). This article reviews these various complications connected to multiple myeloma, examining their various causes and possible treatment.

The advent of new therapies for multiple myeloma brings new hope for patients but also new side effects. Emerging information about the risks of supportive care therapies, including long-term, high-intensity bisphosphonate use and erythropoiesis-stimulating agents, is examined. As the number of drugs in the myeloma armamentarium grows, so does the list of possible side effects and interactions. With current progress, not only are there more complications to consider but patients are also living longer and the risk for delayed complications is becoming more relevant. The author provides perspective about the risks for the most active and commonly used single-agent and combination myeloma therapies.

HEMATOLOGY/ONCOLOGY CLINICS
OF NORTH AMERICA

ELSEVIER
SAUNDERS

HEMATOLOGY/ONCOLOGY CLINICS
OF NORTH AMERICA

Preface

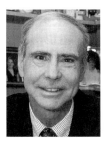

Kenneth C. Anderson, MD

Guest Editor

This issue of *Hematology/Oncology Clinics of North America* highlights the major advances in the biology of multiple myeloma (MM), which have markedly enhanced our understanding of disease pathogenesis and led to improved treatments and patient outcomes. Dr. Giovanni Tonon describes advances in our understanding of molecular pathogenesis, which have allowed for improved diagnosis, prognosis, and targeted therapies. Drs. Constantine Mitsiades and Suzanne Lentzsch review characterization of the role of the bone marrow (BM) microenvironment in tumor cell growth, survival, and drug resistance, and in mechanisms of bone disease in MM. These advances have allowed for development of in vitro models of the MM cell in its BM microenvironment, which have facilitated identification and validation of novel therapies targeting the MM cell, MM cell-host interaction, and BM milieu, as reviewed by Dr. Teru Hideshima. Finally, Dr. Mitsiades highlights advances in the genomics of MM in the BM, which have allowed for the generation of novel genetically-based preclinical in vivo models of MM.

Dr. Robert A. Kyle describes these advances in the oncogenomics of MM that have translated rapidly from the bench to bedside, which permit delineation of the pattern of genetic and clinical changes correlating with progression from normal to monoclonal gammopathy of undetermined significance to MM. These advances also have provided the framework for novel prognostic staging systems within MM, which are summarized by Dr. Rafael Fonseca. Novel therapies targeting the tumor cell in its BM microenvironment, including thalidomide, lenalidomide, and bortezomib, have now been validated in preclinical models and rapidly evaluated in derived clinical trials culminating in their Federal Drug Administration approval. Dr. S. Vincent Rajkumar summarizes how, already, these models have been integrated into the treatment

0889-8588/07/$ – see front matter
doi:10.1016/j.hoc.2007.08.012

paradigm of MM and have improved the extent and frequency of response in
initial therapy in elderly patients who have MM. Importantly, Dr. Jean-Luc
Harousseau describes their use as initial therapy prior to transplant and as
maintenance treatment to prolong progression free and overall survival posttransplant. Dr. Efstathios Kastritis updates the use of these agents alone and
in combination, and novel targeted therapies in the treatment of relapsed/
refractory MM. Dr. Nikhil Munshi describes the advances in oncogenomics
that also have allowed for improved immune therapies for MM, including both
vaccine and adoptive immunotherapy. Finally, Drs. Joan Bladé and Angela
Dispenzieri review advances in the recognition and mechanisms of disease
complications, which have allowed for improved strategies for their avoidance
and treatment.

This new biologically-based treatment paradigm targeting the tumor cell in
its microenvironment has great promise to markedly improve patient outcome
not only in MM, but also in other hematologic cancers and solid tumors as
well.

Kenneth C. Anderson, MD
Jerome Lipper Multiple Myeloma Center
Department of Medical Oncology
Dana-Farber Cancer Institute
Harvard Medical School
44 Binney Street
Boston, MA 02115, USA

E-mail address: kenneth_anderson@dfci.harvard.edu

Hematol Oncol Clin N Am 21 (2007) 985–1006

HEMATOLOGY/ONCOLOGY CLINICS
OF NORTH AMERICA

Molecular Pathogenesis of Multiple Myeloma

Giovanni Tonon, MD, PhD

Medical Oncology, Dana Farber Cancer Institute, Harvard Medical School,
Mayer Building, Rm.417, 44 Binney Street, Boston, MA 02115, USA

Multiple myeloma (MM) is a hematologic tumor characterized by clonal proliferation of neoplastic plasma cells in the bone marrow in association with elevated serum or urine monoclonal paraprotein levels. MM is associated, particularly in the most advanced forms, with increasingly severe clinical manifestations, including lytic bone lesions, anemia, immunodeficiency, and renal impairment. MM accounts for more than 10% of all hematologic malignancies and is the second most frequent hematologic cancer in the United States after non-Hodgkin lymphoma. MM is typically, but not always, preceded by an age-progressive condition termed monoclonal gammopathy of undetermined significance (MGUS), a condition present in 1% of adults older than 25 years of age, that progresses to malignant MM at a rate of 0.5% to 3% per year [1–5].

MM remains incurable despite conventional high-dose chemotherapy with stem cell support. Novel agents, such as thalidomide, the immunoregulatory drug Revlimid, and the proteasome inhibitor bortezomib, can achieve responses in patients who have relapsed and refractory MM; however, the median survival remains at 6 years, with only 10% of patients surviving at 10 years [6–8].

OVERVIEW OF THE GENETIC LESIONS PRESENT IN MULTIPLE MYELOMA

In the last decade significant progress has been made in understanding the pathogenesis of MM, attributable to new conceptual breakthroughs and the availability of new technologies, such as spectral karyotyping, fluorescence in situ hybridization (FISH), expression profiling, and most recently array comparative genomic hybridization (aCGH).

This work was supported by the International Myeloma Foundation (Brian D. Novis Research Award) and by the Fund to Cure Myeloma. Giovanni Tonon is a Special Fellow of the Leukemia and Lymphoma Society.

E-mail address: giovanni_tonon@dfci.harvard.edu

0889-8588/07/$ – see front matter
doi:10.1016/j.hoc.2007.08.004

MM as it is conceived now is a disease characterized by a peculiar constellation of specific genetic lesions that include specific chromosome gains or losses and Ig-related chromosomal translocation. Moreover, gains or losses of small chromosomal segments and genetic and epigenetic changes affecting single genes have been reported. Although several aspects on the pathogenesis of MM remain to be elucidated, a conceptual framework for a classification of MM is now possible based on whole chromosome gains and losses, chromosomal translocations, transcription profiling, and the specific expression of cyclin D genes [5,9–12]. This pattern of genetic changes is unique in MM and has no similarities in any other tumor, either of hematologic, mesenchymal, or epithelial origin, with the possible exception of ALL [13] (see later discussion).

A first major distinction is between hyperdiploid (HD) versus non-hyperdiploid (NHD) MM (Fig. 1). Following up on previous observations [14,15], Smadja and colleagues [12] proposed in 1998 a distinction between patients presenting a hyperdiploid karyotype (number of chromosomes from 48 to 74) with concomitant gains of several odd chromosomes, such as 3, 5, 7, 9, 11, 15, 19, 21, in various combinations, and a second NHD group, with hypodiploid, pseudodiploid, near-diploid, or tetraploid karyotypes. HD MM includes 50% to 60% of patients and presents a more favorable prognosis [16,17]. This distinctive pattern is present also in MGUS [18] and rarely changes during disease progression [19]. An unsupervised approach to aCGH data using non-negative matrix factorization (NMF) [20] has confirmed the existence of these two groups within patients who have MM [10].

Alongside chromosomal gains and losses, MM often presents specific chromosomal translocations affecting the immunoglobulin locus, called primary

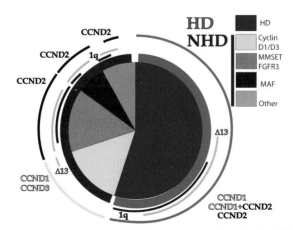

Fig. 1. Classification of multiple myeloma based on cytogenetic, expression arrays, and aCGH. This representation is oversimplified; in particular the frequency of gains of 1q and deletions of chromosome 13 and the degree of overlapping between the two lesions in the different groups is under active investigation.

translocations because they are usually present from the inception of the disease [5,21]. These translocations, which involve the immunoglobulin H (IgH) locus (at 14q32.3) [22] and less frequently the IgL locus (2p12, kappa or 22q11, lambda) [23], juxtapose strong Ig enhancers to various genes leading to their expression dysregulation [21]. These rearrangements seem in general to be mutually exclusive, although in 5% of MGUS and 25% of advanced MM cases two independent translocations can be found in the same patient [9]. Among the most recurrent rearrangements, two directly increase the expression of cyclins: t(11;14)(q13;q32), which occurs in 15% to 20% of patients who have MM, induces cyclin D1 overexpression [24–28]; and t(6;14)(p21;q32), present in 2% to 3% of MM cases, increases the expression of cyclin D3 [29]. Another translocation, t(4;14)(p16.3;q32), is present in approximately 15% of patients [30–32] and dysregulates the expression of the Wolf-Hirschhorn syndrome candidate 1 gene (*WHSC1*, also known as multiple myeloma set domain [*MMSET*]), which encodes a protein with homology to histone methyltransferases; and the receptor tyrosine kinase fibroblast growth factor receptor 3 (*FGFR3*) gene. A small subset of t(4;14) patients develops activating mutations of FGFR3 [33,34] (see later discussion). Finally, the t(14;16)(q32;q23) dysregulates the oncogene *MAF*, a basic leucine zipper transcription factor, in 5% to 10% of patients [35]; and the t(14;20) affects another member of this family, *MAFB*, in 2% to 5% of cases [5,36]. Subsequent studies [17,37] have uncovered a strong association between these primary translocations and NHD [17]. It is therefore possible to distinguish patients who have MM into two major groups, HD and NHD, and within the NHD further subdivide them based on the presence of primary chromosomal translocations (see Fig. 1). It should be emphasized that this distinction, useful as it is, it is nevertheless an oversimplification, because primary translocations are present also in the HD group, at a frequency of approximately 10%.

Recent comprehensive surveys of expression profiling have provided a strong support for this framework and added important insights into the pathogenesis of the different groups [9,11]. In one study, unsupervised hierarchical clustering on 414 patients has identified seven groups of patients [11]. Among these, five very closely recapitulated the HD category and within the NHD, the *c-MAF* and *MAFB*, *CCND1*, and *CCND3* (in two separate but close clusters including both genes), and t(4;14) translocation subsets. Another cluster, defined as low bone disease (LB) included in the "other" group in Fig. 1, did not present any expression features reminiscent of hallmark genetic lesions, and was characterized by low incidence of osteolytic lesions. Finally, the seventh group included patients who had the poorest overall and event-free survival and was characterized by overexpression of proliferation-associated genes, often mapping to the long arm of chromosome 1. Intriguingly, a subset of patients included in this cluster presented, alongside the overexpression of genes associated with proliferation, overexpression of genes distinctive of the HD or of the primary translocation groups. These findings suggest that patients presenting with primary lesions could progress toward a more aggressive disease, after the acquisition of additional genetic lesions, potentially including 1q gains/amplifications or 1p losses/deletions.

This classification based on genetic lesions and expression profiling matches closely with a recent classification centered on the expression of cyclins in MM (TC classification) [9]. HD patients usually show overexpression of cyclin D1, alone or in combination with overexpression of cyclin D2 (D1 and D1+D2 groups according to the TC classification), albeit at levels much lower than the ones present in the t(11;14). A subset of HD patients instead produces cyclin D2 alone. In addition to overexpression of cyclin D1 and D3 in patients who have t(11;14) and t(6;14), respectively, patients who have t(4;14), t(14;16), and t(14;20) often present cyclin D2 overexpression that in the t(14;16) and t(14;20) patients has been directly linked to c-MAF/MAFB dysregulation (see Fig. 1) [9].

Over this general framework, additional genetic or epigenetic modifications are present in the MM genome, sometimes preferentially linked to specific groups of patients or endowed with prognostic relevance. These lesions involve chromosomal regions (such as the short and long arm of chromosome 1, chromosome 13, or the short arm of chromosome 17, where the tumor suppressor TP53 is located), or single genes (such as mutations of oncogenes like members of the RAS family and FGFR3, or mutations of members of the RB1 family); chromosomal rearrangements affecting c-MYC; dysregulated expression of DKK1 and other genes; and finally focal gains/amplifications or losses/deletions, whose mechanistic, pathogenetic, and clinical relevance has not been established as yet.

THE MOLECULAR BASIS OF THE EVOLUTION FROM MONOCLONAL GAMMOPATHY OF UNDETERMINED SIGNIFICANCE TO MULTIPLE MYELOMA

The mechanisms underlying the progression from MGUS to MM are still incompletely understood. From a genetic standpoint the two conditions are remarkably similar. Both present a similar incidence of HD/NHD karyotypes [1] and of IgH/IgL chromosomal translocations, along with deletion of chromosome 13 [38–40]. Also at the expression level, the two conditions are remarkably similar. Several studies have failed to identify significantly different patterns of expression between MGUS and MM [41,42]. Interestingly, Zhan and colleagues [43] have been able to show how a subset of MM, featuring a better prognosis, had an expression signature similar to MGUS. On the other hand, a small subset of MGUS clustered together with MM, pointing to a subset of MGUS patients potentially more prone to evolve into MM.

Among the few genetic changes reported in MM and not present (or present with a lower incidence) in MGUS, two members of RAS family (NRAS and KRAS) are mutated at codons 12, 13, and 61 in 40% to 55% of patients who have MM versus only 5% in MGUS [44–49], suggesting a major role for the activation of the mitogen-activated protein kinase (MAPK) pathway in the progression from MGUS to MM. The t(4;14) seems to be more often present in

MM than in MGUS [9,39,43,50–52], albeit one study has found similar frequencies between the two conditions [38].

HYPERDIPLOID MULTIPLE MYELOMA

Little is known about the mechanisms driving oncogenesis in this group. Analyses of expression data have shown how HD presents a consistent over-expression of cyclin D1 or D2, albeit a clear pathogenetic role of these cyclins in this subgroup is lacking [9]. The pattern of odd chromosome gains suggests a gene dosage effect resulting in the concomitant dysregulation of several oncogenic pathways. Indeed, expression profiling comparisons between HD versus NHD have suggested increased expression of genes involved in protein synthesis and defective protein catabolism and transport in this group of patients [53,54].

Overall, this group presents a better prognosis when compared with NHD MM [16,55,56]. Recent studies, however, have identified subgroups of HD patients presenting with prognosis comparable with NHD patients [10,57]. For example, gNMF have identified a subgroup of patients within the HD group characterized, in addition to gains of odd-number chromosomes, by loss of chromosome 13 or gains in 1q [10]. Moreover, this group presented less frequently gains on chromosome 11. These patients presented a significantly worse event-free survival, and a trend toward worse overall survival when compared with HD patients without 1q gains/amplifications or 13 loss. Other recent studies have corroborated these findings. In a recent report using FISH and expression arrays, unsupervised clustering has confirmed the existence of two groups within the HD, one presenting preferential gains on chromosome 11 and the second one with losses of chromosome 13 and gains of 1q [53], with enrichment for genes mapping to 11 and 1q, respectively, in each group. This group of patients may represent an evolution of HD toward a more aggressive, high-proliferative disease, as suggested by Zhan and colleagues [11]. Another study has identified four subgroups within HD [54]. Of particular interest was cluster 1, associated with high proliferation and poor prognosis when compared with the other clusters and enriched for genes mapping to chromosome 1q. Although the prognostic relevance of 1q gains/amplifications in this subgroup of patients seems to be relatively solid, the prognostic significance of the deletion of chromosome 13 in the context of HD remains controversial [16,55,57]. Other genetic lesions in HD have been linked to poor prognosis in this group, as for example IgH translocations, especially those involving unknown partners [57]. These additional translocations, along with monosomies, are likely arising later in tumor development [58].

NON-HYPERDIPLOID MULTIPLE MYELOMA

FISH, expression array analyses, and more recently aCGH, have been able to classify these patients into several different groups, closely matching the presence of translocations and dysregulated expression of the genes at the breakpoints and members of the cyclin family (TC classification). An oversimplified but nevertheless useful classification of this group of patients could therefore be inferred from the presence of chromosomal translocations (see Fig. 1).

The presence of chromosomal abnormalities in MM has been recognized for a long time, since the 1980s, but a coherent model for their pathogenetic relevance in MM was lacking. In the early 1990s, a few seminal papers identified conclusively the most recurrent translocations and elucidated their anatomy. In particular, it was shown that chromosomal translocations in mouse plasmacytomas affected the immunoglobulin heavy chain (IgH) switch regions [59]. Bergsagel and colleagues [22] demonstrated that a similar mechanism was present also in the human disease. One of the hallmark features of B-cell tumors, including MM, versus other hematologic disease is the almost exclusive pattern of translocations, which does not involve the formation of fusion chimeric proteins as seen in several leukemias and lymphomas, but leads to the dysregulated expression of oncogenes induced by the juxtaposition of the oncogene promoters with Ig regulatory elements. Indeed, the B cell–specific mechanisms of switch recombination and somatic hypermutation have been implicated in the generation of these translocations in MM, in various degrees [5,21]. Shortly thereafter, several oncogenes whose expression was dysregulated by chromosomal translocations were identified. It should be emphasized, however, that with the exception of FGFR3 and MAF the oncogenic role of the genes dysregulated by the different chromosomal translocations have not been experimentally proven (see later discussion).

Translocations Affecting Cyclins

The t(11;14)(q13;q32) dysregulates the expression of the cyclin D1 gene [24–27], with an incidence of approximately 15% in MGUS [38,39] and in MM [50,60]. Another translocation, t(6;14)(p21;q32), induces the dysregulation of cyclin D3 in 2% to 3% of patients who have MM [29]. In a recent expression survey, Zhan and colleagues [11] have shown how cyclin D1 and D3 tumors tend to cluster together. Among the patients who had these translocations two clusters were present, each presenting t(11;14) and t(6;14) translocations. No difference in clinical parameters or survival between the two groups was evident, and the pathogenetic and clinical implications of this distinction are still unclear. Overall, patients who have cyclin D translocations tend to present a better prognosis than NHD patients who have t(4;14), t(14;16), and t(14;20). The pathogenetic consequences of these translocations remain unclear.

t(4;14) and Fibroblast Growth Factor Receptor 3 and Multiple Myeloma Set Domain

Another translocation, t(4;14), affects approximately 15% of patients [51,61] and presents a peculiar anatomy, as a result of an error in IgH switch recombination ([30–32] and [62] for a recent and comprehensive review on t(4;14) in MM). As a result of the translocation, the enhancers, 5' Eμ and 3' Eα are separated and dysregulate the expression of the juxtaposed genes on both derivative chromosomes, at der(4) and der(14). On der(14), the 3′ Ea enhancer dysregulates the expression of the receptor tyrosine kinase FGFR3 gene. On der(4), the 5′ Em enhancer drives the expression of the *WHSC1* gene, also called *MMSET*, which encodes a protein with homology to histone methyltransferases. Approximately 10% of the patients who have t(4;14) also develop activating mutations on FGFR3 [33,34].

Although MMSET is almost always up-regulated in patients presenting with t(4;14) [63], FGFR3 is not overexpressed in up to 25% of patients [11,51,64–66] suggesting that in patients who have t(4;14) the prominent oncogenic role is exerted by MMSET and not by FGFR3. On the other hand, several preclinical studies have demonstrated the oncogenic potential of the activated form of FGFR3 (present in less than 10% of the t(4;14) patients). Gain-of-function studies have consistently demonstrated the oncogenic potential of most of the mutated forms of FGFR3. Ligand-stimulated interleukin-6 (IL-6)–dependent murine B9 cells expressing wild-type FGFR3 proliferated in the absence of IL-6, whereas the growth of B9 cells transfected with mutant FGFR3 was independent from the presence of either FGF or IL-6 [67]. Most mutated forms of FGFR3, but not the wild type, were able to induce the formation of foci and tumors in nude mice after transfection of NIH3T3 cells [33,68]. Irradiated mice injected with bone marrow hematopoietic cells infected with mutant forms of FGFR3 developed transplantable tumors within 6 weeks, whereas WT FGFR3 induced the appearance of tumors only after 1 year [69]. Specific FGFR3 inhibitors have been shown to reduce proliferation and increase apoptosis in t(4;14) MM cell lines with activated FGFR3 [70–73] and in patients who have t(4;14). The usefulness of FGFR3 inhibitors in the treatment of t(4;14) patients in the absence of activated FGFR3 therefore remains to be established.

No studies have so far firmly established the role of MMSET in MM pathogenesis. MMSET interacts with and is likely involved in pathways with a clear relevance in carcinogenesis. For example, the helix-loop-helix transcription factor inhibitor of differentiation 1 (ID-1) has been identified as a target of MMSET [66], and different isoforms of MMSET interact with HDAC1 and Sin3b [74]. The two homologs of MMSET have strong links to cancers. Specifically, WHSC1L1 is involved in a chromosomal translocation in acute myeloid leukemia, t(8;11)(p11.2;p15) [75], is amplified in breast cancer [76] and in lung cancer, and is endowed with oncogenic activity ([77] and Giovanni Tonon, MD, PhD, unpublished data, 2005). The other homolog, NSD1, has been implicated in acute myeloid leukemia [78].

The t(4;14) has been clearly linked to poor prognosis in several studies [51,79–83].

MAF and MAFB Translocations

The t(14;16)(q32.3;q23) is present in approximately 5% to 10% of patients who have MM [5,84] and induces overexpression of the oncogene c-MAF [35], whereas the (14;20)(q32;q11) has been reported in 2% to 5% of MM cases and affects the homolog MAFB [5,36]. Both translocations are associated with a similar expression signature [11], suggesting a shared repository of downstream targets. Surprisingly, overexpression of c-MAF has been reported even in the absence of the translocation [85,86], albeit the mechanism remains unclear. The oncogenic role of c-MAF has been clearly established. Forced overexpression of c-MAF enhances myeloma proliferation, likely through one of its target genes, cyclin D2, that is consistently overexpressed in this group of patients [9]. Inhibition of c-maf blocked tumor formation in immunodeficient mice. Another target of c-maf, integrin b7, was able to increase myeloma adhesion to bone marrow stroma and increased production of VEGF. It seems, therefore, that c-MAF is able to stimulate cell cycle progression and alter bone marrow stromal interactions. An additional report has proposed ARK5, an AMP-activated protein kinase (AMPK)–related protein kinase mediating Akt signals, as a target of c-MAF and MAFB signaling [87].

Previous reports have shown a reduced incidence of bone disease in this group of patients [9,11]. Recent publications point to two genes potentially responsible for this phenotype. The gene DKK1, whose overexpression has been implicated in MM-related bone disease [88], is significantly down-regulated in this group of patients [11]. Moreover Robbiani and colleagues [89] have recently reported that the gene osteopontin (OPN) inversely correlates with MM bone disease and is specifically overexpressed in patients who have translocations affecting the MAF genes.

Although not as clearly as in the case of t(4;14), translocations affecting MAF have also been linked to poor prognosis [11,79].

ADDITIONAL FOCAL GENETIC LESIONS

aCGH studies have identified focal, recurrent, high-amplitude copy number aberrations (CNAs) in cell lines and primary MM tumors [10,90–92]. For example, in a recent study [10], 87 minimal common regions (MCRs) were identified, based on the criteria of presence in primary tumors and occurrence of at least one high-amplitude event: 47 amplifications and 40 deletions, spanning a median size of 0.89 Mb with an average of 12 known genes. Among these lesions, MCRs of known pathogenetic relevance, such as deletion of a region including the TP53 tumor suppressor and focal amplifications of areas including the hepatocyte growth factor (HGF) gene and the MYC and ABL1 oncogenes, were included. As copy number alterations function to alter expression of resident genes, a gene weight measure was conducted merging aCGH results and expression profiling for the genes residing within the amplicons. A similar analysis was attempted also for the deleted loci; however, based on the behavior of TP53 that showed a variable level of overexpression in the presence of hemizygous deletions, as expected in cases presenting with TP53 mutations, genes residing within deletions were excluded from the analysis. For the amplified MCRs, the algorithm was modeled after the behavior of c-MYC, which demonstrated overexpression in patients with and without amplification when compared with the expression level in plasma cells from healthy donors, confirming that its expression is dysregulated by mechanisms other than gene dosage alteration. For each gene residing within an amplified MCR, therefore, only genes (Affymetrix probes) showing overexpression in the presence or the absence of amplification survived the screening. Genes showing this oncogene-like expression pattern were considered high-probability candidates targeted for amplification in these MCRs during MM development. By such criteria, only approximately 30% of the 2151 Affymetrix probes residing in the amplified MCRs survived this screening, including genes with established roles in MM pathogenesis, such as MYC, MCL1, IL6R, HGF, and ABL1, and many functionally diverse genes with no known link to MM development. Stringent validation studies are needed to demonstrate the relevance and validate the oncogenic potential of the candidate genes emerging from aCGH studies, but, as in other diseases, aCGH merged with expression data and compared with the expression level of appropriate controls seems to provide an important tool for uncovering novel tumorigenic genes and pathways.

OTHER GENETIC LESIONS PRESENT IN MULTIPLE MYELOMA ASSOCIATED WITH PROGRESSION AND PROGNOSIS

HD and NHD, along with specific chromosomal translocations, have been linked to prognosis (see previous discussion). Several other chromosomal aberrations and lesions affecting single genes have been reported to be linked with poor prognosis. Additionally, some lesions, prominent among them gains/amplification on 1q, drive increased proliferation, a pattern that has been long recognized in all cancers [93]. In MM, according to a recent study by Zhan and colleagues [11], patients characterized by different translocations and patients in the HD group could evolve toward a pattern characterized by expression of genes associated with high proliferation and poor prognosis. It should be emphasized that any consideration of prognostic markers depends heavily on the treatment regimen. Most of the studies assessing the prognostic relevance of genetic lesions included patients treated with high-dose chemotherapy, eventually associated with bone marrow transplant. In a recent study conducted in patients treated with bortezomib several of the most well-established genetic prognostic markers failed to show any correlation with prognosis in patients treated with this drug [94].

1q Gains/Amplifications

Gains and amplifications in the long arm of chromosome 1 have been identified in several studies [92,95–98], with a frequency of approximately 30% to 40% [99,100]. Jumping translocations, possibly related to highly decondensed pericentromeric heterochromatin, have been proposed as a potential mechanism leading to this aberration [96,101,102]. Gains/amplifications of 1q are associated with t(4;14), t(14;16), and possibly with chromosome 13 deletion [10,99], and associated with more proliferative disease [103]. Several studies have proposed an association between gains/amplification of this region and poor prognosis, based on cytogenetic analysis [104], FISH [37], expression profiling [103], and aCGH [10]. Importantly, Shaughnessy colleagues [105] have shown that among a list of 70 genes linked to early disease-related death, there was an enrichment for overexpressed genes mapping to chromosome 1q. Other studies, however, have questioned the prognostic relevance of this region [99,100]. Gains/amplifications of 1q have been associated with a subgroup of HD patients presenting with poor prognosis (see previous discussion).

The protein kinase CKS1B has been proposed as one of the genes residing in this region that could be the target of this amplification [106]. No focal amplifications or translocations that selectively target this gene have been reported; indeed the region amplified on 1q21 is usually rather extended, spanning several megabases ([10,92] and Giovanni Tonon, MD, PhD, unpublished data, 2006). On the other hand, gain-of-function studies based on the overexpression of CKS1B, and conversely loss-of-function studies with shRNA [106], suggest a role for CKS1B as one of the most promising targets of the amplification in 1q- positive MM cases.

Chromosome 13 Deletions

Tricot and colleagues [107] have for the first time highlighted the high incidence of deletions of chromosome 13 (Δ13) in MM and its potential role in prognosis. Subsequent studies have established that Δ13s are most often hemizygous, tend to affect the whole chromosome 13 in more than 85% to 90% of the patients [92,108,109], and are present in MGUS and MM with a similar overall incidence of around 50% [38,39,79,110–113]. Moreover, there seems to be a strong correlation between the presence of Δ13 and other genetic lesions [50,114], including t(4;14), t(14;16), NHD, and in a subset of HD characterized by poor prognosis, gains of 1q [10] (albeit not all the samples with 1q gains presented Δ13 and vice versa, Giovanni Tonon, MD, PhD, unpublished data, 2006). In less than 10% of patients, focal deletions have been reported in the region corresponding to 13q14 [92,108–110], where the tumor suppressor gene RB1 is located. Interestingly, no focal genetic MCRs were present in this region in any of the primary tumors and cell lines analyzed in the aCGH study by Carrasco and colleagues [10]. Comparison of the expression levels of genes residing in the whole chromosome 13 in the two HD clusters (that is, good-prognosis HD versus poor-prognosis HD, characterized by 1q gains and Δ13) highlighted a region, corresponding to 13q14, as enriched for genes significantly down-regulated in HD with 1q and 13 losses when compared with HD without these lesions. These findings suggest that the expression of genes residing in this specific region is preferentially silenced, by mechanisms that are still unclear, in Δ13 patients. Although RB1 was included in this region, it was not included among the genes whose expression was significantly down-regulated in HD with Δ13. Indeed the role of RB1 in MM has been questioned for a long time, because inactivating mutations of this gene have not been identified among the patients who have hemizygous deletions of chromosome 13 [5]. Either the candidate tumor suppressor gene in this region is indeed RB1, through a mechanism of haploinsufficiency, or other genes are involved. Among the potential candidates is TRIM13 (alias RFP2), a gene that has been proposed as the elusive tumor suppressor gene in the cases with deletion of chromosome 13 in chronic lymphatic leukemia [115]. TRIM13, but not RB1, was located within the boundaries of an MCR identified by Elnenaei and colleagues [116] in patients who had MM with Δ13; it was also included among the genes significantly down-regulated in HD with Δ13 versus HD without Δ13 in the aCGH study [10]; and it is the only gene residing on chromosome 13 included in the list of 70 genes associated with early death in the recent study of Shaughnessy and colleagues [105].

Several studies have proposed Δ13 as an independent poor prognostic factor [39,50,55,79,107,111,112,117–119]. Recent studies have conclusively demonstrated, however, that Δ13 represents a proxy for hypodiploidy, and not an independent prognostic factor [80,120].

Minimal Common Regions Linked to Poor Survival

aCGH analysis has identified MCRs associated with poor survival (hereafter designated as PS-MCRs) (Table 1). This list included an amplification on chromosome 8 (including MYC), amplification in 1q, and a deletion on ch17 (including TP53)– genetic events that have been previously linked to poor prognosis in MM. Of the remaining amplified PS-MCRs, two resided in novel MM loci. The first novel amplified PS-MCR defined a ch8q24 region spanning 6 Mb with 37 genes (distinct from MYC) and was notable for its association with a poor clinical outcome and tumor recurrence in other human cancer types [77]. The second novel amplified PS-MCR targets a ch20q region (43 genes) that is associated with disease progression and metastases in prostate cancer [121], esophageal squamous cell carcinoma, and gastric and colorectal adenocarcinoma [122]. Among the 10 deleted PS-MCRs, four discrete regions mapped to chromosome 1p that resided within a relatively large area on 1p as defined by FISH, previously implicated in poor prognosis in patients who had MM [23,104,123]. The remaining deleted PS-MCRs include 3 on ch16, 2 on ch17 (one of them harboring TP53) and 2 on ch20. Among these, the 16q12 region (45 genes) includes the tumor suppressor CYLD, a gene critical for the NF-kB pathway that is proving to be increasingly important in MM. The prognostic relevance of these lesions needs to be validated in prospective studies of adequate sample size, but provides a valuable entry point for gene discovery and the identification of potentially important clinical correlates.

TP53 Deletion and Mutations

Mutations in the TP53 tumor suppressor gene have been reported in MM, with a frequency ranging from 2% to 20% [124–127]. The frequency of TP53 mutations in MGUS has been reported to be low [127] but increases with progression of the disease, approaching 80% in MM cell lines [128]. Chng and colleagues [129] have shown a strong association of mutations of TP53 with poor prognosis. Moreover, in the same study, TP53 mutations

Table 1
Minimal common regions associated with poor prognosis

Cytogenetic band	MCRs Position (Mb)	Size (Mb)	Max/min value	No. genes	Candidate genes
Amplifications					
1q21.1–1q22	142.60–152.10	9.5	2.5	228	MCL1, IL6R, PSMD4, PSMB4, UBE2Q, UBAP2L, RBM8A, RPS27, PIAS3, POLR3C, HIST2H2AA, LASS2, MRPL9, JTB, HAX1, SHC1, APH-1A, BCL9, ZNF364
8q24.12–8q24.13	120.50–126.52	6.0	0.8	37	DEPDC6, MRPL13, DERL1, ZHX1, TATDN1, RNF139, FBXO32
8q24.21–8q24.3	128.50–146.20	17.7	2.5	127	MYC, PVT1
20q12–20q13.12	39.14–43.39	4.3	1.3	43	TDE1, SFRS6, YWHAB, PPIA
Deletions					
1p36.22	10.41–10.62	0.2	−1.0	4	DFFA
1p35.2	30.86–31.04	0.2	−1.0	4	LAPTM5
1p32.3–1p32.2	54.23–57.13	2.9	−0.9	23	SSBP3, USP24
1p13.3–1p12	111.49–118.21	6.7	−1.0	71	DENND2D, DDX20, ST7L, PPP2CZ, LRIG2, PTPN22, CD58, IGSF2
16q11.2–16q12.2	45.17–52.87	7.7	−1.7	45	DNAJA2, SIAH1, PAPD5, NKD1, CARD15, RBL2, FTS, CYLD
16q13	56.23–56.57	0.1	−1.1	9	GPR56, KATNB1, KIFC3, CNGB1
16q24.3	88.23–88.63	0.4	−1.3	19	GAS8
17p13.2	3.31–4.79	1.5	−1.3	43	TAX1BP3, GSG2
17p13.1–17p12	6.45–13.92	7.5	−1.0	125	TP53, TNFSF12, TNFSF13
20p12.1	13.08–17.41	4.3	−0.9	21	OTOR
20q13.12	43.97–44.11	0.1	−1.1	6	PCIF1

were significantly more frequent in patients who had t(4;14) and t(14;16), but no association was reported with HD and Δ13. Finally, although the results should be taken cautiously because of the small number of cases with mutations, patients who have these translocations show a worse prognosis if they present in addition to mutations in TP53.

Other studies have used deletions in 17p13 (mostly hemizygous) as a surrogate for the inactivation of the TP53 pathway and reported a frequency that in most cases is around 10% [79,80,130,131], with a strong association with poor prognosis [10,79,80,131,132]. Chng and colleagues [129] have reported that half of patients who have MM with TP53 mutations had concomitant hemizygous losses at 17p13; and, conversely, only 16% of patients who have 17p13 hemizygous deletions have mutations in the remaining copy of TP53. It is still unclear, therefore, whether the TP53 pathway is silenced in MM cases with hemizygous 17p13 deletions when no mutations are detected in the remaining copy of TP53. Moreover, whether deletions on 17p13 are indeed a surrogate of TP53 inactivation or are associated with other, yet undetermined, tumor suppressor pathways is still unclear.

RAS Mutations

Two genes belonging to the Ras family (NRAS and KRAS) are mutated with a higher frequency in patients who have MM than in those who have MGUS [44–48]. RAS mutations have been linked to increased levels of cyclin D1 expression, but not to t(4;14) [49].

MYC Alterations

Aberrant expression of c-MYC in MM has been known for many years [133–135] and has shown a strong correlation with progression of the disease [133,136]. More recently, the anatomy of the rearrangements underlying MM presenting with overexpression of c-MYC has been delineated [137–139]. These rearrangements in 25% of cases juxtapose c-MYC with an IgH or IgL locus [140], with a pattern that is more complex than the classic reciprocal translocations present in the primary translocations [21,140]. In other cases, amplifications, deletions, inversions, and insertions without apparent translocations [10,91,138,140], or translocations not involving Ig loci [138,139], have been identified. In a large patient population, rearrangements affecting c-MYC have been reported with a frequency of 3% in MGUS and 10% to 16% in MM [137,140]. The data available on plasma cell leukemias (PCLs) are less consistent among studies, with Fabris and colleagues [137] showing c-MYC rearrangements in 3 of 4 patients who had PCL, whereas Avet-Loiseau and colleagues [140] found only 3 MYC aberrations in 23 patients. In contrast, MM cell lines have more frequent rearrangements of the c-MYC locus, ranging from 55% [140] to more than 90%, depending on the study [137,138]. No significant association has been reported between primary translocations and chromosome 13 deletions, whereas a direct correlation with the levels of beta-2 microglobulin have been noted [140], suggesting a potential impact of c-MYC rearrangements on prognosis. The MCR including c-MYC was among the PS-MCR in the recent aCGH survey [10], although the link between c-MYC rearrangements and prognosis has been questioned [80].

P18 and Other Members of the RB1 Pathway

In addition to cyclin D dysregulation, other members of the RB1 pathway have been reported to be altered, but the pathogenetic and clinical relevance of these changes has not been fully elucidated. For example, the tumor suppressor

CDKN2A (p16) is usually not deleted in MM [10,90–92,141], but is frequently methylated in MGUS and MM (between 20%–30%) [142–146]. No apparent association of this phenotype with the most common genetic lesions or prognosis has been found [143–146], with the exception of two studies that have identified a link with proliferative disease [147,148]. On the other hand, the role of CDKN4C, p18, is well established in MM. Overexpression of p18 in MM cell lines lacking p18 reduces proliferation, whereas it has no effect in a cell line where p18 is normally expressed [149]. p18 is homozygously deleted in up to 38% of MM cell lines and in 2% of MM tumors, but this percentage goes up to 10% in tumors with highest proliferation, as evaluated with an expression profiling signature surrogate [149,150]. Intriguingly, p18 is often overexpressed in the most proliferative MM [149].

SUMMARY

The general outline of the early events in MM has been greatly elucidated in the past decade, but several questions of critical importance for the understanding of the pathogenesis of this disease remain to be addressed.

For example, little is known about the role of the primary events, including cyclin D overexpression and MMSET activity in the early pathogenesis of the disease. The additional lesions that promote the progression of MGUS to MM, and progression within MM toward a more aggressive and proliferative disease, are only starting to emerge. The heterotypic relationship between the stroma and the MM plasma cells has also not been fully explored. Finally, the understanding of the biology of MM cancer stem cells and of the pathways driving their maintenance, proliferation, and differentiation is still in its infancy [151,152]. It is possible that the pattern that is emerging in acute leukemias, in which an ordered succession of genetic events dysregulates the proliferation and the differentiation of cancer stem cell [153], will also emerge in MM and thereby provide a more effective pathogenetic and therapeutic framework for tackling this deadly disease.

Acknowledgments

I thank Dr. Michael Kuehl and Dr. Kenneth Anderson for revising this manuscript and for enlightening discussions. I also thank Dr. Ronald DePinho and all the members of his laboratory for stimulating discussions. I gratefully acknowledge Dr. Silvia Guerzoni for her continuous support and encouragement.

References

[1] Mitsiades CS, Mitsiades N, Munshi NC, et al. Focus on multiple myeloma. Cancer Cell 2004;6(5):439–44.

[2] Kyle RA, Rajkumar SV. Monoclonal gammopathies of undetermined significance: a review. Immunol Rev 2003;194:112–39.

[3] Kyle RA, Rajkumar SV. Multiple myeloma. N Engl J Med 2004;351(18):1860–73.

[4] Anderson KC, Shaughnessy JD Jr, Barlogie B, et al. Multiple myeloma. Hematology Am Soc Hematol Educ Program 2002;214–40.

[5] Kuehl WM, Bergsagel PL. Multiple myeloma: evolving genetic events and host interactions. Nat Rev Cancer 2002;2(3):175–87.

[6] Richardson PG, Barlogie B, Berenson J, et al. Clinical factors predictive of outcome with bortezomib in patients with relapsed, refractory multiple myeloma. Blood 2005;106(9): 2977–81.

[7] Richardson PG, Mitsiades CS, Hideshima T, et al. Novel biological therapies for the treatment of multiple myeloma. Best Pract Res Clin Haematol 2005;18(4):619–34.

[8] Barlogie B, Shaughnessy J, Tricot G, et al. Treatment of multiple myeloma. Blood 2004;103(1):20–32.

[9] Bergsagel PL, Kuehl WM, Zhan F, et al. Cyclin D dysregulation: an early and unifying pathogenic event in multiple myeloma. Blood 2005;106(1):296–303.

[10] Carrasco DR, Tonon G, Huang Y, et al. High-resolution genomic profiles define distinct clinico-pathogenetic subgroups of multiple myeloma patients. Cancer Cell 2006;9(4): 313–25.

[11] Zhan F, Huang Y, Colla S, et al. The molecular classification of multiple myeloma. Blood 2006;108(6):2020–8.

[12] Smadja NV, Fruchart C, Isnard F, et al. Chromosomal analysis in multiple myeloma: cytogenetic evidence of two different diseases. Leukemia 1998;12(6):960–9.

[13] Pui CH, Relling MV, Downing JR. Acute lymphoblastic leukemia. N Engl J Med 2004;350(15):1535–48.

[14] Sawyer JR, Waldron JA, Jagannath S, et al. Cytogenetic findings in 200 patients with multiple myeloma. Cancer Genet Cytogenet 1995;82(1):41–9.

[15] Lai JL, Zandecki M, Mary JY, et al. Improved cytogenetics in multiple myeloma: a study of 151 patients including 117 patients at diagnosis. Blood 1995;85(9):2490–7.

[16] Smadja NV, Bastard C, Brigaudeau C, et al. Hypodiploidy is a major prognostic factor in multiple myeloma. Blood 2001;98(7):2229–38.

[17] Fonseca R, Debes-Marun CS, Picken EB, et al. The recurrent IgH translocations are highly associated with nonhyperdiploid variant multiple myeloma. Blood 2003;102(7): 2562–7.

[18] Chng WJ, Van Wier SA, Ahmann GJ, et al. A validated FISH trisomy index demonstrates the hyperdiploid and nonhyperdiploid dichotomy in MGUS. Blood 2005;106(6): 2156–61.

[19] Chng WJ, Winkler JM, Greipp PR, et al. Ploidy status rarely changes in myeloma patients at disease progression. Leuk Res 2006;30(3):266–71.

[20] Brunet JP, Tamayo P, Golub TR, et al. Metagenes and molecular pattern discovery using matrix factorization. Proc Natl Acad Sci U S A 2004;101(12):4164–9.

[21] Bergsagel PL, Kuehl WM. Chromosome translocations in multiple myeloma. Oncogene 2001;20(40):5611–22.

[22] Bergsagel PL, Chesi M, Nardini E, et al. Promiscuous translocations into immunoglobulin heavy chain switch regions in multiple myeloma. Proc Natl Acad Sci U S A 1996;93(24): 13931–6.

[23] Debes-Marun CS, Dewald GW, Bryant S, et al. Chromosome abnormalities clustering and its implications for pathogenesis and prognosis in myeloma. Leukemia 2003;17(2): 427–36.

[24] Seto M, Yamamoto K, Iida S, et al. Gene rearrangement and overexpression of PRAD1 in lymphoid malignancy with t(11;14)(q13;q32) translocation. Oncogene 1992;7(7): 1401–6.

[25] Chesi M, Bergsagel PL, Brents LA, et al. Dysregulation of cyclin D1 by translocation into an IgH gamma switch region in two multiple myeloma cell lines. Blood 1996;88(2): 674–81.

[26] Akiyama N, Tsuruta H, Sasaki H, et al. Messenger RNA levels of five genes located at chromosome 11q13 in B-cell tumors with chromosome translocation t(11;14)(q13;q32). Cancer Res 1994;54(2):377–9.

[27] Kobayashi H, Saito H, Kitano K, et al. Overexpression of the PRAD1 oncogene in a patient with multiple myeloma and t(11;14)(q13;q32). Acta Haematol 1995;94(4):199–203.

[28] Gabrea A, Bergsagel PL, Chesi M, et al. Insertion of excised IgH switch sequences causes overexpression of cyclin D1 in a myeloma tumor cell. Mol Cell 1999;3(1):119–23.

[29] Shaughnessy J Jr, Gabrea A, Qi Y, et al. Cyclin D3 at 6p21 is dysregulated by recurrent chromosomal translocations to immunoglobulin loci in multiple myeloma. Blood 2001;98(1):217–23.

[30] Chesi M, Nardini E, Brents LA, et al. Frequent translocation t(4;14)(p16.3;q32.3) in multiple myeloma is associated with increased expression and activating mutations of fibroblast growth factor receptor 3. Nat Genet 1997;16(3):260–4.

[31] Richelda R, Ronchetti D, Baldini L, et al. A novel chromosomal translocation t(4;14)(p16.3; q32) in multiple myeloma involves the fibroblast growth-factor receptor 3 gene. Blood 1997;90(10):4062–70.

[32] Chesi M, Nardini E, Lim RS, et al. The t(4;14) translocation in myeloma dysregulates both FGFR3 and a novel gene, MMSET, resulting in IgH/MMSET hybrid transcripts. Blood 1998;92(9):3025–34.

[33] Chesi M, Brents LA, Ely SA, et al. Activated fibroblast growth factor receptor 3 is an oncogene that contributes to tumor progression in multiple myeloma. Blood 2001;97(3): 729–36.

[34] Intini D, Baldini L, Fabris S, et al. Analysis of FGFR3 gene mutations in multiple myeloma patients with t(4;14). Br J Haematol 2001;114(2):362–4.

[35] Chesi M, Bergsagel PL, Shonukan OO, et al. Frequent dysregulation of the c-maf protooncogene at 16q23 by translocation to an Ig locus in multiple myeloma. Blood 1998; 91(12):4457–63.

[36] Hanamura I, Iida S, Akano Y, et al. Ectopic expression of MAFB gene in human myeloma cells carrying (14;20)(q32;q11) chromosomal translocations. Jpn J Cancer Res 2001;92(6):638–44.

[37] Smadja NV, Leroux D, Soulier J, et al. Further cytogenetic characterization of multiple myeloma confirms that 14q32 translocations are a very rare event in hyperdiploid cases. Genes Chromosomes Cancer 2003;38(3):234–9.

[38] Fonseca R, Bailey RJ, Ahmann GJ, et al. Genomic abnormalities in monoclonal gammopathy of undetermined significance. Blood 2002;100(4):1417–24.

[39] Avet-Loiseau H, Facon T, Daviet A, et al. 14q32 translocations and monosomy 13 observed in monoclonal gammopathy of undetermined significance delineate a multistep process for the oncogenesis of multiple myeloma. Intergroupe Francophone du Myelome. Cancer Res 1999;59(18):4546–50.

[40] Kaufmann H, Ackermann J, Baldia C, et al. Both IGH translocations and chromosome 13q deletions are early events in monoclonal gammopathy of undetermined significance and do not evolve during transition to multiple myeloma. Leukemia 2004;18(11):1879–82.

[41] Hardin J, Waddell M, Page CD, et al. Evaluation of multiple models to distinguish closely related forms of disease using DNA microarray data: an application to multiple myeloma. Stat Appl Genet Mol Biol 2004;3:[article10].

[42] Zhan F, Hardin J, Kordsmeier B, et al. Global gene expression profiling of multiple myeloma, monoclonal gammopathy of undetermined significance, and normal bone marrow plasma cells. Blood 2002;99(5):1745–57.

[43] Zhan F, Barlogie B, Arzoumanian V, et al. Gene-expression signature of benign monoclonal gammopathy evident in multiple myeloma is linked to good prognosis. Blood 2007;109(4):1692–700.

[44] Paquette RL, Berenson J, Lichtenstein A, et al. Oncogenes in multiple myeloma: point mutation of N-ras. Oncogene 1990;5(11):1659–63.

[45] Neri A, Murphy JP, Cro L, et al. Ras oncogene mutation in multiple myeloma. J Exp Med 1989;170(5):1715–25.

[46] Bezieau S, Devilder MC, Avet-Loiseau H, et al. High incidence of N and K-Ras activating mutations in multiple myeloma and primary plasma cell leukemia at diagnosis. Hum Mutat 2001;18(3):212–24.

[47] Liu P, Leong T, Quam L, et al. Activating mutations of N- and K-ras in multiple myeloma show different clinical associations: analysis of the Eastern Cooperative Oncology Group Phase III Trial. Blood 1996;88(7):2699–706.

[48] Corradini P, Ladetto M, Voena C, et al. Mutational activation of N- and K-ras oncogenes in plasma cell dyscrasias. Blood 1993;81(10):2708–13.

[49] Rasmussen T, Kuehl M, Lodahl M, et al. Possible roles for activating RAS mutations in the MGUS to MM transition and in the intramedullary to extramedullary transition in some plasma cell tumors. Blood 2005;105(1):317–23.

[50] Avet-Loiseau H, Facon T, Grosbois B, et al. Oncogenesis of multiple myeloma: 14q32 and 13q chromosomal abnormalities are not randomly distributed, but correlate with natural history, immunological features, and clinical presentation. Blood 2002;99(6): 2185–91.

[51] Keats JJ, Reiman T, Maxwell CA, et al. In multiple myeloma, t(4;14)(p16;q32) is an adverse prognostic factor irrespective of FGFR3 expression. Blood 2003;101(4):1520–9.

[52] Malgeri U, Baldini L, Perfetti V, et al. Detection of t(4;14)(p16.3;q32) chromosomal translocation in multiple myeloma by reverse transcription-polymerase chain reaction analysis of IGH-MMSET fusion transcripts. Cancer Res 2000;60(15):4058–61.

[53] Agnelli L, Fabris S, Bicciato S, et al. Upregulation of translational machinery and distinct genetic subgroups characterise hyperdiploidy in multiple myeloma. Br J Haematol 2007;136(4):565–73.

[54] Chng WJ, Kumar S, Vanwier S, et al. Molecular dissection of hyperdiploid multiple myeloma by gene expression profiling. Cancer Res 2007;67(7):2982–9.

[55] Fassas AB, Spencer T, Sawyer J, et al. Both hypodiploidy and deletion of chromosome 13 independently confer poor prognosis in multiple myeloma. Br J Haematol 2002;118(4): 1041–7.

[56] Calasanz MJ, Cigudosa JC, Odero MD, et al. Hypodiploidy and 22q11 rearrangements at diagnosis are associated with poor prognosis in patients with multiple myeloma. Br J Haematol 1997;98(2):418–25.

[57] Chng WJ, Santana-Davila R, Van Wier SA, et al. Prognostic factors for hyperdiploid-myeloma: effects of chromosome 13 deletions and IgH translocations. Leukemia 2006;20(5): 807–13.

[58] Chng WJ, Ketterling RP, Fonseca R. Analysis of genetic abnormalities provides insights into genetic evolution of hyperdiploid myeloma. Genes Chromosomes Cancer 2006;45(12): 1111–20.

[59] Potter M, Wiener F. Plasmacytomagenesis in mice: model of neoplastic development dependent upon chromosomal translocations. Carcinogenesis 1992;13(10):1681–97.

[60] Fonseca R, Blood EA, Oken MM, et al. Myeloma and the t(11;14)(q13;q32); evidence for a biologically defined unique subset of patients. Blood 2002;99(10):3735–41.

[61] Avet-Loiseau H, Li JY, Facon T, et al. High incidence of translocations t(11;14)(q13;q32) and t(4;14)(p16;q32) in patients with plasma cell malignancies. Cancer Res 1998;58 (24):5640–5.

[62] Keats JJ, Reiman T, Belch AR, et al. Ten years and counting: so what do we know about t(4;14)(p16;q32) multiple myeloma. Leuk Lymphoma 2006;47(11):2289–300.

[63] Keats JJ, Maxwell CA, Taylor BJ, et al. Overexpression of transcripts originating from the MMSET locus characterizes all t(4;14)(p16;q32)-positive multiple myeloma patients. Blood 2005;105(10):4060–9.

[64] Santra M, Zhan F, Tian E, et al. A subset of multiple myeloma harboring the t(4;14)(p16;q32) translocation lacks FGFR3 expression but maintains an IGH/MMSET fusion transcript. Blood 2003;101(6):2374–6.

[65] Stewart JP, Thompson A, Santra M, et al. Correlation of TACC3, FGFR3, MMSET and p21 expression with the t(4;14)(p16.3;q32) in multiple myeloma. Br J Haematol 2004;126(1): 72–6.

[66] Hudlebusch HR, Theilgaard-Monch K, Lodahl M, et al. Identification of ID-1 as a potential target gene of MMSET in multiple myeloma. Br J Haematol 2005;130(5):700–8.

[67] Plowright EE, Li Z, Bergsagel PL, et al. Ectopic expression of fibroblast growth factor receptor 3 promotes myeloma cell proliferation and prevents apoptosis. Blood 2000;95(3): 992–8.

[68] Ronchetti D, Greco A, Compasso S, et al. Deregulated FGFR3 mutants in multiple myeloma cell lines with t(4;14): comparative analysis of Y373C, K650E and the novel G384D mutations. Oncogene 2001;20(27):3553–62.

[69] Li Z, Zhu YX, Plowright EE, et al. The myeloma-associated oncogene fibroblast growth factor receptor 3 is transforming in hematopoietic cells. Blood 2001;97(8):2413–9.

[70] Grand EK, Chase AJ, Heath C, et al. Targeting FGFR3 in multiple myeloma: inhibition of t(4;14)-positive cells by SU5402 and PD173074. Leukemia 2004;18(5):962–6.

[71] Trudel S, Ely S, Farooqi Y, et al. Inhibition of fibroblast growth factor receptor 3 induces differentiation and apoptosis in t(4;14) myeloma. Blood 2004;103(9):3521–8.

[72] Trudel S, Li ZH, Wei E, et al. CHIR-258, a novel, multitargeted tyrosine kinase inhibitor for the potential treatment of t(4;14) multiple myeloma. Blood 2005;105(7):2941–8.

[73] Trudel S, Stewart AK, Rom E, et al. The inhibitory anti-FGFR3 antibody, PRO-001, is cytotoxic to t(4;14) multiple myeloma cells. Blood 2006;107(10):4039–46.

[74] Todoerti K, Ronchetti D, Agnelli L, et al. Transcription repression activity is associated with the type I isoform of the MMSET gene involved in t(4;14) in multiple myeloma. Br J Haematol 2005;131(2):214–8.

[75] Rosati R, La Starza R, Veronese A, et al. NUP98 is fused to the NSD3 gene in acute myeloid leukemia associated with t(8;11)(p11.2;p15). Blood 2002;99(10):3857–60.

[76] Angrand PO, Apiou F, Stewart AF, et al. NSD3, a new SET domain-containing gene, maps to 8p12 and is amplified in human breast cancer cell lines. Genomics 2001;74(1):79–88.

[77] Tonon G, Wong KK, Maulik G, et al. High-resolution genomic profiles of human lung cancer. Proc Natl Acad Sci U S A 2005;102(27):9625–30.

[78] Jaju RJ, Fidler C, Haas OA, et al. A novel gene, NSD1, is fused to NUP98 in the t(5;11)(q35;p15.5) in de novo childhood acute myeloid leukemia. Blood 2001;98(4): 1264–7.

[79] Fonseca R, Blood E, Rue M, et al. Clinical and biologic implications of recurrent genomic aberrations in myeloma. Blood 2003;101(11):4569–75.

[80] Avet-Loiseau H, Attal M, Moreau P, et al. Genetic abnormalities and survival in multiple myeloma: the experience of the Intergroupe Francophone du Myelome. Blood 2007;109(8): 3489–95.

[81] Chang H, Sloan S, Li D, et al. The t(4;14) is associated with poor prognosis in myeloma patients undergoing autologous stem cell transplant. Br J Haematol 2004;125(1):64–8.

[82] Winkler JM, Greipp P, Fonseca R. t(4;14)(p16.3;q32) is strongly associated with a shorter survival in myeloma patients. Br J Haematol 2003;120(1):170–1.

[83] Moreau P, Facon T, Leleu X, et al. Recurrent 14q32 translocations determine the prognosis of multiple myeloma, especially in patients receiving intensive chemotherapy. Blood 2002;100(5):1579–83.

[84] Rasmussen T, Knudsen LM, Dahl IM, et al. C-MAF oncogene dysregulation in multiple myeloma: frequency and biological relevance. Leuk Lymphoma 2003;44(10):1761–6.

[85] Hurt EM, Wiestner A, Rosenwald A, et al. Overexpression of c-maf is a frequent oncogenic event in multiple myeloma that promotes proliferation and pathological interactions with bone marrow stroma. Cancer Cell 2004;5(2):191–9.

[86] Lombardi L, Poretti G, Mattioli M, et al. Molecular characterization of human multiple myeloma cell lines by integrative genomics: insights into the biology of the disease. Genes Chromosomes Cancer 2007;46(3):226–38.

[87] Suzuki A, Iida S, Kato-Uranishi M, et al. ARK5 is transcriptionally regulated by the Large-MAF family and mediates IGF-1-induced cell invasion in multiple myeloma: ARK5 as a new molecular determinant of malignant multiple myeloma. Oncogene 2005;24(46): 6936–44.

[88] Tian E, Zhan F, Walker R, et al. The role of the Wnt-signaling antagonist DKK1 in the development of osteolytic lesions in multiple myeloma. N Engl J Med 2003;349(26): 2483–94.

[89] Robbiani DF, Colon K, Ely S, et al. Osteopontin dysregulation and lytic bone lesions in multiple myeloma. Hematol Oncol 2007;25(1):16–20.

[90] Largo C, Saez B, Alvarez S, et al. Multiple myeloma primary cells show a highly rearranged unbalanced genome with amplifications and homozygous deletions irrespective of the presence of immunoglobulin-related chromosome translocations. Haematologica 2007;92(6):795–802.

[91] Largo C, Alvarez S, Saez B, et al. Identification of overexpressed genes in frequently gained/amplified chromosome regions in multiple myeloma. Haematologica 2006;91(2):184–91.

[92] Walker BA, Leone PE, Jenner MW, et al. Integration of global SNP-based mapping and expression arrays reveals key regions, mechanisms, and genes important in the pathogenesis of multiple myeloma. Blood 2006;108(5):1733–43.

[93] Whitfield ML, George LK, Grant GD, et al. Common markers of proliferation. Nat Rev Cancer 2006;6(2):99–106.

[94] Mulligan G, Mitsiades C, Bryant B, et al. Gene expression profiling and correlation with outcome in clinical trials of the proteasome inhibitor bortezomib. Blood 2007;109(8): 3177–88.

[95] Avet-Loiseau H, Andree-Ashley LE, Moore D 2nd, et al. Molecular cytogenetic abnormalities in multiple myeloma and plasma cell leukemia measured using comparative genomic hybridization. Genes Chromosomes Cancer 1997;19(2):124–33.

[96] Sawyer JR, Tricot G, Mattox S, et al. Jumping translocations of chromosome 1q in multiple myeloma: evidence for a mechanism involving decondensation of pericentromeric heterochromatin. Blood 1998;91(5):1732–41.

[97] Gutierrez NC, Garcia JL, Hernandez JM, et al. Prognostic and biologic significance of chromosomal imbalances assessed by comparative genomic hybridization in multiple myeloma. Blood 2004;104(9):2661–6.

[98] Cremer FW, Bila J, Buck I, et al. Delineation of distinct subgroups of multiple myeloma and a model for clonal evolution based on interphase cytogenetics. Genes Chromosomes Cancer 2005;44(2):194–203.

[99] Fonseca R, Van Wier SA, Chng WJ, et al. Prognostic value of chromosome 1q21 gain by fluorescent in situ hybridization and increase CKS1B expression in myeloma. Leukemia 2006;20(11):2034–40.

[100] Chang H, Qi X, Trieu Y, et al. Multiple myeloma patients with CKS1B gene amplification have a shorter progression-free survival post-autologous stem cell transplantation. Br J Haematol 2006;135(4):486–91.

[101] Le Baccon P, Leroux D, Dascalescu C, et al. Novel evidence of a role for chromosome 1 pericentric heterochromatin in the pathogenesis of B-cell lymphoma and multiple myeloma. Genes Chromosomes Cancer 2001;32(3):250–64.

[102] Sawyer JR, Tricot G, Lukacs JL, et al. Genomic instability in multiple myeloma: evidence for jumping segmental duplications of chromosome arm 1q. Genes Chromosomes Cancer 2005;42(1):95–106.

[103] Chang H, Yeung J, Xu W, et al. Significant increase of CKS1B amplification from monoclonal gammopathy of undetermined significance to multiple myeloma and plasma cell leukaemia as demonstrated by interphase fluorescence in situ hybridisation. Br J Haematol 2006;134(6):613–5.

[104] Wu KL, Beverloo B, Lokhorst HM, et al. Abnormalities of chromosome 1p/q are highly associated with chromosome 13/13q deletions and are an adverse prognostic factor for the outcome of high-dose chemotherapy in patients with multiple myeloma. Br J Haematol 2007;136(4):615–23.

[105] Shaughnessy JD Jr, Zhan F, Burington BE, et al. A validated gene expression model of high-risk multiple myeloma is defined by deregulated expression of genes mapping to chromosome 1. Blood 2007;109(6):2276–84.

[106] Zhan F, Colla S, Wu X, et al. CKS1B, overexpressed in aggressive disease, regulates multiple myeloma growth and survival through SKP2- and p27Kip1-dependent and -independent mechanisms. Blood 2007;109(11):4995–5001.

[107] Tricot G, Barlogie B, Jagannath S, et al. Poor prognosis in multiple myeloma is associated only with partial or complete deletions of chromosome 13 or abnormalities involving 11q and not with other karyotype abnormalities. Blood 1995;86(11):4250–6.

[108] Avet-Louseau H, Daviet A, Sauner S, et al. Chromosome 13 abnormalities in multiple myeloma are mostly monosomy 13. Br J Haematol 2000;111(4):1116–7.

[109] Fonseca R, Oken MM, Harrington D, et al. Deletions of chromosome 13 in multiple myeloma identified by interphase FISH usually denote large deletions of the q arm or monosomy. Leukemia 2001;15(6):981–6.

[110] Shaughnessy J, Tian E, Sawyer J, et al. High incidence of chromosome 13 deletion in multiple myeloma detected by multiprobe interphase FISH. Blood 2000;96(4):1505–11.

[111] Facon T, Avet-Loiseau H, Guillerm G, et al. Chromosome 13 abnormalities identified by FISH analysis and serum beta2-microglobulin produce a powerful myeloma staging system for patients receiving high-dose therapy. Blood 2001;97(6):1566–71.

[112] Zojer N, Konigsberg R, Ackermann J, et al. Deletion of 13q14 remains an independent adverse prognostic variable in multiple myeloma despite its frequent detection by interphase fluorescence in situ hybridization. Blood 2000;95(6):1925–30.

[113] Konigsberg R, Ackermann J, Kaufmann H, et al. Deletions of chromosome 13q in monoclonal gammopathy of undetermined significance. Leukemia 2000;14(11):1975–9.

[114] Fonseca R, Oken MM, Greipp PR. The t(4;14)(p16.3;q32) is strongly associated with chromosome 13 abnormalities in both multiple myeloma and monoclonal gammopathy of undetermined significance. Blood 2001;98(4):1271–2.

[115] Mertens D, Wolf S, Schroeter P, et al. Down-regulation of candidate tumor suppressor genes within chromosome band 13q14.3 is independent of the DNA methylation pattern in B-cell chronic lymphocytic leukemia. Blood 2002;99(11):4116–21.

[116] Elnenaei MO, Hamoudi RA, Swansbury J, et al. Delineation of the minimal region of loss at 13q14 in multiple myeloma. Genes Chromosomes Cancer 2003;36(1):99–106.

[117] Desikan R, Barlogie B, Sawyer J, et al. Results of high-dose therapy for 1000 patients with multiple myeloma: durable complete remissions and superior survival in the absence of chromosome 13 abnormalities. Blood 2000;95(12):4008–10.

[118] Fonseca R, Harrington D, Oken MM, et al. Biological and prognostic significance of interphase fluorescence in situ hybridization detection of chromosome 13 abnormalities (delta13) in multiple myeloma: an eastern cooperative oncology group study. Cancer Res 2002;62(3):715–20.

[119] Shaughnessy J, Jacobson J, Sawyer J, et al. Continuous absence of metaphase-defined cytogenetic abnormalities, especially of chromosome 13 and hypodiploidy, ensures long-term survival in multiple myeloma treated with total therapy I: interpretation in the context of global gene expression. Blood 2003;101(10):3849–56.

[120] Gutierrez NC, Castellanos MV, Martin ML, et al. Prognostic and biological implications of genetic abnormalities in multiple myeloma undergoing autologous stem cell transplantation: t(4;14) is the most relevant adverse prognostic factor, whereas RB deletion as a unique abnormality is not associated with adverse prognosis. Leukemia 2007;21(1):143–50.

[121] Wullich B, Riedinger S, Brinck U, et al. Evidence for gains at 15q and 20q in brain metastases of prostate cancer. Cancer Genet Cytogenet 2004;154(2):119–23.

[122] Fujita Y, Sakakura C, Shimomura K, et al. Chromosome arm 20q gains and other genomic alterations in esophageal squamous cell carcinoma, as analyzed by comparative genomic hybridization and fluorescence in situ hybridization. Hepatogastroenterology 2003;50(54):1857–63.

[123] Panani AD, Ferti AD, Papaxoinis C, et al. Cytogenetic data as a prognostic factor in multiple myeloma patients: involvement of 1p12 region an adverse prognostic factor. Anticancer Res 2004;24(6):4141–6.

[124] Neri A, Baldini L, Trecca D, et al. p53 gene mutations in multiple myeloma are associated with advanced forms of malignancy. Blood 1993;81(1):128–35.

[125] Preudhomme C, Facon T, Zandecki M, et al. Rare occurrence of P53 gene mutations in multiple myeloma. Br J Haematol 1992;81(3):440–3.

[126] Portier M, Moles JP, Mazars GR, et al. p53 and RAS gene mutations in multiple myeloma. Oncogene 1992;7(12):2539–43.

[127] Corradini P, Inghirami G, Astolfi M, et al. Inactivation of tumor suppressor genes, p53 and Rb1, in plasma cell dyscrasias. Leukemia 1994;8(5):758–67.

[128] Mazars GR, Portier M, Zhang XG, et al. Mutations of the p53 gene in human myeloma cell lines. Oncogene 1992;7(5):1015–8.

[129] Chng WJ, Price-Troska T, Gonzalez-Paz N, et al. Clinical significance of TP53 mutation in myeloma. Leukemia 2007;21(3):582–4.

[130] Avet-Loiseau H, Li JY, Godon C, et al. P53 deletion is not a frequent event in multiple myeloma. Br J Haematol 1999;106(3):717–9.

[131] Chang H, Qi C, Yi QL, et al. p53 gene deletion detected by fluorescence in situ hybridization is an adverse prognostic factor for patients with multiple myeloma following autologous stem cell transplantation. Blood 2005;105(1):358–60.

[132] Gertz MA, Lacy MQ, Dispenzieri A, et al. Clinical implications of t(11;14)(q13;q32), t(4;14)(p16.3;q32), and -17p13 in myeloma patients treated with high-dose therapy. Blood 2005;106(8):2837–40.

[133] Skopelitou A, Hadjiyannakis M, Tsenga A, et al. Expression of C-myc p62 oncoprotein in multiple myeloma: an immunohistochemical study of 180 cases. Anticancer Res 1993;13(4):1091–5.

[134] Palumbo AP, Pileri A, Dianzani U, et al. Altered expression of growth-regulated protooncogenes in human malignant plasma cells. Cancer Res 1989;49(17):4701–4.

[135] Selvanayagam P, Blick M, Narni F, et al. Alteration and abnormal expression of the c-myc oncogene in human multiple myeloma. Blood 1988;71(1):30–5.

[136] Pope B, Brown R, Luo XF, et al. Disease progression in patients with multiple myeloma is associated with a concurrent alteration in the expression of both oncogenes and tumour suppressor genes and can be monitored by the oncoprotein phenotype. Leuk Lymphoma 1997;25(5–6):545–54.

[137] Fabris S, Storlazzi CT, Baldini L, et al. Heterogeneous pattern of chromosomal breakpoints involving the MYC locus in multiple myeloma. Genes Chromosomes Cancer 2003;37(3): 261–9.

[138] Shou Y, Martelli ML, Gabrea A, et al. Diverse karyotypic abnormalities of the c-myc locus associated with c-myc dysregulation and tumor progression in multiple myeloma. Proc Natl Acad Sci U S A 2000;97(1):228–33.

[139] Hollis GF, Gazdar AF, Bertness V, et al. Complex translocation disrupts c-myc regulation in a human plasma cell myeloma. Mol Cell Biol 1988;8(1):124–9.

[140] Avet-Loiseau H, Gerson F, Magrangeas F, et al. Rearrangements of the c-myc oncogene are present in 15% of primary human multiple myeloma tumors. Blood 2001;98(10):3082–6.

[141] Elnenaei MO, Gruszka-Westwood AM, A'Hernt R, et al. Gene abnormalities in multiple myeloma; the relevance of TP53, MDM2, and CDKN2A. Haematologica 2003;88(5): 529–37.

[142] Ng MH, Chung YF, Lo KW, et al. Frequent hypermethylation of p16 and p15 genes in multiple myeloma. Blood 1997;89(7):2500–6.

[143] Gonzalez-Paz N, Chng WJ, McClure RF, et al. Tumor suppressor p16 methylation in multiple myeloma: biological and clinical implications. Blood 2007;109(3):1228–32.

[144] Dib A, Barlogie B, Shaughnessy JD Jr, et al. Methylation and expression of the p16INK4A tumor suppressor gene in multiple myeloma. Blood 2007;109(3):1337–8.

[145] Ribas C, Colleoni GW, Felix RS, et al. p16 gene methylation lacks correlation with angiogenesis and prognosis in multiple myeloma. Cancer Lett 2005;222(2):247–54.

[146] Kramer A, Schultheis B, Bergmann J, et al. Alterations of the cyclin D1/pRb/p16(INK4A) pathway in multiple myeloma. Leukemia 2002;16(9):1844–51.

[147] Sarasquete ME, Garcia-Sanz R, Armellini A, et al. The association of increased p14ARF/p16INK4a and p15INK4a gene expression with proliferative activity and the clinical course of multiple myeloma. Haematologica 2006;91(11):1551–4.

[148] Mateos MV, Garcia-Sanz R, Lopez-Perez R, et al. Methylation is an inactivating mechanism of the p16 gene in multiple myeloma associated with high plasma cell proliferation and short survival. Br J Haematol 2002;118(4):1034–40.

[149] Dib A, Peterson TR, Raducha-Grace L, et al. Paradoxical expression of INK4c in proliferative multiple myeloma tumors: bi-allelic deletion vs increased expression. Cell Div 2006;1:23.

[150] Tasaka T, Berenson J, Vescio R, et al. Analysis of the p16INK4A, p15INK4B and p18INK4C genes in multiple myeloma. Br J Haematol 1997;96(1):98–102.

[151] Matsui W, Huff CA, Wang Q, et al. Characterization of clonogenic multiple myeloma cells. Blood 2004;103(6):2332–6.

[152] Peacock CD, Wang Q, Gesell GS, et al. Hedgehog signaling maintains a tumor stem cell compartment in multiple myeloma. Proc Natl Acad Sci U S A 2007;104(10):4048–53.

[153] Huntly BJ, Gilliland DG. Leukaemia stem cells and the evolution of cancer-stem-cell research. Nat Rev Cancer 2005;5(4):311–21.

Hematol Oncol Clin N Am 21 (2007) 1007–1034

HEMATOLOGY/ONCOLOGY CLINICS
OF NORTH AMERICA

The Role of the Bone Marrow Microenvironment in the Pathophysiology of Myeloma and Its Significance in the Development of More Effective Therapies

Constantine S. Mitsiades, MD, PhD*, Douglas W. McMillin, PhD, Steffen Klippel, PhD, Teru Hideshima, MD, PhD, Dharminder Chauhan, PhD, Paul G. Richardson, MD, Nikhil C. Munshi, MD, Kenneth C. Anderson, MD

Jerome Lipper Myeloma Center, Department of Medical Oncology, Dana-Farber Cancer Institute, Harvard Medical School, 44 Binney Street, Boston, MA 02115, USA

The functional interplay between malignant cells and their local microenvironment has been proposed to be a feature of many different neoplasias. Several studies over the years in hematologic malignancies and solid tumors (for instance [1–4]) have provided evidence supporting the notion that proliferation, survival, and drug resistance of tumor cells can be modulated by the nonmalignant cells that surround them. In fact, even as early as the late nineteenth century, Stephen Paget had proposed the "seed and soil" hypothesis, according to which the site of development of metastatic disease was influenced by the interaction of tumor cells (the seed) with the local microenvironment of the organs (the soil) where the neoplastic cells are deposited [5]. When the soil of a particular tissue constitutes fertile ground for survival and proliferation of tumor cells, the latter are more likely to form metastatic sites that may ultimately lead to clinical manifestations. Conversely, in those particular organs where the soil does not provide the context for optimal growth of the seed, metastatic tumor foci are more likely to develop slowly, if at all.

In the context of this hypothesis, the pronounced osteotropism of multiple myeloma (MM) [6] was deemed to similarly reflect a protective role of the bone marrow (BM) milieu on MM cells. Through extensive studies on this topic over the last decade or so, MM is currently viewed as a prototypical disease model for the characterization of tumor–microenvironment interactions (as reviewed in [7]).

*Corresponding author. E-mail address: constantine_mitsiades@dfci.harvard.edu (C.S. Mitsiades).

0889-8588/07/$ – see front matter
doi:10.1016/j.hoc.2007.08.007

For instance, it is established that the response of MM cells to conventional therapies, such as glucocorticoids or cytotoxic chemotherapeutics, is attenuated by the presence of BMSCs [7–10]. Conversely, the three new anti-MM agents (bortezomib, thalidomide, and lenalidomide) that were approved in recent years by the FDA not only exhibit direct anti-MM properties but are also capable of overcoming the protective effects of the BMSCs, further supporting the notion that comprehensive understanding of how MM cells interact with their BM milieu could allow for further progress in the therapeutic management of this disease.

In this article, we discuss the recent progress in the studies of MM–BM milieu interactions. We specifically highlight the mechanisms whereby the normal cellular constituents of the BM, including BMSCs, endothelial cells, and osteoclasts, enhance the capacity of MM cells to resist conventional anti-MM treatments, through cell adhesion- and cytokine-mediated cascades. We also describe how current research efforts in this direction have provided new promising leads for future therapeutic interventions that may lead to improved clinical outcome for patients who have MM.

THE CELLULAR CONSTITUENTS AND EXTRACELLULAR COMPONENTS OF THE BONE MARROW MICROENVIRONMENT IN MYELOMA

The microenvironment of the BM includes a broad spectrum of cellular and extracellular components that can influence the biologic behavior of MM cells. For instance, extracellular matrix (ECM) proteins, including fibronectin, collagen, and laminin, provide an architectural meshwork on which diverse cellular components can reside and exert their biologic functions. These cellular constituents include MM cells themselves, cells from various stages of differentiation of normal hematopoietic lineages, BMSCs, endothelial cells, and bone cells, such as osteoclasts and osteoblasts. Subsequent sections of this article describe how physical interactions of MM cells with accessory cells and ECM proteins in the BM influence MM pathophysiology [11–14], either through secreted cytokines and growth factors, including interleukin-6 (IL-6), insulin-like growth factor-1 (IGF-1), vascular endothelial growth factor (VEGF), B-cell activating factor, fibroblast growth factors (FGFs), stromal cell–derived factor (SDF)–1α, and tumor necrosis factor (TNF)–α [9,13–28], or through the functional consequences of direct interaction of MM cells with accessory cells [7,29]. Particular emphasis is placed on the functional networks whereby these interactions activate signaling cascades triggering proliferation, survival, and drug resistance of MM cells [29–31], along with increased bone resorption [32,33] and MM-associated neovascularization of the BM [34,35].

THE INTERACTION OF MULTIPLE MYELOMA CELLS WITH BONE MARROW STROMAL CELLS

BMSCs are considered to have a key role in the entire nexus of functional interactions between MM cells and the BM microenvironment. In the MM literature, BMSCs are typically identified descriptively as a heterogeneous population of mesenchymal cells that are morphologically reminiscent of fibroblasts (as reviewed in [7]). In the context of normal BM physiology, BMSCs are believed to function as an accessory cell population that supports the survival, cell division, and differentiation of normal hematopoietic stem cells and progenitors [36–39]. It is therefore plausible that the stimulatory effect of BMSCs on the proliferation, viability, and drug resistance of MM cells may represent an unfavorable and abnormal reprise of their constitutive role to support normal hematopoietic lineages. It is conceivable that BMSCs use similar molecular mediators (eg, cytokines, growth factors, adhesion molecules) for their interactions with normal hematopoietic cells and MM cells. Unlike normal hematopoietic cells, however, which respond to these stimuli by progressing through the different stages of normal hematopoietic differentiation, MM cells respond to the supportive milieu of the BMSCs not by cell differentiation/maturation but by increase in their malignant potential, through increase in their proliferation rate and resistance to the diverse proapoptotic stimuli [7]. An example of how the same BMSC-derived stimuli can have differential functional consequences in MM cells versus normal hematopoietic cells pertains to IL-6: although IL-6 primarily promotes differentiation of the normal B-cell lineage cells and leads to increased production of immunoglobulin by plasma cells, it stimulates increased proliferation and drug resistance of malignant plasma cells in MM [9,40–48].

MM cell adhesion to BMSCs by way of ICAM-1, VLA-4 [49,50], or other adhesion molecules stimulates MM cell proliferation and enhances survival through diverse interdependent cascades, including direct, cell adhesion–mediated activation of intracellular signal transduction pathways in MM cells and increased paracrine (BMSC-derived) or autocrine (MM cell–derived) production of growth factors/cytokines in the BM microenvironment [7,16,49,50]. In the context of in vitro interaction of BMSCs with MM cells, secretion of cytokines is preceded by adhesion-triggered antiapoptotic signaling events. Eventually, however, the events triggered by cytokine secretion cooperate with those stimulated by direct MM–BMSCs adhesion [51] and it is conceivable that at the in vivo level, the impact of cytokines, growth factors, and adhesion-mediated events are intertwined functionally and temporally.

An unanswered question about BMSCs is whether they include distinct subpopulations that play different functional roles in supporting the MM cell population. Furthermore, although it is likely that BMSCs synergize with other normal cell populations of the BM milieu in providing support to the MM cell population, this plausible hypothesis has not been formally studied so far. Further evaluation of the biologic and phenotypic characteristics of BMSCs should clarify some of these questions and yield new information about possible new therapeutic targets.

INTERACTIONS OF MULTIPLE MYELOMA CELLS WITH MULTIPLE MYELOMA–ASSOCIATED BONE MARROW ENDOTHELIAL CELLS

Neoangiogenesis plays a critical role in the establishment of solid tumors, which typically cannot grow beyond a limited size of a few millimeters [52] without the so-called "angiogenic switch." This event is critical for solid tumors because it allows them to recruit blood vessels that allow them to overcome the growth restrictions imposed by intratumor hypoxia [52,53]. In the context of BM-localized hematologic neoplasias, such as MM, the functional relevance of increased tumor-associated angiogenesis is less intuitive: MM cells grow in the sinusoids of the BM, where there is ready access to O_2 and nutrients from the general circulation. Furthermore, MM cells typically infiltrate the BM in the form of sheets of malignant plasma cells [54], which correspond to larger total surface area (compared with the typical pattern of growth of solid tumors) and thus are even more likely to offer access to sufficient blood supply for MM cells. Several studies, however, have reported increased BM microvascular density (MVD) in MM compared with monoclonal gammopathy have unknown significance or normal BM; higher MVD in advanced MM or PCL compared with early-stage disease; and a correlation of higher MVD with adverse clinical outcome (as reviewed in [55]). A working hypothesis to explain these observations holds that even if the increased BM neovascularization in MM does not provide MM cells with increased access to nutrients and O_2, it could still contribute to their increased proliferation, survival, and drug resistance through paracrine and cell adhesion–mediated interactions similar to those between MM cells and BMSCs. This hypothesis is supported by in vitro data indicating that endothelial cells derived from BM aspirates of patients who have MM (MMECs) and human umbilical vein endothelial cells can trigger increased proliferation of MM cell lines and primary MM cells [56]. Further studies are necessary to identify which cytokines, growth factors, or cell adhesion molecules are specifically responsible for these proliferative effects of endothelial cells on MM cells in vitro and whether these effects also account for the presence of increase microvascular density in the BM of MM patients.

The anti-MM activity exhibited by thalidomide [57] (a known antiangiogenic agent [58] that inhibits bone marrow endothelial cell (BMEC)-mediated secretion of VEGF, bFGF, and HGF), BMEC proliferation and capillarogenesis in patients who have MM [34,59,60], and accumulating pieces of evidence on the antiangiogenic properties of bortezomib [56] further support the notion that there is a link between MMECs and MM biology in vivo. It is difficult to dissect, based on current data, whether this link is etiologically linked to increased access of MM cells to O_2 and nutrients or if it is mainly related to supportive effects of the increased mass of MMECs on MM cells in the BM niche. Similarly, although the use of thalidomide for the treatment of MM was originally based on the hypothesis that its antiangiogenic properties [58] would lead to clinical responses in MM and other tumors, the precise contribution of these effects to the clinical activity of this agent is not easy to quantify. The current view in the MM field is that probably the inhibition of neoangiogenesis by thalidomide cooperates with its other effects (stimulation of immune effectors cells, modulation of tumor–stromal interactions, and direct proapoptotic effects on tumor cells) to lead to its in vivo anti-MM activity [61].

Interestingly, studies in non-MM models have shown that CXCR4 expressed in BM endothelial cells can allow them to internalize circulating SDF-1 resulting in its translocation into the BM, which can in turn lead to increased homing of transplanted human CD34(+) hematopoietic progenitors to the BM [62]. Although more studies are needed to address this point in the MM field, it is plausible that MMECs provide a local pool of SDF-1, which serves to promote the homing of MM cells to the BM. This explanation would be consistent with data from different MM groups (eg, [23,63]), which have shown that SDF-1 stimulates MM cell chemotaxis.

The precise mechanism whereby MMECs are recruited in the MM–BM milieu are probably multifactorial, as evidenced by data emerging from studies in MM models, and from extrapolation of data from other disease settings: MM cell adhesion to BMSCs has been reported to trigger increased production (mostly from the BMSCs) of angiogenic cytokines, such as VEGF [64]. Furthermore, constitutive genetic events in MM or other tumor cells (eg, p53 mutations [65] or myc amplification [66]) and activation of signaling cascades (eg, the IGFs/IGF-1R/Akt cascade [16,67,68]) can lead to increased production of VEGF by tumor cells. These genetic lesions are known to be present in MM cells. Furthermore, inhibition of IGF-1R/Akt signaling in MM cells suppresses VEGF secretion [16]. Taken together these results suggest that in the BM milieu, MM cells and BMSCs can be sources of proangiogenic cytokines, which can contribute to the recruitment of MMECs.

OSTEOCLAST–MULTIPLE MYELOMA CELL INTERACTIONS

Normal bone is being continuously remodeled to respond to changes in applied pressure. In this process, osteoclasts resorb old bone, which is replaced by deposition of new bone by osteoblasts (reviewed in [69]). A substantial difference of the new versus the old bone is that the newly deposited bone components should be architecturally oriented to optimize stress-bearing capacity. Otherwise, bone remodeling should normally create no major net change in bone mass, because new bone deposition by osteoblasts is regulated to equal the quantity of bone resorbed by osteoclasts [69]. In the context of MM, however, bone resorption by osteoclasts is uncoupled from new bone formation by osteoblasts [70,71]. This uncoupling involves up-regulated activity of osteoclasts without corresponding increase in new bone deposition by osteoblasts [70,71]. This disparity is caused by concomitant activation of diverse cascades that increased osteoclast differentiation and function and suppression of several negative regulators of bone resorption or positive regulators of bone formation [72]. The composite effect of these events is the development of focal lytic bone lesions or diffuse osteopenia. A key functional component of this process involves the RANKL/RANK axis. RANK (receptor activator of nuclear factor [NF]–κB) is expressed on osteoclasts and its engagement by the cognate ligand RANKL (RANK ligand) stimulates osteoclast differentiation and activity [73,74]. It has been proposed that MM cells can trigger increased RANK signaling in osteoclasts by stimulating RANKL expression by BMSCs [75];

suppressing production (by BMSCs [76]) of osteoprotegerin (OPG), an endogenous antagonist of RANKL binding to RANK [77]; and triggering production of multiple pro-osteoclastogenic mediators in the BM milieu. These factors include IL-6, IL-1α, IL-1β, and IL-11; chemokines such as MIP-1α; TNF superfamily members, such as TNF-α and TNF-β (lymphotoxin-α); and other soluble mediators, including M-CSF, VEGF, or PTHrP [50,72,78–86].

Among these mediators of MM osteoclastogenesis, considerable attention has been placed on macrophage inflammatory protein-1α (MIP-1α), which potently stimulates osteoclast formation independently of RANKL and increases RANKL- and IL-6–stimulated formation of osteoclasts [87]. MIP-1α levels in plasma from BM aspirates of patients who have MM are higher compared with healthy controls and correlate with the degree of osteolytic lesions [85]. The functional significance of MIP-1α has been credentialed by studies in which antisense oligonucleotide against MIP-1α decreases bone destruction in vivo, and by MM cell adherence to BMSCs in vitro by way of decreased expression of the alpha(5)beta(1) integrin [87], suggesting an MIP-1α–mediated link between bone resorption and BMSC-mediated MM cell proliferation/survival. This link is further supported by data indicating that MIP-1α binds to CCR1 on OCL and CCR5 on MM cells and that inhibition of either CCR1 or CCR5 inhibits OCL formation and MM cell adhesion to BMSCs, respectively [88]. TGF-β is also proposed to play an important role in MM bone disease. TGF-β produced by MM cells augments IL-6 secretion from BMSCs [89] and osteoblasts [90], further triggering increased osteoclast activity.

INTERACTIONS OF MULTIPLE MYELOMA CELLS WITH OSTEOBLASTS

The focal lytic bone lesions or diffuse osteopenia of MM is related not only to the increased activity of osteoclasts but also to the lack of an appropriate compensatory osteoblastic response. The differentiation of mesenchymal stem cells to osteoblastic cells requires the transcriptional activity of Runx2/Cbfa1 [91,92]. The direct cell-to-cell contact of osteoprogenitor cells with MM cells inhibits Runx2/Cbfa1 activity in osteoprogenitor cells. This event is mediated by binding of MM cell VLA-4 to VCAM-1 on osteoblast progenitors [93]. Furthermore, MM cells release factors, such as DKK1 (Dickkopf 1) and IL-7, which also contribute to decreased Runx2/Cbfa1 activity and osteoblast differentiation. DKK1, an inhibitor of the Wnt pathway, is overexpressed at the transcriptional level in MM cells of approximately one third of patients (compared with normal plasma cells) and is detected in the serum of approximately one fourth of patients who have extensive osteolytic bone lesions [94]. Canonical Wnt signaling mediates differentiation of osteoblast progenitor cells, which indicates that high levels of DKK1 released by MM cells in the BM milieu may contribute to the osteoblast differentiation and function in MM bone [94]. This notion is further supported by studies in which recombinant human DKK1 or serum of BM aspirates containing high concentrations of DKK1 inhibited the in vitro differentiation of osteoblast precursor cells [94]. In addition, the soluble Wnt inhibitor Frizzled-related protein 2 (sFRP-2), which also suppresses osteoblast differentiation, is constitutively produced by at least a subset of MM cell lines and primary MM tumor cells [95].

Interleukin-3 (IL-3) stimulates the activity of osteoclasts, but recent reports indicate that it also inhibits bone morphogenic protein-2 (BMP-2)–stimulated osteoblast formation [96,97]. HGF directly inhibits osteoblastogenesis in vitro, and its serum levels in MM patients are increased and correlated inversely with bone-specific alkaline phosphatase, a marker of osteoblast activity [98]. Interestingly, the functional uncoupling of bone resorption and bone formation in MM may perhaps be further facilitated by osteoblasts themselves. In response to TGF-β produced by MM cells, osteoblasts (similar to the response of BMSCs to this growth factor [89]) increase their production of IL-6 [90], which further fuels the increased bone resorption by way of the osteoclasts and the increased proliferation of MM cells. The imbalance in the functional interaction of osteoclasts versus osteoblasts in MM is therefore not likely to be mediated by a single cascade, and instead is most likely due to a multitude of cytokine/growth factor networks [99].

For reasons that are not clearly understood, reduction of tumor burden in MM does not necessarily lead to significant improvement in bone homeostasis; in many cases of patients who achieve complete remission (as identified by studies of conventional serologic parameters of MM) after treatment with conventional anti-MM therapies, pre-existing osteolytic lesions may not heal. This finding suggests that in MM, the relationship of disease activity in tumor cell burden versus bone homeostasis is complex and significant suppression of the MM cell population may not be sufficient to allow for resolution of bone lesions. From a therapeutic standpoint, identifying treatment strategies that not only abrogate bone resorption but also stimulate new bone formation will be useful toward improving the long-term outcome of patients who have MM. In contrast to conventional agents, such as glucocorticoids or cytotoxic chemotherapeutics, the proteasome inhibitor bortezomib has the distinct property of not only targeting the MM cells but also suppressing osteoclast function (likely through the suppression of NF-κB activity, which is an important regulator of osteoclast function) and of stimulating osteoblast activity [100–102], as evidenced by increases in osteocalcin and bone-specific alkaline phosphatase levels in bortezomib-treated patients who have MM [102–104].

This effect of bortezomib not only distinguishes it from conventional anti-MM therapies but also perhaps from other novel ones; intriguing recent data from preclinical models have suggested that the teratogenic effect of thalidomide is associated with up-regulation of DKK1, leading to inhibition of canonical Wnt/β-catenin signaling and increased cell death in the limbs. Conversely, inhibition of DKK1 counteracted thalidomide-induced limb truncations and microphthalmia [105]. If further studies confirm that thalidomide also increases DKK1 expression in the adult bone of patients who have MM, then given the proposed association of increased DKK1 levels with decreased osteoblast function, it is plausible to extrapolate that thalidomide may lead to divergent in vivo effects on MM tumor cell population versus bone homeostasis. Although it is effective in decreasing MM cell burden (through one or more of its proposed mechanisms of anti-MM action), its effect on increasing DKK-1 may contribute to a sustained suppression of osteoblast function. Future studies should determine if this hypothesis is correct and if it has clinically relevant implications for the design of thalidomide-containing regimens for MM treatment.

THE PROCESS OF MULTIPLE MYELOMA CELL HOMING TO THE BONE MARROW

In the early stages of the natural history of MM, malignant plasma cells are not readily detectable in the peripheral blood with routine hematologic analyses. Investigational studies with highly sensitive (eg, PCR-based) studies (eg, [106–110]) suggest presence of clonotypic cells in the systemic circulation. It is therefore plausible to hypothesize that the pathophysiology of MM involves, even in the absence of overt plasma cell leukemia, a compartment of circulating cells that may home to different sites of the skeleton and cause the multifocal distribution of bone disease of MM. A key question that remains unanswered is whether the predilection of MM cells for establishing lesions in the bones compared with other organs is predominantly because the bone and BM are a more fertile soil for MM or because the BM microenvironment attracts MM cells more than other tissues do. These questions have not been addressed yet, in part because the molecular signals that attract MM cells to the bone have not been fully characterized.

Among those factors that are considered as key candidates for such a role, stromal cell–derived factor 1 (SDF-1) has a prominent position. SDF-1 interacts with its receptor CXCR4 on MM cells to trigger increased motility and migration in vitro [23,63]. It is currently proposed that high levels of SDF-1 produced by the BM milieu attract MM cells to migrate to the BM. Other factors that are known to stimulate MM cell migration in vitro and are considered to contribute to MM cell homing to the BM in vivo include VEGF [21,22,111], HGF [112], MIP-1α [23,63], and IGF-1 [17,113,114]. When the MM cells are attracted to the BM, they then interact with ECM proteins or BMSCs by way of several adhesion molecules. For instance, CD44, VLA-4 (very late antigen-4, CD49d), VLA-5 (CD49e), LFA-1 (leukocyte function-associated antigen-1, CD11a), NCAM (neuronal adhesion molecule, CD56), ICAM-1 (intercellular adhesion molecule, CD54), syndecan-1 (CD138), and MPC-1 (CD49e) all contribute to MM cell adhesion to the ECM or BMSCs [11,49,115–118]. VLA-4 is expressed on MM cells and binds fibronectin and VCAM-1 (CD106) of ECM and BMSCs, respectively. Binding to fibronectin increases in MM cells the levels of p27^{Kip1} and induces NF-κB activation [119], which in turn triggers cell adhesion–mediated resistance to conventional chemotherapeutics [11,120–122]. Furthermore, MM cell adhesion to ECM by way of binding syndecan-1 to type I collagen (or by other adhesion molecules) triggers release of matrix metalloproteinases (MMP), such as MMP-1, which promotes bone resorption and tumor invasion [123].

From a translational standpoint, inhibition of CXCR4 signaling has been evaluated preclinically [23,63] and experience from the context of use of AMD3100 in stem cell mobilization in patients who have MM scheduled to undergo autologous stem cell transplantation [124] suggests that it can be safely administered in these patients and can increase the number of mobilized CD34+ cells, which can facilitate prompt and durable engraftment of mobilized cells without mobilizing tumor cells from the BM. This latter feature, which is favorable in potential uses of CXCR4 inhibitors to improve mobilization of hematopoietic stem cells for the purposes of autologous stem cell transplantation in MM, is not the outcome that would be expected from the role of CXCR4 in MM cell homing to BM. It suggests that CXCR4 inhibition per se may not be sufficient to expel MM cells from the BM milieu, perhaps because CXCR4 function in MM cells may be important for their initial homing to the BM, but not for their continued presence there or because inhibition of other chemokine-mediated signaling cascades may be important for mobilizing MM cells out of the BM milieu. This hypothesis would be plausible, given the pleiotropic nature of mediators of other pathophysiologic processes governing MM cell behavior in the BM (eg, bone resorption and decreased osteoblast activity). If it is indeed further confirmed that MM cell homing to the BM involves a constellation of factors, rather than merely SDF-1/CXCR4 signaling, CXCR4 targeting may be only one of several different strategies that should combine to comprehensively target the homing of MM tumor cells to the BM.

AN INTEGRATED VIEW OF FUNCTIONAL NETWORKS OF CYTOKINES/MITOGENS AND THEIR RECEPTORS MEDIATING THE INTERACTIONS BETWEEN TUMOR AND STROMA IN MULTIPLE MYELOMA LESIONS

Mutations of individual genes along with amplifications, deletions, or rearrangements of entire chromosomal regions are key determinants of the biologic behavior of neoplastic cells. The pathophysiology of MM is not influenced exclusively by the genetic composition of MM tumor cells but is also affected by how the MM cells interact with their local microenvironment. Although the MM cells perturb normal bone remodeling and lead to establishment of osteolytic bone disease [72,125], the BM microenvironment offers MM cells a supportive stroma, access to vascular networks, and locally produced growth factors and cytokines, which all contribute, through diverse mechanisms, to attenuated in vivo responsiveness of MM cells to proapoptotic stimuli [16,99], such as conventional therapies, including steroids, DNA-damaging agents, and irradiation.

In the BM milieu of patients who have MM, the presence of the MM tumor cells leads, directly or indirectly, to functional uncoupling of new bone formation from resorption [71,81,86]. This event has multifaceted implications in the pathophysiology of MM. The decreased bone density at sites of MM involvement compromises the weight-bearing capacity and capacity of the skeleton, predisposes to spontaneous fractures, and increases calcium release from the resorbed bone, which, without appropriate treatment, can lead to significant hypercalcemia and ensuing medical complications in renal function and status of fluids and electrolytes. At the same time, increased resorptive activity not only compromises the mechanical stability of the bone but also releases high levels of cytokines/growth factors, some of which (with IL-6, IL-1α, IL-1β, MIP-1α, IGFs, and TNF-α as main examples [7,50,72,78–86]) support MM cell viability, proliferation, and resistance to treatments. These events apply not only for MM but also for other malignancies and may explain, at least in part, why breast, prostate, or other epithelial cancers exhibit a propensity for formation of bone metastases [126]. As the fertile soil of the BM facilitates the increased burden of MM cells, they in turn trigger more bone resorption, generating a vicious cycle of bone resorption and tumor growth.

The bone microenvironment-derived in vivo resistance of MM cells to various therapies applies to other neoplasias also (as reported in [127–135]). It does not exclude other mechanisms proposed to explain the de novo or acquired resistance of tumors to treatments (eg, selection of clones with genetically-determined refractoriness to various anticancer treatments or the concept of tumor stem cells [136,137]). For example, although more data may be needed to delineate the role of the proposed "MM stem cell," studies from other fields, including those on normal hematopoietic stem cells [138], point out that hematopoietic stem cells, malignant or nonmalignant, do not function independently of their local milieu but respond to their stimuli and significantly depend on it [139].

SIGNALING PATHWAYS STIMULATED IN MULTIPLE MYELOMA CELLS DURING THEIR INTERACTION WITH THEIR LOCAL MICROENVIRONMENT

The direct contact of MM cells to ECM proteins, BMSCs, and other cells of the BM milieu (including osteoblasts, endothelial cells, and hematopoietic cells) [11,119,140] and the resulting induction of autocrine/paracrine release of cytokines/growth factors [9,16,50] triggers in MM cells a pleiotropic spectrum of proliferative/antiapoptotic signaling pathways, including PI-3K/Akt/mTOR/ p70S6K [16,141], IKK-α/NF-κB [16,142], Ras/Raf/MAPK [16], and JAK/ STAT3 [143–146]. These signaling pathways can be activated by binding of growth factors/cytokines (eg, IL-6, IGFs, IL-1, IL-21, HGF, and so forth) to their respective receptors or by direct stimulation of intracellular signaling (eg, by integrin-linked kinase and focal adhesion kinase) because of the binding of cell adhesion molecules on the surface of MM cells with their counterparts on accessory cells of the BM milieu or with ECM molecules [16,114,141–146]. Growth factor– and adhesion molecule–triggered signaling can lead to similar functional sequelae, because they activate overlapping downstream cascades, including PI-3K/Akt/mTOR/p70S6K, Ras/Raf/MAPK, and IKK-α/NF-κB pathways. PI-3K/Akt activation triggers phosphorylation and cytoplasmic sequestration of proapoptotic members of the Forkhead transcription factor family [16]; increased D-type cyclin expression [16]; up-regulation of caspase inhibitors, such as FLIP or cIAP-2; and up-regulation of antiapoptotic Bcl-2 family members, including Mcl-1 [16]. Cytokine/adhesion-triggered signaling can also activate telomerase function (thereby enhancing the replicative potential of MM cells) and stimulate HIF-1a and its effects in helping the recruitment by tumor cells of new blood vessels [16,141,147].

Each of the diverse mitogens/survival factors released in the BM milieu of MM patients (eg, IL-6, IGFs, HGF, IL-1α, IL-1β, TNF-α, VEGF, Notch family members, and so forth [9,16,30,40,42,147,148]) can trigger multiple, and often overlapping, signaling pathways. The biologic sequelae of each of these cytokines can be distinct for various reasons, including the differential targeting of specific accessory cells of the BM milieu. For instance, IL-6 not only potently stimulates MM cell proliferation, but also triggers osteoclasts to increase bone resorption, a property also exhibited by IL-1 and VEGF [78,82,83,86,125,149]. TNF-α is reported to directly trigger MM cell proliferation and resistance to apoptosis [150], but can also modulate, through activation of NF-κB, the expression of diverse cell adhesion molecules on the surface of BMSCs and MM cells [151], thus further facilitating MM-BMSC adhesion and ensuing cytokine production [151]. SDF-1/CXCL12 signaling through its receptor CXCR4 has modest, if any, direct mitogenic/antiapoptotic activity on MM cells [63] by promoting MM cell homing to the BM milieu [30], which is more conducive to increased viability and expansion of the tumor cell population.

THE RELATIVE IMPORTANCE OF IL-6, IGFS AND OTHER CYTOKINES IN THE BIOLOGIC BEHAVIOR OF MULTIPLE MYELOMA CELLS IN THE BONE MARROW MILIEU

IL-6 has been historically viewed as a major, if not the major, growth factor in the pathophysiology of MM. Although IL-6 promotes differentiation of normal B-lineage cells to normal plasma cells [152], its effects on the malignant plasma cells of MM involve stimulation of proliferation and increased resistance to dexamethasone and other conventional therapeutics [48,153–157] by way of IL-6R–mediated activation of PI-3K/Akt, MAPK, and JAK/STAT3 cascades [48,141,145,146,158]; IL-6 also stimulates osteoclastogenesis [159], linking the increased in MM tumor burden in the BM with bone resorption.

IL-6 cannot by itself explain all aspects of MM pathophysiology and its selective therapeutic targeting is not likely to offer curative anti-MM responses. Indeed, only a subset of MM cell lines responds to IL-6 stimulation in vitro (and usually at levels considerably higher than those detected in peripheral blood samples of MM patients [16]), and even fewer of them depend on exogenous IL-6 stimulation for their sustained in vitro survival.

In clinical trials of anti–IL-6 neutralizing antibodies in MM, decreased levels of C-reactive protein, a surrogate marker for IL-6 bioactivity, were detected [160]. Major clinical responses were not observed [161], however, in contrast to what would have been expected based on the preclinical hypothesis on the significance of IL-6 for MM cells. Aside from the pharmacodynamic and pharmacokinetic reasons that may explain these results [162,163], it is unlikely that IL-6 inhibition can alone achieve significant clinical responses in MM. On one hand, MM cells probably depend on a multitude of BM cytokines/growth factors for the biologic behavior and the redundancy between their signaling pathways can allow them to survive even when a significant pathway, such as the IL-6/IL-6R cascade, has been abrogated. On the other hand, patients enrolled in clinical trials for MM often have advanced disease, at which stage the malignant cells may have become independent from IL-6 and perhaps several other cytokines of the BM [7,16,31]. This phenomenon can perhaps explain why MM cell lines, which are most often derived from samples of patients who have plasma cell leukemia or extramedullary plasmacytomas, in most cases do not depend on, or are even unresponsive to, IL-6. Recently established new classes of anti-MM drugs, such as bortezomib, thalidomide, and lenalidomide, which overcome the effects of IL-6 on MM cells, have moved in the clinical applications from the relapsed/refractory setting [57,164–166] to newly diagnosed patients [167–170] (ie, the clinical setting in which anti–IL-6 therapeutic strategies would be expected to be more successful). It therefore remains to be determined whether optimizations in IL-6 inhibition strategies may allow this class of agents to provide any added benefit to the clinical activity of existing anti-MM therapies.

The concern that IL-6 inhibition alone is not sufficient to achieve major clinical responses in MM has fueled further interest in other growth factors/cytokines that may complement IL-6 signaling, compensate for its inhibition, or drive proliferation and survival of IL-6–independent MM cells in the context of advanced disease. One signaling pathway that meets these criteria involves insulin-like growth factors (IGFs) and their receptor IGF-1R (CD221) [16]. Extensive, yet sporadic, prior studies in diverse neoplasias had shown that IGFs and IGF-1R are implicated in the biology of many types of solid tumors; increased levels of circulating IGF-1 have been associated with higher risk for diverse forms of epithelial cancers (eg, [171–173]). IGF-1R expression is necessary for normal cells to undergo malignant transformation in vitro by a series of oncogenes [174–176]. Extensive studies (reviewed in [177]), including studies with human MM cell lines, have reported increased proliferation of neoplastic cell lines, including MM lines, on in vitro stimulation with IGF-1. For many years, however, this pathway was not viewed as an attractive target for anticancer drug development; the extensive homology to insulin receptor (InsR) [178] and the widespread expression of IGF-1R in normal tissues and at levels often comparable to those present in their malignant counterparts [178] suggested that perhaps selective small-molecule IGF-1R inhibitors might not be feasible to synthesize or that other therapeutics (eg, specific anti–IGF-1R monoclonal antibodies [179–182]) that could achieve this goal might be too toxic for clinical use. These obstacles were addressed in part by studies initially focused on MM models, which showed that certain aminopyrrolopyrimidine's small molecules could selectively inhibit the IGF-1R kinase activity, could be administered orally and safely (for instance no significant hyperglycemia was observed in the studies of these inhibitors) in preclinical animal models, had in vitro antitumor activity against a broad spectrum of drug-resistant MM cell lines and primary MM cells and tumor cells from other neoplasias, and had in vivo anti-MM activity in models of diffuse MM bone lesions as single agents and in combination with other anti-MM therapeutics [16,183]. These observations confirmed that small molecule kinase inhibitors with sufficient selectivity against IGF-1R versus IR can achieve in vivo antitumor responses with acceptable side effect profile [16,183] and validated the importance of IGF-1R as a therapeutic target for MM and other malignancies, also providing a framework for preclinical and clinical studies of other strategies to selectively target this pathway (eg, for mAbs against IGF-1R and other chemical classes of IGF-1R kinase inhibitors [184–186]).

The potent effects of IGF-1R inhibitor against MM cells in particular, and tumor cells more generally, can be attributed to IGF-1R functioning for neoplastic cells as a key regulator of many pathways critical for the malignant phenotype. Specifically, IGF-1R activation stimulates the telomerase and proteasome activities [16]; up-regulates anti-apoptotic caspase inhibitors [16], thus conferring resistance against dexamethasone, cytotoxic chemotherapeutics, and, in part, proteasome inhibitors; enhances the ability of MM cells to respond to other cytokines (eg, IL-6); and stimulates the production of proangiogenic cytokines (eg, VEGF) [16]. These pleiotropic molecular sequelae of IGF-1R signaling, may explain, at least in part, why IGF-1R inhibition can enhance the antitumor activity of other anticancer agents [16], and most likely the use of this class of agents as sensitizers administered intermittently to improve antitumor activity of other established therapies would be an effective strategy to improve outcome and prevent the emergence of drug resistance, while limiting potential adverse events.

The IGF-1R cascade is not the only growth factor/cytokine signaling system that features such a pleiotropicity of molecular events, nor the only cytokine-driven pathway that can support the MM cell viability or proliferation. In fact, many signaling effectors downstream of IGF-1R can also be stimulated by other mitogens/survival factors (eg, PI-3K/Akt activation is also triggered by IL-6, HGF, and several other cytokines implicated in MM biology) [112,141,187]. Primary tumor cells from advanced MM patients (eg, at the stage of plasma cell leukemia or extramedullary plasmacytomas) can survive in short-term in vitro cultures independently of certain BM-derived cytokines, such as IL-6, but generally remain responsive to IGF-1R inhibition [16]. This finding suggests that in advanced MM (ie, the clinical stages that generally constitute the testing ground for investigational therapies) inhibition of IGF inhibition represents a viable therapeutic option, apparently because the function of this target remains important for MM cell survival. This phenomenon can perhaps be explained, at least in part, by in vitro data suggesting that, whereas other cytokines/growth factors of the BM milieu may activate some of the same cascades activated by IGFs (eg, PI-3K/Akt, IKK/NF-κB), IGFs trigger more potent or protracted activation of these pathways [16]. Furthermore, compared with several other cytokines implicated in the pathophysiology of MM, tumor cells are exposed to high levels of IGF-1, which are not only present in serum but are also produced locally in the BM milieu by various types of normal cells, including osteoblasts and BMSCs [16]. These considerations may explain why even MM cells derived from patients who have advanced disease can remain responsive to IGF-1R inhibition. Taken together, these observations on the biology of the IGFs/IGF-1R cascade in MM indicate that this target merits further consideration for more efforts toward clinical translation.

THE GENETIC SUBSTRATE OF TUMOR–MICROENVIRONMENT INTERACTIONS IN MULTIPLE MYELOMA

The bidirectional interactions of MM cells with their BM milieu have important clinical sequelae, which include increased bone resorption and MM cell resistance to conventional chemotherapeutic agents, even in the absence of genetic lesions that would otherwise confer constitutive resistance [7,99]. It is currently viewed that the biologic behavior of MM cells is determined by the composite effect of their own constitutive genetic features and of the stimuli that they are exposed to in their local BM milieu. Importantly, genetic lesions of MM cells may influence the nature of their interaction with their BM milieu and its functional consequences. For example, MM cells harboring the t(14;16) translocation overexpress the transcription factor c-maf, which activates cyclin D2 expression and increases MM cell proliferation [188]. Furthermore, c-maf up-regulates β7-integrin expression and MM cell adhesion to BMSCs [188]. In addition, MM cells with hyperdiploid karyotypes seem to uniquely depend on their interaction with the BM microenvironment, which is proposed to trigger (through yet-undefined mechanisms) increased expression of cyclin D1, despite the absence of primary immunoglobulin gene translocations involving the cyclin D1 gene [189]. These examples support the notion that the genetics of MM cells and their interactions with the BM milieu are not completely independent of each other. Instead, they functionally interact to influence the biologic and clinical behavior of the disease.

FUTURE DIRECTIONS IN THE THERAPEUTIC TARGETING OF TUMOR–STROMAL INTERACTIONS

The interaction of MM cells with their BM milieu is unfavorable from a pathophysiologic and clinical standpoint because it directly interferes with the process of bone remodeling, leads to skeletal lesions (which in turn can lead to further clinical complications, such as spontaneous fractures), and can attenuate the response of MM cell to therapies [16,141]. Even in early stages of MM, when its neoplastic cells perhaps do not yet harbor all the genetic defects necessary for constitutive establishment of drug resistance, it is conceivable that the protective effect of the BM milieu may allow at least some of the MM cells to survive sufficiently long to acquire additional genetic lesions critical for their resistance to treatment. The clinical activity that novel therapies, such as thalidomide, lenalidomide, and bortezomib, can achieve even in steroid- or chemo-refractory MM [57,164–166,190–192], combined with that the ability of these agents to overcome the protective effects of BMSCs on MM cells, further supports the notion that the MM–BM microenvironment interaction constitutes an important parameter that needs to be taken into consideration for the design of investigational anti-MM therapeutics. These MM–BM milieu interactions can be viewed per se as legitimate targets for development of novel therapeutic strategies.

The therapeutic interventions oriented toward the tumor–microenvironment interactions in MM can target, in principle, any individual molecular components and cellular compartments participating in, mediating, or facilitating these interactions; BMSCs and other accessory cells in the BM milieu are bone fide therapeutic targets that have already been targeted, at least in part, at a clinical level with novel agents, such as thalidomide, lenalidomide, and proteasome inhibitors. For instance, thalidomide and lenalidomide have antiangiogenic properties in vivo [58,193–195] and can target the MM-associated endothelium. The proteasome inhibitor bortezomib has been shown not only to have direct anti-MM activity but also to perturb the function of MMECs [56]. Bisphosphonates are proposed to have direct antitumor activity in preclinical models [196,197], but their principal anti-MM action in vivo is to inhibit the bone resorptive action of osteoclasts, thereby indirectly abrogating other sequelae of osteoclast function, including the increased local production of cytokines [149]. BMSCs and their biologic effects are considered therapeutic targets, particularly in view of their support for MM cell proliferation and viability. A theoretic limitation of the therapeutic targeting of BMSCs is the potential scenario that the functional perturbation of the BMSCs would not only affect the biology of the MM cells but also compromise the support that the BM stroma provided to normal hematopoietic cells [198]. One potential strategy to address this issue is to focus on targeting the functional networks of cytokines and growth factors that mediate the support of BMSCs on MM cells. For instance, such approaches would aim at decreasing the production and release of these mediators from the BMSCs, other cells of the host microenvironment, or perhaps MM cells themselves (in those cases of growth factors/cytokines that may also be produced in an autocrine fashion by MM cells), or suppressing the local bioavailability of these factors in the BM microenvironment. One possible example of how this can be achieved at a clinical level involves the drug class of histone deacetylase (HDAC) inhibitors. HDAC inhibitors, such as the first-in-class FDA-approved agent vorinostat (SAHA), not only exhibit direct anti-MM activity [199,200] but also can decrease the production of IL-6 by BMSCs cocultured with MM cells [200]. RANK-Fc constructs or osteoprotegerin (OPG) can inhibit osteoclast activation and bone resorption [201,202]. Antibodies against cytokines/growth factors (eg, VEGF, HGF, DKK-1); soluble forms of their respective receptors; and small-molecule inhibitors of downstream signaling pathways can also be used not only to inhibit MM cell proliferation directly but also to perturb tumor-associated recruitment of blood vessels and bone resorption [94,112,203].

Another approach aiming at abrogating tumor–microenvironmental interactions involves the targeting of the mechanisms whereby MM cells communicate with their microenvironment: this can involve alteration in the patterns of adhesive interactions of MM cells with other cells of the BM microenvironment or with the ECM, and inhibition of the ability of MM cells to receive or respond to the proliferative/antiapoptotic cues provided to them by growth factors/cytokines of the BM milieu [99]. For example, monoclonal antibodies against those cell adhesion molecules that mediate MM-BMSC binding have been explored in preclinical MM models as potential therapeutic agents; a monoclonal antibody against α4 integrin was used to treat mice bearing murine MM cells and decreased MM tumor burden, suppressed the number of osteoclasts and the extent of bone resorption, and prolonged the overall survival of the mice [204].

A broad range of molecular targets on MM cells and a wide constellation of corresponding investigational agents can target the capability of MM tumor cells to sense survival cues from their environment and respond to them at a preclinical and clinical level. Receptors for cytokine/growth factors and their downstream pathways have attracted particular interest in recent years, including studies of IGF-1R inhibitors [16], FGF-R3 inhibitors [205–207], inhibitors of Ras farnesylation [208–211], small molecule inhibitors of IKK [142] or other inhibitors of IKK/NF-κB signaling (eg, the cell permeable peptide SN-50, which blocks the nuclear translocation and transcriptional activity of NF-κB [212]), diverse inhibitors of the PI-3K/Akt/mTOR axis (eg, small molecule mTOR inhibitors, such as rapamycin or RAD-001) [213–217], or inhibitors of telomerase activity [218,219]. Of particular interest are agents that can simultaneously perturb the function of multiple signaling cascades, often at multiple molecular levels for one or more of these pathways. Multitargeted kinase inhibitors (eg, [220,221]) fall into that category of agents; they are composed of single chemical entities that are capable of simultaneously inhibiting the function of multiple kinases with structurally similar kinase domains. Another class of drugs that can achieve a similar multitargeted effect, but through different molecular mechanisms, involves the heat shock protein 90 (hsp90) inhibitors, including the geldanamycin analog 17-AAG. Hsp90 is a molecular chaperone that regulates the three-dimensional conformation and function of a wide range of proteins that regulate the proliferation of neoplastic cells and their resistance to apoptosis [222]. When hsp90 function is inhibited, its client proteins cannot assume their proper conformation and their functional capacity is perturbed by their misfolding, which also triggers their ubiquitination and eventual proteasomal degradation. Interestingly, many mutated or chimeric oncoproteins that drive the proliferation/survival of neoplastic cells are more sensitive to hsp90 inhibition than their wild-type counterparts in nonmalignant cells [222], which may explain, at least in part, the differential sensitivity of malignant versus normal cells to hsp90 inhibition. 17-AAG and other hsp90 inhibitors of the ansamycin family bind to the ATP-binding pocket of hsp90, which is critical for the chaperoning function and leads to misfolding and inhibition of function of multiple hsp90 client proteins, including the PI-3K/Akt, Ras/Raf/MAPK, mTOR/p70S6K, and IKK/NF-κB cascades. Preclinical studies in MM have shown that hsp90 inhibitors are active against MM cells in vitro and in vivo [223–225] and ongoing clinical trials have shown that the KOS-953 formulation of 17-AAG can be safely administered in phase I trials of patients who have MM [226] and can enhance the anti-MM activity of bortezomib [227].

SUMMARY

The three recently FDA-approved anti-MM agents (bortezomib, thalidomide, and lenalidomide) abrogate, at least in part, the protection that the BM microenvironment can confer to MM cells against cytotoxic chemotherapy and dexamethasone. The clinical success of these three agents suggests that further improvements in the therapeutic management for MM may also come through the identification of other classes of anti-MM drugs that share a common property of overcoming the protective effects of the BM milieu on MM cells. The multitude of cellular compartments with which MM cells interact in the BM milieu, and the broad constellation of cytokines, growth factors, and adhesion molecules that mediate MM–BM milieu interactions, may pose some translational challenges. It is likely that targeting of any individual molecular or cellular mediator of the MM–BM milieu interactions will not be sufficient to achieve curative responses because of the functional redundancy of the cascades triggering MM cell survival and drug resistance. It is hoped that currently available preclinical models for MM cell interactions with the BM microenvironment will offer insight into the functional hierarchy of molecular events that are essential for the survival of MM cells in the bone milieu and provide the rationale for combination therapies that will achieve, without significant toxicities, comprehensive abrogation of all essential tumor–microenvironment interactions that are posing barriers to curative therapies for this disease.

References

[1] Mitsiades CS, Koutsilieris M. Molecular biology and cellular physiology of refractoriness to androgen ablation therapy in advanced prostate cancer. Expert Opin Investig Drugs 2001;10(6):1099–115.

[2] van Kempen LC, Ruiter DJ, van Muijen GN, et al. The tumor microenvironment: a critical determinant of neoplastic evolution. Eur J Cell Biol 2003;82(11):539–48.

[3] Munk Pedersen I, Reed J. Microenvironmental interactions and survival of CLL B-cells. Leuk Lymphoma 2004;45(12):2365–72.

[4] Zhou J, Mauerer K, Farina L, et al. The role of the tumor microenvironment in hematological malignancies and implication for therapy. Front Biosci 2005;10:1581–96.

[5] Paget S. The distribution of secondary growths in cancer of the breast. Lancet 1889;1: 571–3.

[6] Bataille R, Harousseau JL. Multiple myeloma. N Engl J Med 1997;336(23):1657–64.

[7] Mitsiades CS, Mitsiades N, Munshi NC, et al. Focus on multiple myeloma. Cancer Cell 2004;6(5):439–44.

[8] Chauhan D, Uchiyama H, Urashima M, et al. Regulation of interleukin 6 in multiple myeloma and bone marrow stromal cells. Stem Cells 1995;13(Suppl 2):35–9.

[9] Chauhan D, Uchiyama H, Akbarali Y, et al. Multiple myeloma cell adhesion-induced interleukin-6 expression in bone marrow stromal cells involves activation of NF-kappa B. Blood 1996;87(3):1104–12.

[10] Hideshima T, Richardson P, Chauhan D, et al. The proteasome inhibitor PS-341 inhibits growth, induces apoptosis, and overcomes drug resistance in human multiple myeloma cells. Cancer Res 2001;61(7):3071–6.

[11] Damiano JS, Cress AE, Hazlehurst LA, et al. Cell adhesion mediated drug resistance (CAM-DR): role of integrins and resistance to apoptosis in human myeloma cell lines. Blood 1999;93(5):1658–67.

[12] Akiyama M, Hideshima T, Hayashi T, et al. Cytokines modulate telomerase activity in a human multiple myeloma cell line. Cancer Res 2002;62(13):3876–82.

[13] Chauhan D, Li G, Hideshima T, et al. Blockade of ubiquitin-conjugating enzyme CDC34 enhances anti-myeloma activity of bortezomib/proteasome inhibitor PS-341. Oncogene 2004;23(20):3597–602.

[14] Hideshima T, Catley L, Yasui H, et al. Perifosine, an oral bioactive novel alkylphospholipid, inhibits Akt and induces in vitro and in vivo cytotoxicity in human multiple myeloma cells. Blood 2006;107(10):4053–62.

[15] Freund GG, Kulas DT, Mooney RA. Insulin and IGF-1 increase mitogenesis and glucose metabolism in the multiple myeloma cell line, RPMI 8226. J Immunol 1993;151(4):1811–20.

[16] Mitsiades CS, Mitsiades NS, McMullan CJ, et al. Inhibition of the insulin-like growth factor receptor-1 tyrosine kinase activity as a therapeutic strategy for multiple myeloma, other hematologic malignancies, and solid tumors. Cancer Cell 2004;5(3):221–30.

[17] Vanderkerken K, Asosingh K, Braet F, et al. Insulin-like growth factor-1 acts as a chemoattractant factor for 5T2 multiple myeloma cells. Blood 1999;93(1):235–41.

[18] Asosingh K, Gunthert U, Bakkus MH, et al. In vivo induction of insulin-like growth factor-I receptor and CD44v6 confers homing and adhesion to murine multiple myeloma cells. Cancer Res 2000;60(11):3096–104.

[19] Podar K, Anderson KC. The pathophysiologic role of VEGF in hematologic malignancies: therapeutic implications. Blood 2005;105(4):1383–95.

[20] Podar K, Catley LP, Tai YT, et al. GW654652, the pan-inhibitor of VEGF receptors, blocks the growth and migration of multiple myeloma cells in the bone marrow microenvironment. Blood 2004;103(9):3474–9.

[21] Podar K, Tai YT, Davies FE, et al. Vascular endothelial growth factor triggers signaling cascades mediating multiple myeloma cell growth and migration. Blood 2001;98(2):428–35.

[22] Podar K, Tai YT, Lin BK, et al. Vascular endothelial growth factor-induced migration of multiple myeloma cells is associated with beta 1 integrin- and phosphatidylinositol 3-kinase-dependent PKC alpha activation. J Biol Chem 2002;277(10):7875–81.

[23] Hideshima T, Chauhan D, Hayashi T, et al. The biological sequelae of stromal cell-derived factor-1alpha in multiple myeloma. Mol Cancer Ther 2002;1(7):539–44.

[24] Otsuki T, Yamada O, Yata K, et al. Expression of fibroblast growth factor and FGF-receptor family genes in human myeloma cells, including lines possessing t(4;14)(q16.3;q32. 3) and FGFR3 translocation. Int J Oncol 1999;15(6):1205–12.

[25] Chauhan D, Catley L, Li G, et al. A novel orally active proteasome inhibitor induces apoptosis in multiple myeloma cells with mechanisms distinct from bortezomib. Cancer Cell 2005;8(5):407–19.

[26] Novak AJ, Darce JR, Arendt BK, et al. Expression of BCMA, TACI, and BAFF-R in multiple myeloma: a mechanism for growth and survival. Blood 2004;103(2):689–94.

[27] Moreaux J, Legouffe E, Jourdan E, et al. BAFF and APRIL protect myeloma cells from apoptosis induced by IL-6 deprivation and dexamethasone. Blood 2004;103(8):3148–57.

[28] Tai YT, Li XF, Breitkreutz I, et al. Role of B-cell-activating factor in adhesion and growth of human multiple myeloma cells in the bone marrow microenvironment. Cancer Res 2006;66(13):6675–82.

[29] Hideshima T, Anderson KC. Molecular mechanisms of novel therapeutic approaches for multiple myeloma. Nat Rev Cancer 2002;2(12):927–37.

[30] Hideshima T, Bergsagel PL, Kuehl WM, et al. Advances in biology of multiple myeloma: clinical applications. Blood 2004;104(3):607–18.

[31] Kuehl WM, Bergsagel PL. Multiple myeloma: evolving genetic events and host interactions. Nat Rev Cancer 2002;2(3):175–87.

[32] Roodman GD. Pathogenesis of myeloma bone disease. Blood Cells Mol Dis 2004;32(2): 290–2.

[33] Roodman GD. Myeloma bone disease: pathogenesis and treatment. Oncology (Williston Park) 2005;19(8):983–4, 986.

[34] Ribatti D, Nico B, Vacca A. Importance of the bone marrow microenvironment in inducing the angiogenic response in multiple myeloma. Oncogene 2006;25(31):4257–66.

[35] Ribatti D, Scavelli C, Roccaro AM, et al. Hematopoietic cancer and angiogenesis. Stem Cells Dev 2004;13(5):484–95.

[36] Werts ED, DeGowin RL, Knapp SK, et al. Characterization of marrow stromal (fibroblastoid) cells and their association with erythropoiesis. Exp Hematol 1980;8(4):423–33.

[37] Greenberg BR, Wilson FZ, Woo L. Granulopoietic effects of human bone marrow fibroblastic cells and abnormalities in the "granulopoietic microenvironment". Blood 1981;58(3): 557–64.

[38] Reincke U, Hannon EC, Rosenblatt M, et al. Proliferative capacity of murine hematopoietic stem cells in vitro. Science 1982;215(4540):1619–22.

[39] Kaneko S, Motomura S, Ibayashi H. Differentiation of human bone marrow-derived fibroblastoid colony forming cells (CFU-F) and their roles in haemopoiesis in vitro. Br J Haematol 1982;51(2):217–25.

[40] Kawano M, Hirano T, Matsuda T, et al. Autocrine generation and requirement of BSF-2/IL-6 for human multiple myelomas. Nature 1988;332(6159):83–5.

[41] Kawano M, Kuramoto A, Hirano T, et al. Cytokines as autocrine growth factors in malignancies. Cancer Surv 1989;8(4):905–19.

[42] Kawano M, Tanaka H, Ishikawa H, et al. Interleukin-1 accelerates autocrine growth of myeloma cells through interleukin-6 in human myeloma. Blood 1989;73(8):2145–8.

[43] Shimizu S, Yoshioka R, Hirose Y, et al. Establishment of two interleukin 6 (B cell stimulatory factor 2/interferon beta 2)-dependent human bone marrow-derived myeloma cell lines. J Exp Med 1989;169(1):339–44.

[44] Klein B, Zhang XG, Jourdan M, et al. Interleukin-6 is the central tumor growth factor in vitro and in vivo in multiple myeloma. Eur Cytokine Netw 1990;1(4):193–201.

[45] Barut BA, Zon LI, Cochran MK, et al. Role of interleukin 6 in the growth of myeloma-derived cell lines. Leuk Res 1992;16(10):951–9.

[46] Urashima M, Chauhan D, Uchiyama H, et al. CD40 ligand triggered interleukin-6 secretion in multiple myeloma. Blood 1995;85(7):1903–12.

[47] Urashima M, Ogata A, Chauhan D, et al. Interleukin-6 promotes multiple myeloma cell growth via phosphorylation of retinoblastoma protein. Blood 1996;88(6):2219–27.

[48] Chauhan D, Kharbanda S, Ogata A, et al. Interleukin-6 inhibits Fas-induced apoptosis and stress-activated protein kinase activation in multiple myeloma cells. Blood 1997;89(1): 227–34.

[49] Uchiyama H, Barut BA, Chauhan D, et al. Characterization of adhesion molecules on human myeloma cell lines. Blood 1992;80(9):2306–14.

[50] Uchiyama H, Barut BA, Mohrbacher AF, et al. Adhesion of human myeloma-derived cell lines to bone marrow stromal cells stimulates interleukin-6 secretion. Blood 1993;82(12):3712–20.

[51] Nefedova Y, Landowski TH, Dalton WS. Bone marrow stromal-derived soluble factors and direct cell contact contribute to de novo drug resistance of myeloma cells by distinct mechanisms. Leukemia 2003;17(6):1175–82.

[52] Folkman J. Role of angiogenesis in tumor growth and metastasis. Semin Oncol 2002; 29(6 Suppl 16):15–8.

[53] Naumov GN, Bender E, Zurakowski D, et al. A model of human tumor dormancy: an angiogenic switch from the nonangiogenic phenotype. J Natl Cancer Inst 2006;98(5): 316–25.

[54] Nawab RA, Azar HA. The laboratory diagnosis of plasma cell myeloma and related disorders. Orthop Clin North Am 1979;10(2):391–404.

[55] Rajkumar SV, Kyle RA. Angiogenesis in multiple myeloma. Semin Oncol 2001;28(6): 560–4.

[56] Roccaro AM, Hideshima T, Raje N, et al. Bortezomib mediates antiangiogenesis in multiple myeloma via direct and indirect effects on endothelial cells. Cancer Res 2006;66(1): 184–91.

[57] Singhal S, Mehta J, Desikan R, et al. Antitumor activity of thalidomide in refractory multiple myeloma. N Engl J Med 1999;341(21):1565–71.

[58] D'Amato RJ, Loughnan MS, Flynn E, et al. Thalidomide is an inhibitor of angiogenesis. Proc Natl Acad Sci U S A 1994;91(9):4082–5.

[59] Vacca A, Scavelli C, Montefusco V, et al. Thalidomide downregulates angiogenic genes in bone marrow endothelial cells of patients with active multiple myeloma. J Clin Oncol 2005;23(23):5334–46.

[60] Vacca A, Ria R, Semeraro F, et al. Endothelial cells in the bone marrow of patients with multiple myeloma. Blood 2003;102(9):3340–8.

[61] Anderson KC. Moving disease biology from the lab to the clinic. Cancer 2003; 97(3 Suppl):796–801.

[62] Dar A, Goichberg P, Shinder V, et al. Chemokine receptor CXCR4-dependent internalization and resecretion of functional chemokine SDF-1 by bone marrow endothelial and stromal cells. Nat Immunol 2005;6(10):1038–46.

[63] Menu E, Asosingh K, Indraccolo S, et al. The involvement of stromal derived factor 1alpha in homing and progression of multiple myeloma in the 5TMM model. Haematologica 2006;91(5):605–12.

[64] Gupta D, Treon SP, Shima Y, et al. Adherence of multiple myeloma cells to bone marrow stromal cells upregulates vascular endothelial growth factor secretion: therapeutic applications. Leukemia 2001;15(12):1950–61.

[65] Tai YT, Podar K, Gupta D, et al. CD40 activation induces p53-dependent vascular endothelial growth factor secretion in human multiple myeloma cells. Blood 2002;99(4): 1419–27.

[66] Baudino TA, McKay C, Pendeville-Samain H, et al. c-Myc is essential for vasculogenesis and angiogenesis during development and tumor progression. Genes Dev 2002;16(19):2530–43.

[67] Oh JS, Kucab JE, Bushel PR, et al. Insulin-like growth factor-1 inscribes a gene expression profile for angiogenic factors and cancer progression in breast epithelial cells. Neoplasia 2002;4(3):204–17.

[68] Poulaki V, Mitsiades CS, McMullan C, et al. Regulation of vascular endothelial growth factor expression by insulin-like growth factor I in thyroid carcinomas. J Clin Endocrinol Metab 2003;88(11):5392–8.

[69] Tanaka Y, Nakayamada S, Okada Y. Osteoblasts and osteoclasts in bone remodeling and inflammation. Curr Drug Targets Inflamm Allergy 2005;4(3):325–8.

[70] Taube T, Beneton MN, McCloskey EV, et al. Abnormal bone remodelling in patients with myelomatosis and normal biochemical indices of bone resorption. Eur J Haematol 1992;49(4):192–8.

[71] Bataille R, Chappard D, Marcelli C, et al. Mechanisms of bone destruction in multiple myeloma: the importance of an unbalanced process in determining the severity of lytic bone disease. J Clin Oncol 1989;7(12):1909–14.

[72] Ashcroft AJ, Davies FE, Morgan GJ. Aetiology of bone disease and the role of bisphosphonates in multiple myeloma. Lancet Oncol 2003;4(5):284–92.

[73] Sezer O, Heider U, Zavrski I, et al. RANK ligand and osteoprotegerin in myeloma bone disease. Blood 2003;101(6):2094–8.

[74] Hofbauer LC, Schoppet M. Clinical implications of the osteoprotegerin/RANKL/RANK system for bone and vascular diseases. JAMA 2004;292(4):490–5.

[75] Roux S, Meignin V, Quillard J, et al. RANK (receptor activator of nuclear factor-kappaB) and RANKL expression in multiple myeloma. Br J Haematol 2002;117(1):86–92.

[76] Pearse RN, Sordillo EM, Yaccoby S, et al. Multiple myeloma disrupts the TRANCE/osteo-protegerin cytokine axis to trigger bone destruction and promote tumor progression. Proc Natl Acad Sci U S A 2001;98(20):11581–6.

[77] Lacey DL, Timms E, Tan HL, et al. Osteoprotegerin ligand is a cytokine that regulates oste-oclast differentiation and activation. Cell 1998;93(2):165–76.

[78] Kawano M, Yamamoto I, Iwato K, et al. Interleukin-1 beta rather than lymphotoxin as the major bone resorbing activity in human multiple myeloma. Blood 1989;73(6): 1646–9.

[79] Mundy GR. Hypercalcemic factors other than parathyroid hormone-related protein. Endo-crinol Metab Clin North Am 1989;18(3):795–806.

[80] Nakamura M, Merchav S, Carter A, et al. Expression of a novel 3.5-kb macrophage col-ony-stimulating factor transcript in human myeloma cells. J Immunol 1989;143(11): 3543–7.

[81] Bataille R, Chappard D, Klein B. The critical role of interleukin-6, interleukin-1B and mac-rophage colony-stimulating factor in the pathogenesis of bone lesions in multiple myeloma. Int J Clin Lab Res 1992;21(4):283–7.

[82] Nakagawa M, Kaneda T, Arakawa T, et al. Vascular endothelial growth factor (VEGF) di-rectly enhances osteoclastic bone resorption and survival of mature osteoclasts. FEBS Lett 2000;473(2):161–4.

[83] Niida S, Kaku M, Amano H, et al. Vascular endothelial growth factor can substitute for macrophage colony-stimulating factor in the support of osteoclastic bone resorption. J Exp Med 1999;190(2):293–8.

[84] Han JH, Choi SJ, Kurihara N, et al. Macrophage inflammatory protein-1alpha is an osteo-clastogenic factor in myeloma that is independent of receptor activator of nuclear factor kappaB ligand. Blood 2001;97(11):3349–53.

[85] Choi SJ, Cruz JC, Craig F, et al. Macrophage inflammatory protein 1-alpha is a potential osteoclast stimulatory factor in multiple myeloma. Blood 2000;96(2):671–5.

[86] Callander NS, Roodman GD. Myeloma bone disease. Semin Hematol 2001;38(3): 276–85.

[87] Choi SJ, Oba Y, Gazitt Y, et al. Antisense inhibition of macrophage inflammatory protein 1-alpha blocks bone destruction in a model of myeloma bone disease. J Clin Invest 2001;108(12):1833–41.

[88] Oba Y, Lee JW, Ehrlich LA, et al. MIP-1alpha utilizes both CCR1 and CCR5 to induce osteoclast formation and increase adhesion of myeloma cells to marrow stromal cells. Exp Hematol 2005;33(3):272–8.

[89] Urashima M, Ogata A, Chauhan D, et al. Transforming growth factor-beta1: differential effects on multiple myeloma versus normal B cells. Blood 1996;87(5):1928–38.

[90] Franchimont N, Rydziel S, Canalis E. Transforming growth factor-beta increases interleu-kin-6 transcripts in osteoblasts. Bone 2000;26(3):249–53.

[91] Ducy P, Zhang R, Geoffroy V, et al. Osf2/Cbfa1: a transcriptional activator of osteoblast differentiation. Cell 1997;89(5):747–54.

[92] Karsenty G, Ducy P, Starbuck M, et al. Cbfa1 as a regulator of osteoblast differentiation and function. Bone 1999;25(1):107–8.

[93] Giuliani N, Colla S, Morandi F, et al. Myeloma cells block RUNX2/CBFA1 activity in human bone marrow osteoblast progenitors and inhibit osteoblast formation and differen-tiation. Blood 2005;106(7):2472–83.

[94] Tian E, Zhan F, Walker R, et al. The role of the Wnt-signaling antagonist DKK1 in the development of osteolytic lesions in multiple myeloma. N Engl J Med 2003;349(26): 2483–94.

[95] Oshima T, Abe M, Asano J, et al. Myeloma cells suppress bone formation by secreting a sol-uble Wnt inhibitor, sFRP-2. Blood 2005;106(9):3160–5.

[96] Lee JW, Chung HY, Ehrlich LA, et al. IL-3 expression by myeloma cells increases both osteoclast formation and growth of myeloma cells. Blood 2004;103(6):2308–15.

[97] Ehrlich LA, Chung HY, Ghobrial I, et al. IL-3 is a potential inhibitor of osteoblast differentiation in multiple myeloma. Blood 2005;106(4):1407–14.

[98] Standal T, Abildgaard N, Fagerli UM, et al. HGF inhibits BMP-induced osteoblastogenesis: possible implications for the bone disease of multiple myeloma. Blood 2007;109(7): 3024–30.

[99] Mitsiades CS, Mitsiades NS, Munshi NC, et al. The role of the bone microenvironment in the pathophysiology and therapeutic management of multiple myeloma: interplay of growth factors, their receptors and stromal interactions. Eur J Cancer 2006;42(11): 1564–73.

[100] Murray EJ, Bentley GV, Grisanti MS, et al. The ubiquitin-proteasome system and cellular proliferation and regulation in osteoblastic cells. Exp Cell Res 1998;242(2): 460–9.

[101] Garrett IR, Chen D, Gutierrez G, et al. Selective inhibitors of the osteoblast proteasome stimulate bone formation in vivo and in vitro. J Clin Invest 2003;111(11):1771–82.

[102] Heider U, Kaiser M, Muller C, et al. Bortezomib increases osteoblast activity in myeloma patients irrespective of response to treatment. Eur J Haematol 2006;77(3):233–8.

[103] Zangari M, Yaccoby S, Cavallo F, et al. Response to bortezomib and activation of osteoblasts in multiple myeloma. Clin Lymphoma Myeloma 2006;7(2):109–14.

[104] Shimazaki C, Uchida R, Nakano S, et al. High serum bone-specific alkaline phosphatase level after bortezomib-combined therapy in refractory multiple myeloma: possible role of bortezomib on osteoblast differentiation. Leukemia 2005;19(6):1102–3.

[105] Knobloch J, Shaughnessy JD Jr, Ruther U. Thalidomide induces limb deformities by perturbing the Bmp/Dkk1/Wnt signaling pathway. FASEB J 2007;21(7):1410–21.

[106] Bergsagel PL, Masellis Smith A, Belch AR, et al. The blood B-cells and bone marrow plasma cells in patients with multiple myeloma share identical IgH rearrangements. Curr Top Microbiol Immunol 1995;194:17–24.

[107] Bergsagel PL, Smith AM, Szczepek A, et al. In multiple myeloma, clonotypic B lymphocytes are detectable among CD19+ peripheral blood cells expressing CD38, CD56, and monotypic Ig light chain. Blood 1995;85(2):436–47.

[108] Kiel K, Cremer FW, Rottenburger C, et al. Analysis of circulating tumor cells in patients with multiple myeloma during the course of high-dose therapy with peripheral blood stem cell transplantation. Bone Marrow Transplant 1999;23(10):1019–27.

[109] Zojer N, Schuster-Kolbe J, Assmann I, et al. Chromosomal aberrations are shared by malignant plasma cells and a small fraction of circulating CD19+ cells in patients with myeloma and monoclonal gammopathy of undetermined significance. Br J Haematol 2002;117(4):852–9.

[110] Rasmussen T, Lodahl M, Hancke S, et al. In multiple myeloma clonotypic CD38-/CD19+/ CD27+ memory B cells recirculate through bone marrow, peripheral blood and lymph nodes. Leuk Lymphoma 2004;45(7):1413–7.

[111] Lin B, Podar K, Gupta D, et al. The vascular endothelial growth factor receptor tyrosine kinase inhibitor PTK787/ZK222584 inhibits growth and migration of multiple myeloma cells in the bone marrow microenvironment. Cancer Res 2002;62(17):5019–26.

[112] Hov H, Holt RU, Ro TB, et al. A selective c-met inhibitor blocks an autocrine hepatocyte growth factor growth loop in ANBL-6 cells and prevents migration and adhesion of myeloma cells. Clin Cancer Res 2004;10(19):6686–94.

[113] Asosingh K, De Raeve H, Croucher P, et al. In vivo homing and differentiation characteristics of mature (CD45-) and immature (CD45+) 5T multiple myeloma cells. Exp Hematol 2001;29(1):77–84.

[114] Tai YT, Podar K, Catley L, et al. Insulin-like growth factor-1 induces adhesion and migration in human multiple myeloma cells via activation of beta1-integrin and phosphatidylinositol 3'-kinase/AKT signaling. Cancer Res 2003;63(18):5850–8.

[115] Anderson K. Advances in the biology of multiple myeloma: therapeutic applications. Semin Oncol 1999;26(5 Suppl 13):10–22.

[116] Kim I, Uchiyama H, Chauhan D, et al. Cell surface expression and functional significance of adhesion molecules on human myeloma-derived cell lines. Br J Haematol 1994;87(3): 483–93.

[117] Asosingh K. Migration, adhesion and differentiation of malignant plasma cells in the 5T murine model of myeloma. Verh K Acad Geneeskd Belg 2003;65(2):127–34.

[118] Asosingh K, Gunthert U, De Raeve H, et al. A unique pathway in the homing of murine multiple myeloma cells: CD44v10 mediates binding to bone marrow endothelium. Cancer Res 2001;61(7):2862–5.

[119] Landowski TH, Olashaw NE, Agrawal D, et al. Cell adhesion-mediated drug resistance (CAM-DR) is associated with activation of NF-kappa B (RelB/p50) in myeloma cells. Oncogene 2003;22(16):2417–21.

[120] Damiano JS, Dalton WS. Integrin-mediated drug resistance in multiple myeloma. Leuk Lymphoma 2000;38(1–2):71–81.

[121] Hazlehurst LA, Damiano JS, Buyuksal I, et al. Adhesion to fibronectin via beta1 integrins regulates p27kip1 levels and contributes to cell adhesion mediated drug resistance (CAM-DR). Oncogene 2000;19(38):4319–27.

[122] Hazlehurst LA, Enkemann SA, Beam CA, et al. Genotypic and phenotypic comparisons of de novo and acquired melphalan resistance in an isogenic multiple myeloma cell line model. Cancer Res 2003;63(22):7900–6.

[123] Barille S, Akhoundi C, Collette M, et al. Metalloproteinases in multiple myeloma: production of matrix metalloproteinase-9 (MMP-9), activation of proMMP-2, and induction of MMP-1 by myeloma cells. Blood 1997;90(4):1649–55.

[124] Flomenberg N, DiPersio J, Calandra G. Role of CXCR4 chemokine receptor blockade using AMD3100 for mobilization of autologous hematopoietic progenitor cells. Acta Haematol 2005;114(4):198–205.

[125] Roodman GD. Role of the bone marrow microenvironment in multiple myeloma. J Bone Miner Res 2002;17(11):1921–5.

[126] Koutsilieris M, Mitsiades C, Lembessis P, et al. Cancer and bone repair mechanism: clinical applications for hormone refractory prostate cancer. J Musculoskelet Neuronal Interact 2000;1(1):15–7.

[127] Hazlehurst LA, Argilagos RF, Emmons M, et al. Cell adhesion to fibronectin (CAM-DR) influences acquired mitoxantrone resistance in U937 cells. Cancer Res 2006;66(4): 2338–45.

[128] Mougel L, Tarpin M, Albert P, et al. Three-dimensional culture and multidrug resistance: effects on immune reactivity of MCF-7 cells by monocytes. Anticancer Res 2004;24(2B):935–41.

[129] Sherman-Baust CA, Weeraratna AT, Rangel LB, et al. Remodeling of the extracellular matrix through overexpression of collagen VI contributes to cisplatin resistance in ovarian cancer cells. Cancer Cell 2003;3(4):377–86.

[130] Sausville EA. The challenge of pathway and environment-mediated drug resistance. Cancer Metastasis Rev 2001;20(1–2):117–22.

[131] Mudry RE, Fortney JE, York T, et al. Stromal cells regulate survival of B-lineage leukemic cells during chemotherapy. Blood 2000;96(5):1926–32.

[132] Taylor ST, Hickman JA, Dive C. Survival signals within the tumour microenvironment suppress drug-induced apoptosis: lessons learned from B lymphomas. Endocr Relat Cancer 1999;6(1):21–3.

[133] Sethi T, Rintoul RC, Moore SM, et al. Extracellular matrix proteins protect small cell lung cancer cells against apoptosis: a mechanism for small cell lung cancer growth and drug resistance in vivo. Nat Med 1999;5(6):662–8.

[134] Taylor ST, Hickman JA, Dive C. Epigenetic determinants of resistance to etoposide regulation of Bcl-X(L) and Bax by tumor microenvironmental factors. J Natl Cancer Inst 2000;92(1):18–23.

[135] Song S, Wientjes MG, Gan Y, et al. Fibroblast growth factors: an epigenetic mechanism of broad spectrum resistance to anticancer drugs. Proc Natl Acad Sci U S A 2000;97(15): 8658–63.

[136] Huff CA, Matsui W, Smith BD, et al. The paradox of response and survival in cancer therapeutics. Blood 2006;107(2):431–4.

[137] Matsui W, Huff CA, Wang Q, et al. Characterization of clonogenic multiple myeloma cells. Blood 2004;103(6):2332–6.

[138] Lemischka IR. Microenvironmental regulation of hematopoietic stem cells. Stem Cells 1997;15(Suppl 1):63–8.

[139] Bissell MJ, Labarge MA. Context, tissue plasticity, and cancer: are tumor stem cells also regulated by the microenvironment? Cancer Cell 2005;7(1):17–23.

[140] Shain KH, Landowski TH, Dalton WS. Adhesion-mediated intracellular redistribution of c-Fas-associated death domain-like IL-1-converting enzyme-like inhibitory protein-long confers resistance to CD95-induced apoptosis in hematopoietic cancer cell lines. J Immunol 2002;168(5):2544–53.

[141] Hideshima T, Nakamura N, Chauhan D, et al. Biologic sequelae of interleukin-6 induced PI3-K/Akt signaling in multiple myeloma. Oncogene 2001;20(42):5991–6000.

[142] Hideshima T, Chauhan D, Richardson P, et al. NF-kappa B as a therapeutic target in multiple myeloma. J Biol Chem 2002;277(19):16639–47.

[143] De Vos J, Jourdan M, Tarte K, et al. JAK2 tyrosine kinase inhibitor tyrphostin AG490 downregulates the mitogen-activated protein kinase (MAPK) and signal transducer and activator of transcription (STAT) pathways and induces apoptosis in myeloma cells. Br J Haematol 2000;109(4):823–8.

[144] Ogata A, Chauhan D, Urashima M, et al. Blockade of mitogen-activated protein kinase cascade signaling in interleukin 6-independent multiple myeloma cells. Clin Cancer Res 1997;3(6):1017–22.

[145] Ogata A, Chauhan D, Teoh G, et al. IL-6 triggers cell growth via the Ras-dependent mitogen-activated protein kinase cascade. J Immunol 1997;159(5):2212–21.

[146] Berger LC, Hawley TS, Lust JA, et al. Tyrosine phosphorylation of JAK-TYK kinases in malignant plasma cell lines growth-stimulated by interleukins 6 and 11. Biochem Biophys Res Commun 1994;202(1):596–605.

[147] Mitsiades CS, Mitsiades N, Poulaki V, et al. Activation of NF-kappaB and upregulation of intracellular anti-apoptotic proteins via the IGF-1/Akt signaling in human multiple myeloma cells: therapeutic implications. Oncogene 2002;21(37):5673–83.

[148] Nefedova Y, Cheng P, Alsina M, et al. Involvement of Notch-1 signaling in bone marrow stroma-mediated de novo drug resistance of myeloma and other malignant lymphoid cell lines. Blood 2004;103(9):3503–10.

[149] Derenne S, Amiot M, Barille S, et al. Zoledronate is a potent inhibitor of myeloma cell growth and secretion of IL-6 and MMP-1 by the tumoral environment. J Bone Miner Res 1999;14(12):2048–56.

[150] Jourdan M, Tarte K, Legouffe E, et al. Tumor necrosis factor is a survival and proliferation factor for human myeloma cells. Eur Cytokine Netw 1999;10(1):65–70.

[151] Hideshima T, Chauhan D, Schlossman R, et al. The role of tumor necrosis factor alpha in the pathophysiology of human multiple myeloma: therapeutic applications. Oncogene 2001;20(33):4519–27.

[152] Sehgal PB, Walther Z, Tamm I. Rapid enhancement of beta 2-interferon/B-cell differentiation factor BSF-2 gene expression in human fibroblasts by diacylglycerols and the calcium ionophore A23187. Proc Natl Acad Sci U S A 1987;84(11):3663–7.

[153] Juge-Morineau N, Francois S, Puthier D, et al. The gp 130 family cytokines IL-6, LIF and OSM but not IL-11 can reverse the anti-proliferative effect of dexamethasone on human myeloma cells. Br J Haematol 1995;90(3):707–10.

[154] Chauhan D, Pandey P, Ogata A, et al. Dexamethasone induces apoptosis of multiple myeloma cells in a JNK/SAP kinase independent mechanism. Oncogene 1997;15(7):837–43.

[155] Urashima M, Teoh G, Chauhan D, et al. Interleukin-6 overcomes p21WAF1 upregulation and G1 growth arrest induced by dexamethasone and interferon-gamma in multiple myeloma cells. Blood 1997;90(1):279–89.

[156] Chauhan D, Hideshima T, Pandey P, et al. RAFTK/PYK2-dependent and -independent apoptosis in multiple myeloma cells. Oncogene 1999;18(48):6733–40.

[157] Chauhan D, Pandey P, Hideshima T, et al. SHP2 mediates the protective effect of interleukin-6 against dexamethasone-induced apoptosis in multiple myeloma cells. J Biol Chem 2000;275(36):27845–50.

[158] Hideshima T, Chauhan D, Teoh G, et al. Characterization of signaling cascades triggered by human interleukin-6 versus Kaposi's sarcoma-associated herpes virus-encoded viral interleukin 6. Clin Cancer Res 2000;6(3):1180–9.

[159] Lowik CW, van der Pluijm G, Bloys H, et al. Parathyroid hormone (PTH) and PTH-like protein (PLP) stimulate interleukin-6 production by osteogenic cells: a possible role of interleukin-6 in osteoclastogenesis. Biochem Biophys Res Commun 1989;162(3):1546–52.

[160] Bataille R, Barlogie B, Lu ZY, et al. Biologic effects of anti-interleukin-6 murine monoclonal antibody in advanced multiple myeloma. Blood 1995;86(2):685–91.

[161] Klein B, Wijdenes J, Zhang XG, et al. Murine anti-interleukin-6 monoclonal antibody therapy for a patient with plasma cell leukemia. Blood 1991;78(5):1198–204.

[162] Lu ZY, Brailly H, Wijdenes J, et al. Measurement of whole body interleukin-6 (IL-6) production: prediction of the efficacy of anti-IL-6 treatments. Blood 1995;86(8):3123–31.

[163] Montero-Julian FA, Klein B, Gautherot E, et al. Pharmacokinetic study of anti-interleukin-6 (IL-6) therapy with monoclonal antibodies: enhancement of IL-6 clearance by cocktails of anti-IL-6 antibodies. Blood 1995;85(4):917–24.

[164] Richardson PG, Barlogie B, Berenson J, et al. A phase 2 study of bortezomib in relapsed, refractory myeloma. N Engl J Med 2003;348(26):2609–17.

[165] Richardson PG, Schlossman RL, Weller E, et al. Immunomodulatory drug CC-5013 overcomes drug resistance and is well tolerated in patients with relapsed multiple myeloma. Blood 2002;100(9):3063–7.

[166] Richardson PG, Sonneveld P, Schuster MW, et al. Bortezomib or high-dose dexamethasone for relapsed multiple myeloma. N Engl J Med 2005;352(24):2487–98.

[167] Rajkumar SV, Hayman S, Gertz MA, et al. Combination therapy with thalidomide plus dexamethasone for newly diagnosed myeloma. J Clin Oncol 2002;20(21):4319–23.

[168] Weber D, Rankin K, Gavino M, et al. Thalidomide alone or with dexamethasone for previously untreated multiple myeloma. J Clin Oncol 2003;21(1):16–9.

[169] Rajkumar SV, Blood E, Vesole D, et al. A randomized phase III clinical trial of thalidomide plus dexamethasone versus dexamethasone alone in newly diagnosed multiple myeloma: a clinical trial coordinated by the Eastern Cooperative Oncology Group. J Clin Oncol 2006;24(3):431–6.

[170] Rajkumar SV, Hayman SR, Lacy MQ, et al. Combination therapy with lenalidomide plus dexamethasone (Rev/Dex) for newly diagnosed myeloma. Blood 2005;106(13): 4050–3.

[171] Hankinson SE, Willett WC, Colditz GA, et al. Circulating concentrations of insulin-like growth factor-I and risk of breast cancer. Lancet 1998;351(9113):1393–6.

[172] Chan JM, Stampfer MJ, Giovannucci E, et al. Plasma insulin-like growth factor-I and prostate cancer risk: a prospective study. Science 1998;279(5350):563–6.

[173] LeRoith D, Roberts CT. The insulin-like growth factor system and cancer. Cancer Lett 2003;195(2):127–37.

[174] Sell C, Dumenil G, Deveaud C, et al. Effect of a null mutation of the insulin-like growth factor I receptor gene on growth and transformation of mouse embryo fibroblasts. Mol Cell Biol 1994;14(6):3604–12.

[175] Coppola D, Ferber A, Miura M, et al. A functional insulin-like growth factor I receptor is required for the mitogenic and transforming activities of the epidermal growth factor receptor. Mol Cell Biol 1994;14(7):4588–95.

[176] Porcu P, Ferber A, Pietrzkowski Z, et al. The growth-stimulatory effect of simian virus 40 T antigen requires the interaction of insulinlike growth factor 1 with its receptor. Mol Cell Biol 1992;12(11):5069–77.

[177] Mitsiades CS, Mitsiades N. Treatment of hematologic malignancies and solid tumors by inhibiting IGF receptor signaling. Expert Rev Anticancer Ther 2005;5(3):487–99.

[178] Adams TE, Epa VC, Garrett TP, et al. Structure and function of the type 1 insulin-like growth factor receptor. Cell Mol Life Sci 2000;57(7):1050–93.

[179] Chaiken RL, Moses AC, Usher P, et al. Insulin stimulation of aminoisobutyric acid transport in human skin fibroblasts is mediated through both insulin and type I insulin-like growth factor receptors. J Clin Endocrinol Metab 1986;63(5):1181–5.

[180] Flier JS, Usher P, Moses AC. Monoclonal antibody to the type I insulin-like growth factor (IGF-I) receptor blocks IGF-I receptor-mediated DNA synthesis: clarification of the mitogenic mechanisms of IGF-I and insulin in human skin fibroblasts. Proc Natl Acad Sci U S A 1986;83(3):664–8.

[181] Kull FC Jr, Jacobs S, Su YF, et al. Monoclonal antibodies to receptors for insulin and somatomedin-C. J Biol Chem 1983;258(10):6561–6.

[182] Poretsky L, Grigorescu F, Seibel M, et al. Distribution and characterization of insulin and insulin-like growth factor I receptors in normal human ovary. J Clin Endocrinol Metab 1985;61(4):728–34.

[183] Garcia-Echeverria C, Pearson MA, Marti A, et al. In vivo antitumor activity of NVP-AEW541-A novel, potent, and selective inhibitor of the IGF-IR kinase. Cancer Cell 2004;5(3):231–9.

[184] Girnita A, Girnita L, del Prete F, et al. Cyclolignans as inhibitors of the insulin-like growth factor-1 receptor and malignant cell growth. Cancer Res 2004;64(1):236–42.

[185] Stromberg T, Ekman S, Girnita L, et al. IGF-1 receptor tyrosine kinase inhibition by the cyclolignan PPP induces G2/M-phase accumulation and apoptosis in multiple myeloma cells. Blood 2006;107(2):669–78.

[186] Menu E, Jernberg-Wiklund H, Stromberg T, et al. Inhibiting the IGF-1 receptor tyrosine kinase with the cyclolignan PPP: an in vitro and in vivo study in the 5T33MM mouse model. Blood 2006;107(2):655–60.

[187] Holt RU, Baykov V, Ro TB, et al. Human myeloma cells adhere to fibronectin in response to hepatocyte growth factor. Haematologica 2005;90(4):479–88.

[188] Hurt EM, Wiestner A, Rosenwald A, et al. Overexpression of c-maf is a frequent oncogenic event in multiple myeloma that promotes proliferation and pathological interactions with bone marrow stroma. Cancer Cell 2004;5(2):191–9.

[189] Bergsagel PL, Kuehl WM, Zhan F, et al. Cyclin D dysregulation: an early and unifying pathogenic event in multiple myeloma. Blood 2005;106(1):296–303.

[190] Richardson P, Schlossman R, Jagannath S, et al. Thalidomide for patients with relapsed multiple myeloma after high-dose chemotherapy and stem cell transplantation: results of an open-label multicenter phase 2 study of efficacy, toxicity, and biological activity. Mayo Clin Proc 2004;79(7):875–82.

[191] Richardson PG, Blood E, Mitsiades CS, et al. A randomized phase 2 study of lenalidomide therapy for patients with relapsed or relapsed and refractory multiple myeloma. Blood 2006;108(10):3458–64.

[192] Richardson PG, Jagannath S, Avigan DE, et al. Lenalidomide plus bortezomib (Rev-Vel) in relapsed and/or refractory multiple myeloma (MM): final results of a multicenter phase 1 trial. Blood 2006;108(11):124A.

[193] Kenyon BM, Browne F, D'Amato RJ. Effects of thalidomide and related metabolites in a mouse corneal model of neovascularization. Exp Eye Res 1997;64(6):971–8.

[194] D'Amato RJ, Lentzsch S, Anderson KC, et al. Mechanism of action of thalidomide and 3-aminothalidomide in multiple myeloma. Semin Oncol 2001;28(6):597–601.

[195] Stirling DI. The pharmacology of thalidomide. Sem in Hematol 2000;37:5–14.

[196] Shipman CM, Rogers MJ, Apperley JF, et al. Bisphosphonates induce apoptosis in human myeloma cell lines: a novel anti-tumour activity. Br J Haematol 1997;98(3):665–72.

[197] Aparicio A, Gardner A, Tu Y, et al. In vitro cytoreductive effects on multiple myeloma cells induced by bisphosphonates. Leukemia 1998;12(2):220–9.

[198] Uhlman DL, Verfaillie C, Jones RB, et al. BCNU treatment of marrow stromal monolayers reversibly alters haematopoiesis. Br J Haematol 1991;78(3):304–9.

[199] Mitsiades CS, Mitsiades NS, McMullan CJ, et al. Transcriptional signature of histone deacetylase inhibition in multiple myeloma: biological and clinical implications. Proc Natl Acad Sci U S A 2004;101(2):540–5.

[200] Mitsiades N, Mitsiades CS, Richardson PG, et al. Molecular sequelae of histone deacetylase inhibition in human malignant B cells. Blood 2003;101(10):4055–62.

[201] Sordillo EM, Pearse RN. RANK-Fc: a therapeutic antagonist for RANK-L in myeloma. Cancer 2003;97(3 Suppl):802–12.

[202] Vanderkerken K, De Leenheer E, Shipman C, et al. Recombinant osteoprotegerin decreases tumor burden and increases survival in a murine model of multiple myeloma. Cancer Res 2003;63(2):287–9.

[203] Holash J, Davis S, Papadopoulos N, et al. VEGF-Trap: a VEGF blocker with potent antitumor effects. Proc Natl Acad Sci U S A 2002;99(17):11393–8.

[204] Mori Y, Shimizu N, Dallas M, et al. Anti-alpha4 integrin antibody suppresses the development of multiple myeloma and associated osteoclastic osteolysis. Blood 2004;104(7): 2149–54.

[205] Trudel S, Ely S, Farooqi Y, et al. Inhibition of fibroblast growth factor receptor 3 induces differentiation and apoptosis in t(4;14) myeloma. Blood 2004;103(9):3521–8.

[206] Trudel S, Li ZH, Wei E, et al. CHIR-258, a novel, multitargeted tyrosine kinase inhibitor for the potential treatment of t(4;14) multiple myeloma. Blood 2005;105(7):2941–8.

[207] Zhu L, Somlo G, Zhou B, et al. Fibroblast growth factor receptor 3 inhibition by short hairpin RNAs leads to apoptosis in multiple myeloma. Mol Cancer Ther 2005;4(5):787–98.

[208] Sebti SM, Hamilton AD. Farnesyltransferase and geranylgeranyltransferase I inhibitors and cancer therapy: lessons from mechanism and bench-to-bedside translational studies. Oncogene 2000;19(56):6584–93.

[209] Le Gouill S, Pellat-Deceunynck C, Harousseau JL, et al. Farnesyl transferase inhibitor R115777 induces apoptosis of human myeloma cells. Leukemia 2002;16(9):1664–7.

[210] Bolick SC, Landowski TH, Boulware D, et al. The farnesyl transferase inhibitor, FTI-277, inhibits growth and induces apoptosis in drug-resistant myeloma tumor cells. Leukemia 2003;17(2):451–7.

[211] Alsina M, Fonseca R, Wilson EF, et al. Farnesyltransferase inhibitor tipifarnib is well tolerated, induces stabilization of disease, and inhibits farnesylation and oncogenic/tumor survival pathways in patients with advanced multiple myeloma. Blood 2004;103(9): 3271–7.

[212] Mitsiades N, Mitsiades CS, Poulaki V, et al. Biologic sequelae of nuclear factor-kappaB blockade in multiple myeloma: therapeutic applications. Blood 2002;99(11):4079–86.

[213] Frost P, Moatamed F, Hoang B, et al. In vivo antitumor effects of the mTOR inhibitor CCI-779 against human multiple myeloma cells in a xenograft model. Blood 2004;104(13): 4181–7.

[214] Mitsiades NS, McMullan CJ, Poulaki V, et al. The mTOR inhibitor RAD001 (everolimus) is active against multiple myeloma cells in vitro and in vivo. Blood 2004;104(11s):418a.

[215] Raje N, Kumar S, Hideshima T, et al. Combination of the mTOR inhibitor rapamycin and CC-5013 has synergistic activity in multiple myeloma. Blood 2004;104(13):4188–93.

[216] Stromberg T, Dimberg A, Hammarberg A, et al. Rapamycin sensitizes multiple myeloma cells to apoptosis induced by dexamethasone. Blood 2004;103(8):3138–47.

[217] Shi Y, Yan H, Frost P, et al. Mammalian target of rapamycin inhibitors activate the AKT kinase in multiple myeloma cells by up-regulating the insulin-like growth factor

receptor/insulin receptor substrate-1/phosphatidylinositol 3-kinase cascade. Mol Cancer Ther 2005;4(10):1533–40.

[218] Shammas MA, Shmookler Reis RJ, Akiyama M, et al. Telomerase inhibition and cell growth arrest by G-quadruplex interactive agent in multiple myeloma. Mol Cancer Ther 2003;2(9):825–33.

[219] Shammas MA, Shmookler Reis RJ, Li C, et al. Telomerase inhibition and cell growth arrest after telomestatin treatment in multiple myeloma. Clin Cancer Res 2004;10(2):770–6.

[220] Negri J, Mitsiades N, Deng QW, et al. PKC412 is a multi-targeting kinase inhibitor with activity against multiple myeloma in vitro and in vivo. Blood 2005;106(11):75a.

[221] Deng QW, Mitsiades N, Negri J, et al. Dasatinib (BMS-354825): a multi-targeted kinase inhibitor with activity against multiple myeloma. Blood 2005;106(11):451A–451A.

[222] Xu W, Neckers L. Targeting the molecular chaperone heat shock protein 90 provides a multifaceted effect on diverse cell signaling pathways of cancer cells. Clin Cancer Res 2007;13(6):1625–9.

[223] Mitsiades CS, Mitsiades NS, McMullan CJ, et al. Antimyeloma activity of heat shock protein-90 inhibition. Blood 2006;107(3):1092–100.

[224] Chatterjee M, Jain S, Stuhmer T, et al. STAT3 and MAPK signaling maintain overexpression of heat shock proteins 90alpha and beta in multiple myeloma cells, which critically contribute to tumor-cell survival. Blood 2007;109(2):720–8.

[225] Sydor JR, Normant E, Pien CS, et al. Development of 17-allylamino-17-demethoxygeldanamycin hydroquinone hydrochloride (IPI-504), an anti-cancer agent directed against Hsp90. Proc Natl Acad Sci U S A 2006;103(46):17408–13.

[226] Richardson PG, Chanan-Khan AA, Alsina M, et al. Safety and activity of KOS-953 in patients with relapsed refractory multiple myeloma (MM): Interim results of a phase 1 trial. Blood 2005;106(11):109a.

[227] Richardson P, Chanan-Khan A, Lonial S, et al. A multicenter Phase 1 clinical trial of tanespimycin (KOS-953) + Bortezomib (BZ): encouraging activity and manageable toxicity in heavily pre-treated patients with relapsed refractory multiple myeloma (MM). Paper presented at the 2006 Annual Meeting of the American Society of Hematology. Orlando (FL), December 2006.

Hematol Oncol Clin N Am 21 (2007) 1035–1049

HEMATOL■GY/■N■■L■GY ■LINICS
OF NORTH AMERICA

ELSEVIER
SAUNDERS

Pathophysiology of Multiple Myeloma Bone Disease

Suzanne Lentzsch, MD, PhD[a],*, Lori A. Ehrlich, MD, PhD[b],
G. David Roodman, MD, PhD[a,b]

[a]Division of Hematology/Oncology, Department of Medicine, University of Pittsburgh,
5150 Centre Avenue, Pittsburgh, PA 15232, USA
[b]Division of Hematology/Oncology, Veterans Administration Pittsburgh Healthcare System,
Research and Development, 151-U, University Drive C, Pittsburgh, PA 15240, USA

Multiple myeloma (MM) is a plasma cell malignancy characterized by the frequent development of osteolytic bone lesions [1]. Almost all patients who have MM develop osteopenia or osteolytic lesions that result in pathologic fractures or severe bone pain. More than 50% [2] of all patients who have MM develop pathologic fractures frequently resulting in severe debilitation. The development of osteolytic lesions is attributable to increased bone resorption caused by stimulation of osteoclast (OCL) formation and activity [3–5]. This increased OCL activity is accompanied by decreased osteoblast (OBL) function resulting in imbalanced bone remodeling with increased bone resorption and decreased bone formation [6,7]. These data are supported by studies showing that patients who have MM with bone lesions have reduced bone formation markers, such as alkaline phosphatase and osteocalcin, together with increased bone resorption markers [8]. In the last few years, several potential mechanisms involved in this process have been reported. Increased knowledge of the signaling pathways involved in the regulation of OCL/OBL function have provided us with a better understanding of the pathophysiologic mechanisms involved in bone remodeling. In this article the authors discuss potential mechanisms involved in myeloma bone disease to identify the potential therapeutic targets for the treatment of MM bone disease.

NORMAL BONE REMODELING

The skeleton undergoes a continuous turnover and remodels itself through the balanced activity of OCLs and OBLs on trabecular bone surfaces. OCLs are the major mediators of bone resorption arising from hematopoietic precursors

*Corresponding author. Division of Hematology/Oncology, Department of Medicine, University of Pittsburgh, 5150 Centre Avenue, #568, Pittsburgh, PA 15232. *E-mail address:* lentzschs@upmc.edu (S. Lentzsch).

0889-8588/07/$ – see front matter
doi:10.1016/j.hoc.2007.08.009

derived from the macrophage lineage [9]. Activated OCLs resorb bone and are regulated by their formation and activity, systemic hormones, and local factors produced in the bone microenvironment. The bone marrow microenvironment thus plays a critical role in the formation and activation of OCLs. Two major stimulators of OCL formation are macrophage colony stimulating factor (M-CSF) and receptor activator of nuclear factor-κB ligand (RANKL). RANKL is expressed by activated T cells, bone marrow stromal cells (BMSCs), and OBLs, and binds to its receptor RANK, which is expressed by OCL precursors, chondrocytes, and mature OCLs. The binding of RANKL to RANK promotes OCL maturation and activation and prevents apoptosis [10].

RANKL binds the RANK receptor on OCL precursors and induces the formation of OCLs by signaling through the nuclear factor-κB and Jun N-terminal kinase pathways. The secretion of RANKL from BMSCs and OBLs is also induced by most osteotropic factors, such as parathyroid hormone, 1,25-dihydroxyvitamin D_3, and prostaglandins [11,12]. Glucocorticoids, IL-1β, TNF-α, IL-11, and prostaglandin-E2 also induce the expression of RANKL, whereas TGFβ decreases the expression of RANKL. The importance of RANKL for OCL formation was clearly shown by RANKL and RANK knockout mice. These mice lack OCLs and develop severe osteoporosis [13,14]. Osteoprotegerin (OPG) is, like RANKL, a member of the tumor necrosis factor receptor superfamily. It is a soluble decoy receptor for RANKL and thereby inhibits the differentiation and resorption of OCLs [15]. The ratio between OPG and RANKL regulates the activity and formation of OCLs. As a counterpart of RANKL, the overproduction of OPG in transgenic mice caused severe osteopetrosis, whereas in the absence of OPG the mice developed osteopenia (Fig. 1) [16,17].

OCLs induce bone resorption by secreting proteases, dissolving the matrix, and producing acid that releases bone mineral into the extracellular space under the ruffled border of the OCL [18]. The ruffled border forms a tight sealing zone that acts like an extracellular lysosome to degrade bone, which explains why adherence of OCLs to the bone surface is critical for the bone resorptive process. Agents that can affect the adherence of OCLs to bone matrix therefore might be effective for the treatment of lytic bone lesions [19].

INCREASED OSTEOCLAST ACTIVITY IN MULTIPLE MYELOMA

In MM, the destruction of bone is mediated by OCLs rather than by tumor cells [20]. OCLs accumulate only at bone-resorbing surfaces adjacent to MM cells. The number of OCLs is not increased in areas uninvolved with tumor [21]. Although the bone resorption in MM is increased, the bone formation is suppressed so that bone lesions in patients who have MM become purely lytic [22].

Myeloma cells adhere to BMSCs through binding of VLA-4 ($\alpha4\beta1$ integrin), present on the surface of MM cells, to vascular cell adhesion molecule-1 (VCAM-1), which is expressed on stromal cells. The adherence of MM cells to BMSCs and OBLs enhances the production of RANKL, M-CSF, and other

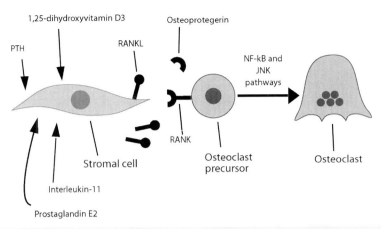

Fig. 1. Osteoclast formation and receptor activator of nuclear factor-jB ligand (RANKL). Expression of RANKL on bone marrow stromal cells is induced by osteotrophic factors, such as 1,25-dihydroxyvitamin D3, PTH, IL-11, and prostaglandin E2. RANKL on stromal cells binds to RANK on osteoclast precursor cells inducing differentiation into mature, multinucleated osteoclasts. (*Adapted from* Roodman GD. Mechanisms of bone metastasis. N Engl J Med 2004; 350(16):1658; with permission.)

cytokines that activate OCL, such as IL-6, IL-11, IL-1β, TNFs, and bFGF. At the same time, the production of OPG, the decoy receptor of RANKL, is suppressed. Several factors have been described that increase OCL activity in MM [23]. The leading candidates are interleukin-6 (IL-6), macrophage inflammatory protein-1 alpha (MIP-1α), RANKL, and interleukin-1beta (IL-1β). IL-1β is a potent stimulator of OCL formation [24], but the levels of IL-1β detected in patients who have MM are very low [25–27]. This observation suggests that IL-1β is probably not a major mediator of MM bone disease (Fig. 2).

Interleukin-6

IL-6 can induce proliferation and block apoptosis of MM cells [28]. It is a potent stimulator of OCL formation and can enhance the effects of parathyroid hormone on the formation of OCL in vivo [29,30]. In addition, adherence of myeloma cells to BMSCs increases the production of IL-6 by BMSCs [31]. This phenomenon suggests that IL-6 plays an important role in enhancing the growth and survival of myeloma cells and stimulating OCL formation. IL-6 levels do not correlate with the extent of bone disease in patients who have MM, however, so the exact role of IL-6 in myeloma bone disease remains to be determined.

Receptor Activator of Nuclear Factor-κB Ligand

The most important factors for the development of OCLs are M-CSF and RANKL. M-CSF expands the pool of OCL precursors and subsequently RANKL stimulates OCL precursors to develop into mature OCL. Stromal

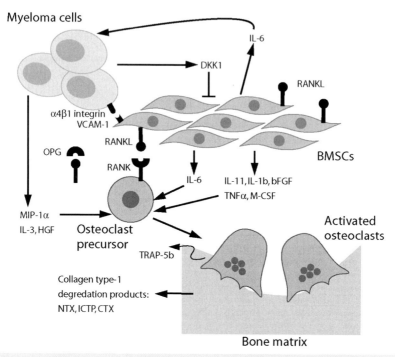

Fig. 2. The myeloma microenvironment. Myeloma cells bind to bone marrow stromal cells though the interaction of VCAM-1 and a4b1 inducing expression of RANKL and IL-6 by the stromal cells. IL-6 acts as a growth factor for myeloma cells. RANKL and IL-6 induce differentiation of osteoclast precursors into mature osteoclasts that resorb bone releasing collagen type-1 degradation products. Other factors secreted by the myeloma cells (MIP-1a, IL-3, and HGF) and stromal cells (IL-11, IL-1b, bFGF, TNF-a, and M-CSF) induce osteoclast differentiation. DKK1 expressed by myeloma cells blocks differentiation of stromal cells into osteoblasts. (*Adapted from* Terpos E, Dimopoulos M-A. Myeloma bone disease: pathophysiology and management. Ann Oncol 2005;16:1224; with permission.)

cells and OBLs express RANKL when stimulated by appropriate cytokines and chemokines.

Myeloma cells also can express and induce RANKL and down-regulate the expression of OPG in preosteoblastic and stromal cell cocultures [32]. RANKL expression is increased in bone marrow biopsies from patients who have MM. RANKL is also overexpressed in stromal cells, OBLs, and activated T cells in areas with high numbers of MM cells [33]. In addition, OPG expression in bone marrow specimens from patients who have MM is reduced and the interaction between myeloma cells and BMSCs inhibits OPG production [32]. In MM, the down-regulation of OPG leads to reduced inhibition of RANKL and increased OCL activation. Consistent with these observations, when serum samples of patients who had MM were evaluated, OPG levels were decreased, whereas serum levels of soluble RANKL and the soluble RANKL/OPG ratio were increased. Further, the RANKL/OPG ratio correlated with the extent of the bone disease and markers of bone resorption [34]. These data confirm that the RANKL/OPG pathway is a major mediator of MM bone disease.

Macrophage Inflammatory Protein-1 alpha

MIP-1α belongs to the RANTES (regulated on activation normal T cell expressed and secreted) family of chemokines and is a chemoattractant and activator of phagocytes [35]. MIP-1α is also a chemotactic factor for OCL precursors and can induce differentiation of OCL progenitors and contributes to OCL formation [36–38]. MIP-1α is produced and secreted by MM cells, and the levels correlate with the severity of MM bone disease [36,39–41]. MIP-1α antibodies or blocking antibodies against the receptor CCR5, and transfection of MM cells with antisense constructs to MIP-1α, could block enhanced bone resorption in murine models of MM bone disease [36,42]. Furthermore, MIP-1α can enhance RANKL expression in stromal cells and thereby indirectly increase osteoclastogenesis [36]. Besides the effects on OCLs, MIP-1α also directly acts on MM cells, because MM cells express the receptor for MIP-1α, CCR1 [36]. It was also shown that MIP-1α promotes growth, survival and migration of MM cells. MIP-1α induced the activation of multiple signaling pathways crucial for MM growth and survival, including the phosphatidylinositol 3-kinase (PI3-K)/AKT and MAPK pathways, leading to increased proliferation and protection against apoptosis in MM [43]. Targeting MIP-1α could thus provide an effective approach in the treatment of MM bone disease.

OSTEOBLAST INHIBITION IN MULTIPLE MYELOMA

When patients who have MM are in remission from their disease with no evidence of malignant cells in the marrow, lytic bone lesions persist [44]. Bisphosphonate treatment inhibits bone resorption without inducing bone repair. Lytic lesions are visible by radiographic imaging or MRI, but bone scanning underestimates the extent of bone disease because it detects reactive bone formation by OBLs after osteoclastic bone resorption. In patients who have MM with impaired OBL function, therefore, bone scans do not readily reveal a defect [45]. The clinical observation that patients who have MM have decreased OBL activity was confirmed in several in vitro and in vivo studies.

Hjorth-Hansen and colleagues [46] show marked osteoblastopenia in a mouse model of MM. When they injected the MM cell line JJN-3 into irradiated SCID mice, this resulted in a 99% reduction in OBL per millimeter bone perimeter and a 70% reduction in bone volume. Silvestris and colleagues [47] showed that OBLs derived from patients who have MM are more susceptible to apoptosis induced by TNF-α. In addition, previous studies also showed that myeloma cells secrete a soluble OBL-inhibiting factor [48]. Little is known about the identity of these agents that can suppress OBL function in MM, however. Possible candidates for OBL inhibitors in MM include DKK1 and other factors that block the Wnt pathway, along with IL-3 and IL-7 (Fig. 3).

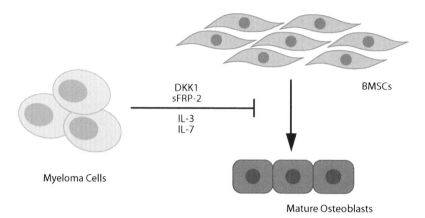

Fig. 3. Proposed osteoblast inhibitors in myeloma. Several soluble factors have been proposed to be osteoblast inhibitors in myeloma. DKK1, sFRP-3, IL-3, and IL-7 are all believed to be secreted from the myeloma cells. Differentiation of mesenchymal stem cells, a subset of the bone marrow stromal cells, into mature osteoblasts may be inhibited by these factors. (*Courtesy of* Lori A. Ehrlich, MD, PhD, Pittsburgh, PA.)

DKK1 and the Wnt Signaling Pathway

The Wnt signaling pathway is important in the growth, development, and function of OBLs and early lymphopoiesis [49]. Classically, Wnt binds to LRP5 or 6, another soluble mediator, and the complex then binds to the frizzled receptor. Signal transduction from the frizzled receptor results in dephosphorylation and stabilization of β-catenin. β-catenin localizes to the nucleus and increases expression of target genes. Activation of the β-catenin pathway leads to activation of OBL differentiation in vitro [50]. There are several soluble inhibitors of the Wnt pathway, including Dickkopf (DKK1) and secreted frizzled receptor-like proteins (sFRP). DKK1 binds to LRP5 and 6, sequestering them from binding to Wnt, thereby inhibiting proper signaling.

Tian and colleagues [51] were the first to investigate the role of DKK1 in OBL inhibition in myeloma. They found that DKK1 was up-regulated in myeloma plasma cells by microarray analysis, and confirmed its expression by ELISA and immunostaining. DKK1 expression was greater in patients who had one or more lytic lesions by MRI compared with patients who had MM with no lytic lesions, indicating a possible role for DKK1 in bone disease. They were not able to show a correlation between DKK1 levels and the severity of myeloma, however. In fact, patients who had more aggressive myeloma did not express DKK1. They then determined if DKK1 could inhibit OBL differentiation. For these studies, they used the murine mesenchymal cell line C2C12, which can be committed to the OBL pathway by the addition of BMP-2. OBL differentiation was measured by alkaline phosphatase expression. Recombinant human DKK1 added to BMP-2–treated C2C12 cultures inhibited ALP expression by the C2C12 cells, suggesting that DKK1 inhibits

OBL formation. Importantly, plasma from patients expressing high levels of DKK1 also blocked ALP expression by these cells, and this inhibition could be reversed by the addition of a neutralizing antibody to DKK1 [51]. Another study by Politou and colleagues [52] also showed that patients who have myeloma have increased serum levels of DKK1. This study found a wide range of DKK1 expression levels in patients who had myeloma, with positive correlation of high DKK1 levels with advanced stages of myeloma.

Contrary to the above findings, Giuliani and colleagues [53] used primary OBL cultures from normal patients and showed that DKK1 did not inhibit OBL formation in early (14 day, colony-forming unit–fibroblast, CFU-F) or late (21 day, colony-forming unit–osteoblast, CFU-OB) cultures. In fact, DKK1 had a slight stimulatory effect on CFU-OB cultures. Similarly, DKK1 did not inhibit Runx2 activity, the primary OBL-specific transcription factor, except for a slight inhibitory effect at high levels of DKK1. These results suggest that DKK1 may not be responsible for OBL inhibition in MM.

The sFRP family proteins are also soluble inhibitors of Wnt signaling. These decoy receptors block binding of Wnt to the membrane-bound receptor, frizzled. sFRP-2 and -3 have also been investigated as possible mediators of OBL inhibition in MM. In preliminary studies, Oshima and colleagues [54] showed that sFRP-2 was secreted by primary myeloma cells and cell lines, and recombinant sFRP-2 inhibited differentiation of the murine OBL-like cell line, MC3T3-E1. Importantly, conditioned media from MM cell lines inhibited mineralization by MC3T3-E1 cells, and this was partially reversed by immunodepletion of sFRP-2. FRZB, also known as sFRP-3, has been shown in two studies to be up-regulated in malignant plasma cells of patients who have MM, but the role of sFRP-3 in MM bone disease has not been clearly defined [55]. In addition, Davies and colleagues [56] also showed a down-regulation of the downstream effector gene, CTNNB1 or β-catenin, in MM. These results suggest that Wnt signaling inhibitors may play a role in inhibiting OBL differentiation in MM, but further studies are necessary to confirm their role in MM bone disease.

Interleukin-3

Interleukin-3 (IL-3) levels are elevated in serum and bone marrow of patients who have myeloma [57,58]. Lee and colleagues [58] reported that 75% of patients who have MM have increased IL-3 levels. This study also determined that IL-3 acts as a myeloma growth factor and stimulates OCL formation in vitro. Recent studies have investigated the role and mechanism of IL-3 inhibition of OBLs in myeloma.

Ehrlich and colleagues [59] showed that OBL differentiation in human and murine cultures was significantly inhibited by IL-3 at levels present in patients who had myeloma. Further, bone marrow plasma from patients who had MM with high IL-3 inhibited OBL differentiation in human CFU-F cultures. The inhibitory effects of plasma from patients who had high IL-3 were partially reversed by the addition of a neutralizing antibody to human IL-3. In contrast, the inhibitory effects of marrow plasma from patients who had normal IL-3 levels were unchanged by the addition of anti–IL-3. This study further shows that IL-3 acts indirectly by way of monocytes/macrophages to inhibit OBL differentiation. Importantly, depletion of the $CD45^+$ hematopoietic cells in primary OBL cultures blocked the capacity of IL-3 to inhibit OBL differentiation. Reconstitution of the $CD45^-$ cultures with $CD45^+$ cells restored the capacity of IL-3 to inhibit OBL differentiation. These studies suggest that IL-3 might contribute to the uncoupling of bone turnover in myeloma because IL-3 stimulates OCLs, increasing bone destruction, and also inhibits OBL differentiation. IL-3 may therefore act as a bifunctional mediator of MM bone disease, increasing OCL formation and suppressing OBL differentiation.

Interleukin-7

Interleukin-7 (IL-7) is another potential inhibitor of OBL differentiation in MM. Estrogen deficiency because of ovariectomy results in loss of bone mass in models of osteoporosis, and Weitzmann and colleagues [60] reported increased levels of IL-7 in mice following ovariectomy. In this report, they showed that IL-7 blocked new bone formation after ovariectomy. In mouse calvarial OBL cultures, OBL activity was suppressed with basal or BMP2 treatment.

Guiliani and colleagues [53] have proposed a role for IL-7 in OBL inhibition in MM. In a recent study, they showed that IL-7 levels were increased in marrow of patients who had MM. IL-7 inhibited OBL differentiation in early (14 days) and late (21 days) OBL cultures in a dose-dependent manner. IL-7 also inhibited Runx2 activity, an important OBL transcription factor, in cultures of human OBLs. Importantly, treatment of BMSCs with a myeloma cell line–conditioned media or plasma from patients who had MM blocked CFU-F formation at 14 days, and this inhibition was partially reversed by the addition of a neutralizing antibody to IL-7. These data suggest that IL-7 may be one of several factors suppressing OBL activity in MM.

BIOCHEMICAL MARKERS OF BONE TURNOVER IN MULTIPLE MYELOMA

The value of biochemical markers of bone turnover for monitoring patients who have bone metastases is still under investigation. Levels of bone-specific alkaline phosphatase, osteocalcin, and a type I procollagen C-propeptide in serum are indicators of OBL activity, whereas serum levels of C-terminal cross-linking telopeptide of type I collagen (CTx or ICTP), tartrate-resistant acid phosphatase (TRAP), and urinary levels of N-terminal cross-linking telopeptide of type I collagen (NTx) are markers of OCL activity. A histomorphometric study of bone biopsies of patients who had MM showed that high urinary NTx levels and serum CTx levels correlate with low bone mineral density [61]. In Cox analysis, CTx showed the highest predictive value. This study further showed that increases in serum CTx levels correlated with the stage of disease and differed significantly between MGUS, MM stage I, and MM in stages II–III ($P<.001$) [62,63]. Furthermore, Jakob and colleagues [64] evaluated serum CTx levels in untreated MM patients who had no skeletal abnormalities on conventional radiographs and correlated these data to MRI findings of the spine. This study showed that serum CTx was significantly increased in patients who had abnormal bone MRIs compared with patients who had normal MRIs. Another study showed that high levels of serum CTx and urinary NTx correlated with increased risk for early progression of bone lesions during standard melphalan-prednisone treatment [61]. In another study of patients receiving zoledronic acid or pamidronate, patients who had MM with high and moderate NTx levels had twofold increases in their risk for skeletal complications and disease progression compared with patients who had low NTx levels [65].

In summary, serum CTx and urinary NTx are the most sensitive tools for estimating the increased bone resorption in MM, and might be clinically useful for identifying patients at increased risk for active bone disease. Because bisphosphonates can have devastating side effects, such as osteonecrosis of the jaw, bone resorption markers will receive more attention in future treatment strategies. Several studies have focused on the role of bone markers to guide treatment of osteolytic lesions with the goal to avoid overtreatment associated with unwanted side effects, such as osteonecrosis of the jaw.

NEW APPROACHES FOR THE TREATMENT OF BONE DISEASE IN MULTIPLE MYELOMA

Bisphosphonate therapy is associated with severe side effects, such as renal toxicity and osteonecrosis of the jaw, which are believed to be associated with drug-induced irreversible cessation of bone remodeling. Additionally, the use of bisphosphonates in the face of significant impairment of renal function is difficult and may be contraindicated. New drugs capable of targeting activated OCLs without completely arresting bone resorption and modeling are needed.

Bortezomib (Velcade) as a Potential Bone Anabolic Agent in Multiple Myeloma

Treatment of patients who have myeloma with bisphosphonates blocks the increased OCL activity but has little effect on stimulating OBLs to repair bone lesions. Preliminary studies of bortezomib indicate that it may increase OBL activity resulting in enhanced new bone formation and potentially repair of lytic bone lesions. Degradation of proteins by the ubiquitin-proteasome pathway has been shown to be critical for myeloma cell survival, and inhibition of the proteasome with bortezomib resulted in an effective anti-myeloma agent as shown in several clinical trials [66]. The proteasome pathway is also an important regulator of OBL differentiation [67] prompting investigators to examine the association between bortezomib treatment and OBL activation.

Two case reports initially showed an increase in alkaline phosphatase, a marker of OBL activation, in patients treated with bortezomib [68,69]. Zangari and colleagues [69] conducted a retrospective analysis of three trials of bortezomib in relapsed myeloma. In all three trials, patients who had a partial response to bortezomib therapy had increased alkaline phosphatase compared with nonresponders. Additionally, patients who responded to bortezomib treatment were compared with those who responded to dexamethasone. The bortezomib-treated group had higher serum levels of alkaline phosphatase than the dexamethasone responders indicating that the increase in the OBL marker is not merely a result of reduced tumor burden.

A prospective study by Heider and colleagues [70] analyzed patients who had relapsed myeloma enrolled in clinical trials using bortezomib (alone or with dexamethasone) compared with other agents. Patients treated with bortezomib had increased levels of bone-specific alkaline phosphatase and osteocalcin, markers of increased OBL activity. The increase in ALP and osteocalcin was observed in patients whose myeloma responded to bortezomib treatment and in nonresponders but was not seen in the other treatment groups regardless of response.

Giuliani and colleagues [71] investigated the in vitro and in vivo effects of bortezomib. In human OBL precursor cultures, bortezomib increased markers of OBL differentiation and OBL-specific transcription factors, which resulted in enhanced bone nodule formation. Bone marrow samples of patients responding to bortezomib had a significantly increased number of osteoblastic cells compared with nonresponders. These studies suggest that bortezomib can stimulate OBLs, despite that the mechanism of action on OBL stimulation has not been fully determined, and further studies are required.

RANKL is responsible for OCL-mediated bone resorption in a broad range of conditions and plays a key role in establishment and propagation of skeletal disease in MM. Denosumab (AMG-162) is a fully human monoclonal antibody that binds RANKL with high affinity and specificity and inhibits RANKL–RANK interaction, mimicking the endogenous effects of osteoprotegerin, a soluble RANKL decoy receptor. A phase 1 clinical trial in healthy postmenopausal women and patients who had MM showed that single and multiple subcutaneous injections of denosumab caused rapid and sustained suppression of markers of osteoclastic bone resorption with a favorable safety profile [72].

Besides directly targeting cytokines or pathways mediating OCL formation and activation, the inhibition of the development of OCLs by inhibiting OCL differentiation might also be an effective approach to control OCL activity. Anderson and colleagues [73] showed that CC-4047 (Actimid), which is a derivative of thalidomide and has similar action as lenalidomide, inhibits OCL development by affecting the lineage commitment of OCL precursors. CC-4047 down-regulated the expression of PU-1, a critical transcription factor for the development of OCLs. The down-regulation of PU-1 in hematopoietic progenitor cells resulted in a shift of lineage development toward granulocytes, accompanied by a complete inhibition of OCL formation with a concomitant accumulation of immature granulocytes.

The new generation of HDAC inhibitors, such as PXD101, is highly effective at inhibiting OCL formation, suggesting that besides inhibition of MM growth these drugs are also effective at inhibiting OCL activity [74]. PXD101 can inhibit OCL formation at clinically achievable doses.

SDX-308 is a nonsteroidal anti-inflammatory drug. It is a non–COX-2–inhibiting indole-pyran analog and is structurally related to SDX-101, an R-enantiomer of etodolac. Recent publications have shown that SDX-308 has a potent anti-myeloma effect and shows synergism in combination with other drugs for the treatment of chronic lymphocytic leukemia. In addition, SDX-308 inhibits OCL formation and activity by blocking nuclear factor-κB activity [75]. Because SDX-308 directly suppresses OCL formation and function and directly targets MM cells, it is a promising candidate for the treatment of MM.

SUMMARY

Lytic bone lesions are among the most debilitating problems in patients who have MM. The molecular mechanisms responsible for the development of bone disease in MM are still under investigation. The activation of OCLs with a concomitant inactivation of OBLs is mediated by a tight interaction between stromal cells, OBLs, OCLs, and MM cells. Increasing understanding of the pathophysiology responsible for bone destruction in MM should provide more specific therapies with fewer side effects for patients who have MM resulting in the highest possible quality of life.

References
[1] Kyle RA, Rajkumar SV. Multiple myeloma. N Engl J Med 2004;351(18):1860–73.
[2] Melton LJ 3rd, Chrischilles EA, Cooper C, et al. How many women have osteoporosis? JBMR Anniversary Classic. JBMR, Volume 7, Number 9, 1992. J Bone Miner Res 2005;20(5): 886–92.
[3] Barille-Nion S, Bataille R. New insights in myeloma-induced osteolysis. Leuk Lymphoma 2003;44(9):1463–7.
[4] Giuliani N, Colla S, Rizzoli V. New insight in the mechanism of osteoclast activation and formation in multiple myeloma: focus on the receptor activator of NF-kappaB ligand (RANKL). Exp Hematol 2004;32(8):685–91.
[5] Roodman GD. Pathogenesis of myeloma bone disease. Blood Cells Mol Dis 2004;32(2): 290–2.
[6] Bataille R, Chappard D, Marcelli C, et al. Mechanisms of bone destruction in multiple myeloma: the importance of an unbalanced process in determining the severity of lytic bone disease. J Clin Oncol 1989;7(12):1909–14.
[7] Bataille R, Chappard D, Marcelli C, et al. Osteoblast stimulation in multiple myeloma lacking lytic bone lesions. Br J Haematol 1990;76(4):484–7.
[8] Vejlgaard T, Abildgaard N, Jans H, et al. Abnormal bone turnover in monoclonal gammopathy of undetermined significance: analyses of type I collagen telopeptide, osteocalcin, bone-specific alkaline phosphatase and propeptides of type I and type III procollagens. Eur J Haematol 1997;58(2):104–8.
[9] Roodman GD. Cell biology of the osteoclast. Exp Hematol 1999;27(8):1229–41.
[10] Hsu H, Lacey DL, Dunstan CR, et al. Tumor necrosis factor receptor family member RANK mediates osteoclast differentiation and activation induced by osteoprotegerin ligand. Proc Natl Acad Sci U S A 1999;96(7):3540–5.

[11] Hofbauer LC, Heufelder AE. Osteoprotegerin and its cognate ligand: a new paradigm of osteoclastogenesis. Eur J Endocrinol 1998;139(2):152–4.

[12] Yasuda H, Shima N, Nakagawa N, et al. Osteoclast differentiation factor is a ligand for osteoprotegerin/osteoclastogenesis-inhibitory factor and is identical to TRANCE/RANKL. Proc Natl Acad Sci U S A 1998;95(7):3597–602.

[13] Dougall WC, Glaccum M, Charrier K, et al. RANK is essential for osteoclast and lymph node development. Genes Dev 1999;13(18):2412–24.

[14] Tsukii K, Shima N, Mochizuki S, et al. Osteoclast differentiation factor mediates an essential signal for bone resorption induced by 1 alpha,25-dihydroxyvitamin D3, prostaglandin E2, or parathyroid hormone in the microenvironment of bone. Biochem Biophys Res Commun 1998;246(2):337–41.

[15] Simonet WS, Lacey DL, Dunstan CR, et al. Osteoprotegerin: a novel secreted protein involved in the regulation of bone density. Cell 1997;89(2):309–19.

[16] Min H, Morony S, Sarosi I, et al. Osteoprotegerin reverses osteoporosis by inhibiting endosteal osteoclasts and prevents vascular calcification by blocking a process resembling osteoclastogenesis. J Exp Med 2000;192(4):463–74.

[17] Mizuno A, Amizuka N, Irie K, et al. Severe osteoporosis in mice lacking osteoclastogenesis inhibitory factor/osteoprotegerin. Biochem Biophys Res Commun 1998;247(3):610–5.

[18] Blair HC, Teitelbaum SL, Ghiselli R, et al. Osteoclastic bone resorption by a polarized vacuolar proton pump. Science 1989;245(4920):855–7.

[19] Horton MA, Dorey EL, Nesbitt SA, et al. Modulation of vitronectin receptor-mediated osteoclast adhesion by Arg-Gly-Asp peptide analogs: a structure-function analysis. J Bone Miner Res 1993;8(2):239–47.

[20] Boyde A, Maconnachie E, Reid SA, et al. Scanning electron microscopy in bone pathology: review of methods, potential and applications. Scan Electron Microsc 1986;(Pt 4):1537–54.

[21] Bataille R, Chappard D, Basle M. Excessive bone resorption in human plasmacytomas: direct induction by tumour cells in vivo. Br J Haematol 1995;90(3):721–4.

[22] Taube T, Beneton MN, McCloskey EV, et al. Abnormal bone remodelling in patients with myelomatosis and normal biochemical indices of bone resorption. Eur J Haematol 1992;49(4):192–8.

[23] Roodman GD. Biology of osteoclast activation in cancer. J Clin Oncol 2001;19(15): 3562–71.

[24] Pfeilschifter J, Chenu C, Bird A, et al. Interleukin-1 and tumor necrosis factor stimulate the formation of human osteoclastlike cells in vitro. J Bone Miner Res 1989;4(1):113–8.

[25] Lust JA, Donovan KA. The role of interleukin-1 beta in the pathogenesis of multiple myeloma. Hematol Oncol Clin North Am 1999;13(6):1117–25.

[26] Sati HI, Greaves M, Apperley JF, et al. Expression of interleukin-1beta and tumour necrosis factor-alpha in plasma cells from patients with multiple myeloma. Br J Haematol 1999;104(2):350–7.

[27] Soutar RL, Dillon JM, Brown D, et al. Cytokine expression in multiple myeloma and monoclonal gammopathy: analysis by reverse transcription/polymerase chain reaction and quantitative PCR. Leuk Lymphoma 1996;24(1–2):111–20.

[28] Cheung WC, Van Ness B. Distinct IL-6 signal transduction leads to growth arrest and death in B cells or growth promotion and cell survival in myeloma cells. Leukemia 2002;16(6): 1182–8.

[29] de la Mata J, Uy HL, Guise TA, et al. Interleukin-6 enhances hypercalcemia and bone resorption mediated by parathyroid hormone-related protein in vivo. J Clin Invest 1995;95(6): 2846–52.

[30] Kurihara N, Bertolini D, Suda T, et al. IL-6 stimulates osteoclast-like multinucleated cell formation in long term human marrow cultures by inducing IL-1 release. J Immunol 1990;144(11): 4226–30.

[31] Teoh G, Anderson KC. Interaction of tumor and host cells with adhesion and extracellular matrix molecules in the development of multiple myeloma. Hematol Oncol Clin North Am 1997;11(1):27–42.

[32] Giuliani N, Bataille R, Mancini C, et al. Myeloma cells induce imbalance in the osteoprotegerin/osteoprotegerin ligand system in the human bone marrow environment. Blood 2001;98(13):3527–33.

[33] Giuliani N, Colla S, Sala R, et al. Human myeloma cells stimulate the receptor activator of nuclear factor-kappa B ligand (RANKL) in T lymphocytes: a potential role in multiple myeloma bone disease. Blood 2002;100(13):4615–21.

[34] Terpos E, Szydlo R, Apperley JF, et al. Soluble receptor activator of nuclear factor kappaB ligand-osteoprotegerin ratio predicts survival in multiple myeloma: proposal for a novel prognostic index. Blood 2003;102(3):1064–9.

[35] Cook DN. The role of MIP-1 alpha in inflammation and hematopoiesis. J Leukoc Biol 1996;59(1):61–6.

[36] Abe M, Hiura K, Wilde J, et al. Role for macrophage inflammatory protein (MIP)-1alpha and MIP-1beta in the development of osteolytic lesions in multiple myeloma. Blood 2002;100(6):2195–202.

[37] Fuller K, Owens JM, Chambers TJ. Macrophage inflammatory protein-1 alpha and IL-8 stimulate the motility but suppress the resorption of isolated rat osteoclasts. J Immunol 1995;154(11):6065–72.

[38] Kukita T, Nomiyama H, Ohmoto Y, et al. Macrophage inflammatory protein-1 alpha (LD78) expressed in human bone marrow: its role in regulation of hematopoiesis and osteoclast recruitment. Lab Invest 1997;76(3):399–406.

[39] Choi SJ, Cruz JC, Craig F, et al. Macrophage inflammatory protein 1-alpha is a potential osteoclast stimulatory factor in multiple myeloma. Blood 2000;96(2):671–5.

[40] Hashimoto T, Abe M, Oshima T, et al. Ability of myeloma cells to secrete macrophage inflammatory protein (MIP)-1alpha and MIP-1beta correlates with lytic bone lesions in patients with multiple myeloma. Br J Haematol 2004;125(1):38–41.

[41] Uneda S, Hata H, Matsuno F, et al. Macrophage inflammatory protein-1 alpha is produced by human multiple myeloma (MM) cells and its expression correlates with bone lesions in patients with MM. Br J Haematol 2003;120(1):53–5.

[42] Choi SJ, Oba Y, Gazitt Y, et al. Antisense inhibition of macrophage inflammatory protein 1-alpha blocks bone destruction in a model of myeloma bone disease. J Clin Invest 2001;108(12):1833–41.

[43] Lentzsch S, Gries M, Janz M, et al. Macrophage inflammatory protein 1-alpha (MIP-1 alpha) triggers migration and signaling cascades mediating survival and proliferation in multiple myeloma (MM) cells. Blood 2003;101(9):3568–73.

[44] Anderson KC, Shaughnessy JD Jr, Barlogie B, et al. Multiple myeloma. Hematology Am Soc Hematol Educ Program 2002;2002:214–40.

[45] Leonard RC, Owen JP, Proctor SJ, et al. Multiple myeloma: radiology or bone scanning? Clin Radiol 1981;32(3):291–5.

[46] Hjorth-Hansen H, Seifert MF, Borset M, et al. Marked osteoblastopenia and reduced bone formation in a model of multiple myeloma bone disease in severe combined immunodeficiency mice. J Bone Miner Res 1999;14(2):256–63.

[47] Silvestris F, Cafforio P, Calvani N, et al. Impaired osteoblastogenesis in myeloma bone disease: role of upregulated apoptosis by cytokines and malignant plasma cells. Br J Haematol 2004;126(4):475–86.

[48] Evans CE, Galasko CS, Ward C. Does myeloma secrete an osteoblast inhibiting factor? J Bone Joint Surg Br 1989;71(2):288–90.

[49] Westendorf JJ, Kahler RA, Schroeder TM. Wnt signaling in osteoblasts and bone diseases. Gene 2004;341:19–39.

[50] Bain G, Muller T, Wang X, et al. Activated beta-catenin induces osteoblast differentiation of C3H10T1/2 cells and participates in BMP2 mediated signal transduction. Biochem Biophys Res Commun 2003;301(1):84–91.

[51] Tian E, Zhan F, Walker R, et al. The role of the Wnt-signaling antagonist DKK1 in the development of osteolytic lesions in multiple myeloma. N Engl J Med 2003;349(26):2483–94.

[52] Politou MC, Heath DJ, Rahemtulla A, et al. Serum concentrations of Dickkopf-1 protein are increased in patients with multiple myeloma and reduced after autologous stem cell transplantation. Int J Cancer 2006;119(7):1728–31.

[53] Giuliani N, Colla S, Morandi F, et al. Myeloma cells block RUNX2/CBFA1 activity in human bone marrow osteoblast progenitors and inhibit osteoblast formation and differentiation. Blood 2005;106:2472–83.

[54] Oshima T, Abe M, Asano J, et al. Myeloma cells suppress osteoblast differentiation by secreting a soluble wnt inhibitor, sFRP-2 [abstract 2356]. Presented at the 46th annual meeting of the American Society of Hematology. San Diego (CA), December 4–7, 2004.

[55] De Vos J, Couderc G, Tarte K, et al. Identifying intercellular signaling genes expressed in malignant plasma cells by using complementary DNA arrays. Blood 2001;98(3):771–80.

[56] Davies FE, Dring AM, Li C, et al. Insights into the multistep transformation of MGUS to myeloma using microarray expression analysis. Blood 2003;102(13):4504–11.

[57] Merico F, Bergui L, Gregoretti MG, et al. Cytokines involved in the progression of multiple myeloma. Clin Exp Immunol 1993;92(1):27–31.

[58] Lee JW, Chung HY, Ehrlich LA, et al. IL-3 expression by myeloma cells increases both osteoclast formation and growth of myeloma cells. Blood 2004;103(6):2308–15.

[59] Ehrlich LA, Chung HY, Ghobrial I, et al. IL-3 is a potential inhibitor of osteoblast differentiation in multiple myeloma. Blood 2005;106(4):1407–14.

[60] Weitzmann MN, Roggia C, Toraldo G, et al. Increased production of IL-7 uncouples bone formation from bone resorption during estrogen deficiency. J Clin Invest 2002;110(11):1643–50.

[61] Abildgaard N, Brixen K, Eriksen EF, et al. Sequential analysis of biochemical markers of bone resorption and bone densitometry in multiple myeloma. Haematologica 2004;89(5):567–77.

[62] Durie BGM, Salmon SE. A clinical staging system for multiple myeloma. Correlation of measured cell mass with presenting clinical features, response to treatment and survival. Cancer 1975;36(3):842–54.

[63] Jakob C, Zavrski I, Heider U, et al. Bone resorption parameters [carboxy-terminal telopeptide of type-I collagen (ICTP), amino-terminal collagen type-I telopeptide (NTx), and deoxypyridinoline (Dpd)] in MGUS and multiple myeloma. Eur J Haematol 2002;69(1):37–42.

[64] Jakob C, Zavrski I, Heider U, et al. Serum levels of carboxy-terminal telopeptide of type-I collagen are elevated in patients with multiple myeloma showing skeletal manifestations in magnetic resonance imaging but lacking lytic bone lesions in conventional radiography. Clin Cancer Res 2003;9(8):3047–51.

[65] Coleman RE, Major P, Lipton A, et al. Predictive value of bone resorption and formation markers in cancer patients with bone metastases receiving the bisphosphonate zoledronic acid. J Clin Oncol 2005;23(22):4925–35.

[66] Kropff M, Bisping G, Wenning D, et al. Proteasome inhibition in multiple myeloma. Eur J Cancer 2006;42(11):1623–39.

[67] Garrett IR, Chen D, Gutierrez G, et al. Selective inhibitors of the osteoblast proteasome stimulate bone formation in vivo and in vitro. J Clin Invest 2003;111(11):1771–82.

[68] Shimazaki C, Uchida R, Nakano S, et al. High serum bone-specific alkaline phosphatase level after bortezomib-combined therapy in refractory multiple myeloma: possible role of bortezomib on osteoblast differentiation. Leukemia 2005;19(6):1102–3.

[69] Zangari M, Esseltine D, Lee CK, et al. Response to bortezomib is associated to osteoblastic activation in patients with multiple myeloma. Br J Haematol 2005;131(1):71–3.

[70] Heider U, Kaiser M, Muller C, et al. Bortezomib increases osteoblast activity in myeloma patients irrespective of response to treatment. Eur J Haematol 2006;77(3):233–8.

[71] Giuliani N, Morandi F, Tagliaferri S, et al. The proteasome inhibitor bortezomib affects osteoblast differentiation in vitro and in vivo in multiple myeloma patients. Blood 2007;110: 334–8.

[72] Mera K, Ito K. [Therapeutic agents for disorders of bone and calcium metabolism—Denosumab, a fully human monoclonal antibody-targeting RANKL as a therapy for cancer-induced bone diseases]. Clin Calcium 2007;17(1):37–46 [in Japanese].

[73] Anderson G, Gries M, Kurihara N, et al. Thalidomide derivative CC-4047 inhibits osteoclast formation by down regulation of PU.1. Blood 2006;107:3098–105.

[74] Feng R, Oton A, Patrene K, et al. Combination of the proteasome inhibitor bortezomib and a histone deacetylase inhibitor PXD101 results in synergistic inhibition of osteoclastogenesis and multiple myeloma growth in vitro and in vivo [abstract 507]. Presented at the American Society of Hematology Annual Meeting. Orlando (FL), December 9–12, 2006.

[75] Feng R, Anderson G, Xiao G, et al. SDX-308, a nonsteroidal anti-inflammatory agent, inhibits NF-{kappa}B activity, resulting in strong inhibition of osteoclast formation/activity and multiple myeloma cell growth. Blood 2007;109(5):2130–8.

Hematol Oncol Clin N Am 21 (2007) 1051–1069

HEMAT●L■GY/ON●●L■GY ■LINICS
OF NORTH AMERICA

Mouse Models of Human Myeloma

Constantine S. Mitsiades, MD, PhD*,
Kenneth C. Anderson, MD, Daniel R. Carrasco, MD, PhD

Jerome Lipper Multiple Myeloma Center, Department of Medical Oncology,
Dana-Farber Cancer Institute, Harvard Medical School, 44 Binney Street, Boston, MA 02115, USA

The preclinical assessment of novel therapies for multiple myeloma (MM), just like for any other neoplasia, relies to a significant extent on in vivo animal models, in which the potential toxicities and antitumor activity of the various candidate treatments are evaluated. This article highlights some of the key in vivo models used in the preclinical evaluation of investigational treatments for MM. The study of novel therapeutics for solid tumors has predominantly involved subcutaneous xenografts into immunocompromised mouse models. These models have also been extensively used in the MM field. The bone marrow (BM) microenvironment plays a critical role in proliferation, viability, and drug resistance of MM cells in vivo (as reviewed in [1]). This important consideration has led to a more pronounced emphasis, within the MM field, in development of animal models in which MM cells can form lesions in the skeleton [2–5]. Animal models that fulfill this feature include the SCID-hu model, models of diffuse MM lesions in SCID/NOD mice, or the 5T series models. These in vivo systems provided valuable insight into the pathophysiology of MM and on the anti-MM properties of several classes of investigational agents. Each in vivo model discussed herein has advantages and limitations. These should all be taken into careful consideration, not only for the decision of which model should be used for preclinical evaluation of a particular agent but also for the interpretation of results obtained from preclinical in vivo studies with each of these models. We also review here the recent advancements in the development of mouse genetic models of multiple myeloma that may afford the community enhanced opportunities in the elucidation of the functional role of specific genetic mutations and the discovery of new MM-relevant genes by genomic technologies.

This work was supported by Multiple Myeloma Research Foundation (CSM) and an NCI SPORE grant Career Developmental Award (CSM). CSM is as Special Fellow of the Leukemia and Lymphoma Society. DRC is supported by a Kimmel Award.

*Corresponding author. E-mail address: constantine_mitsiades@dfci.harvard.edu
(C.S. Mitsiades).

0889-8588/07/$ – see front matter
doi:10.1016/j.hoc.2007.08.003

SUBCUTANEOUS XENOGRAFTS OF MULTIPLE MYELOMA CELL LINES

Similarly to subcutaneous xenograft models for solid tumors, human MM cell lines can be injected subcutaneously in immunocompromised mice (eg, nude, SCID, SCID/NOD, SCID-beige) to allow for establishment of palpable plasmacytoma tumors [6]. In some studies with this approach, MM cells have been injected as a mixture with matrigel, to facilitate the engraftment of MM cells and formation of palpable subcutaneous tumors [7]. Following the random assignment of plasmacytoma-bearing mice to control and drug-treated cohorts, treatment with active drugs versus vehicle begins. In studies using these models, the primary endpoint has typically been the volume of subcutaneous plasmacytomas, calculated with various proposed equations (eg, as in [7]), in which the diameter of the tumor is the key variable. Mice are euthanized when the plasmacytomas reach a predetermined threshold of size (typically a diameter of 2 cm) or when significant compromise in their quality of life (eg, significant weight loss, bleeding, infection, and so forth) is noted.

There is no significant conceptual and practical difference between the subcutaneous xenograft models using MM versus those applied in the context of preclinical evaluation of new therapies for solid tumors. Such models have been used to assess a large spectrum of anti-MM therapeutics. Some of these new therapies eventually translated into FDA-approved anti-MM medications (or others currently tested in clinical trials), including proteasome inhibitors (such as bortezomib, previously known as PS-341 [7]) and NPI-0052 (also known as salinosporamide A) [8], thalidomide, and its immunomodulatory analogs [9]. Classes of investigational anti-MM agents that were tested in subcutaneous xenograft models include heat shock protein (hsp90) inhibitor IPI-504 [10]; the Akt inhibitor perifosine [11]; the anti-FGF-R3 neutralizing antibody PRO-001 [12] or FGF-R3 kinase inhibitors [13,14]; agonists for death receptor, such as Apo2L/TRAIL [15]; inhibitors of antiapoptotic Bcl-2 family members [16]; other kinase inhibitors, including inhibitors of VEGF-R [17] or p38MAPK [18]; epothilone [19]; mTOR inhibitors [20]; or antibodies targeting surface receptors, such as interleukin-6 receptor [21] or surface antigens [22].

Subcutaneous plasmacytoma xenograft models have the advantage that MM lesions can be easily monitored and any changes in their size can be quantified easily with caliper measurements. Quantification of systemic levels of tumor markers or imaging studies may be necessary, if not imperative, for other models in which the MM involvement is systemic or not superficial. They are not needed in the context of subcutaneous plasmacytoma models, however. In addition, plasmacytomas can be easily excised and evaluated for histologic and molecular profiling studies.

A key limitation of the subcutaneous plasmacytoma models is that they place MM cells in a subcutaneous microenvironment and therefore do not take into account the interaction of MM cells with the BM microenvironment or the impact that this interaction has for the proliferation, survival, and drug resistance of MM cells in vivo. Several conventional anti-MM therapeutics (eg, dexamethasone, alkylating agents, anthracyclines) are quite active in vitro against MM cells when they are cultured alone, but considerably less active when MM cells are cocultured with bone marrow stromal cells (BMSCs) (as reviewed in [1,23]). Subcutaneous plasmacytoma models do not include such MM–BMSC interactions; therefore, it is conceivable that an individual thera-peutic may exhibit anti-MM activity in these models but may not overcome the protective effects of the BM milieu. Furthermore, subcutaneous plasmacy-tomas may occasionally reach large volumes, but with modest, if any, impact on the quality of life of their hosts, even though they may otherwise meet stan-dard criteria for euthanasia. Subcutaneous plasmacytomas also do not lead to the characteristic skeletal complications of MM (eg, bone resorption, spontane-ous fractures), which further limits the relevance of overall survival as an effi-cacy endpoint in these models. Collectively, the non-orthotopic nature of subcutaneous plasmacytoma xenografts and the potential dissociation of the overall survival of mice from the pattern and volumes of plasmacytoma growth can lead to overestimations in these models of the in vivo anti-MM activity that an investigational antitumor agent would exhibit in a more orthotopic context, such as the setting of treatment of MM patients.

THE SCID-HU MODEL

The limitations of subcutaneous MM xenografts provided strong impetus for development of SCID-hu model for MM. The SCID-hu mouse was pioneered in the 1980s as a heterochimeric small animal model designed to support hu-man hematopoietic differentiation and function in vivo in xenograft systems. In its original version [24,25], the SCID-hu mouse involved successful engraft-ment of human hematolymphoid cells into immunodeficient C.B-17 SCID mice. The goal was to recapitulate multilineage human hematopoiesis in vivo and overcome species-dependent caveats that presented in the experimental study (eg, the tropism of HIV infection for CD4+ cells of human, but not ro-dent, derivation). The same principle was applied in MM by Urashima and col-leagues [2] who surgically implanted human fetal bone grafts bilaterally in SCID mice, with the intent to use the human bone grafts as a niche where hu-man MM cells can locally interact with a human bone milieu, recapitulating the close interaction of MM cells with the bone microenvironment in human pa-tients who have MM. The rationale behind the application of the SCID-hu model in MM (as opposed to using direct injections of human MM cells into the murine bones) was that the MM–bone microenvironment interaction is me-diated by cytokines and cell adhesion molecules that may operate at least in part in a species-dependent manner [2]. For example, it has been proposed that murine interleukin-6 (IL-6) is a significantly less potent mitogen for human MM cells than human IL-6, and that therefore the optimal growth of human MM cells in vivo would require their exposure to a tissue microenvironment of human origin with local production of human IL-6. In the first report of the SCID-hu MM model, as few as 10,000 human MM cells were injected into the human bone graft and caused extensive BM infiltration with MM cells

[2]. This neoplastic population was confirmed to be of human origin, based on immunohistochemical identification of human light chain expression in the plasma cells of the human bone graft, detection of monoclonal human immunoglobulin and human IL-6 in the peripheral blood serum samples of the mice, and detection of monoclonal Ig light chain deposition in renal tubules. Approximately 12 weeks after injection of human MM cells in one of two human bone grafts, MM cells could be detected in the contralateral, non–MM cell injected bone graft [2].

Since its first application, the SCID-hu MM model has been extensively used in MM studies to evaluate the interactions of human MM cells with the bone milieu and to assess the anti-MM activity of diverse investigational therapeutics. Yaccoby and colleagues [26] used the SCID-hu model to study primary MM cells in vivo and reported that 80% of primary MM tumor samples can be successfully engrafted in this model. These studies also reported that the implanted human bone fragment often presents with resorption, consistent with the bone resorption associated with MM cell growth in the bones of patients [27]. In subsequent studies, the group of Yaccoby and Epstein reported that purified primary CD38 (++) CD45 (−) myeloma cells grew (in eight of nine experiments) in the human bone grafts of the SCDI-hu model and produced typical manifestations of MM. In addition, peripheral blood cell preparations that had not been previously depleted of plasma cells did lead (in four of four cases) to development of MM in the mice, whereas BM or mononuclear cell preparations depleted of plasma cells did not lead to MM lesions [28].

The same SCID-hu model (or variations thereof) has been applied to evaluate the anti-MM activity of thalidomide [29], delineate the mechanisms of MM cell-induced bone resorption [30,31], and evaluate the anti-MM efficacy of candidate investigational agents. These studies were not limited only to strategies targeting the increased bone resorption of MM cells (eg, RANKL antagonists, such as RANK-Fc constructs [30,32]) but also evaluated small molecule inhibitors, such as the IKK inhibitor MLN120B [33] and the farnesyltransferase inhibitor tipifarnib [34], monoclonal antibodies against CD138 [35] or insulin-like growth factors [36], and cytokine superantagonists [37].

A key advantage of the SCID-hu model is that it addresses the concerns that cytokines/adhesion molecules from the murine BM might not interact optimally with human MM cells [2]. As a result, the SCID-hu model has become a very useful model in studying the natural history of MM-associated bone resorption or neovascularization and the anti-MM efficacy of novel therapies. Similarly to the subcutaneous plasmacytoma xenograft models, MM cells injected into the SCID-hu model are located (particularly early after MM cell injection) predominantly in the bone graft. It is therefore relatively easy in this model to obtain samples of the MM-bearing bone graft for further analyses. Unlike subcutaneous xenograft models in which the size of plasmacytomas is an easily measurable endpoint, it is less easy in the SCID-hu model to quantify the tumor burden and its changes with treatment. MM cells, at least in the initial phases of their growth in SCID-hu mice, do not form palpable and measurable plasmacytomas but grow within the bone graft [2]. Even when MM cells have completely infiltrated the bone graft and have started to grow beyond it, the precise volume of the resulting plasmacytoma-like structure cannot be reliably estimated with caliper measurements. As a result, the use of the SCID-hu model generally requires serial measurement of serologic and biochemical markers, such as serum levels for human monoclonal immunoglobulin [38], IL-6, or its soluble receptor (sIL-6R) [37].

The SCID-hu model has limitations, which should not be viewed as reason to ignore its advantages or scientific value. Specifically, the SCID-hu model does not allow MM cells to develop the diffuse and multifocal pattern of lesions that are present in human patients who have MM. Although this model offers a species-compatible platform for the study of MM-associated bone resorption, its pathophysiologic consequences (eg, spontaneous fractures) and their sequelae (eg, hind limb paralysis) cannot be readily evaluated in the SCID-hu model: the transplanted human bone graft is not an essential component of the host's skeleton, but it practically functions as an appendage to the subcutaneous tissue. Consequently, even if the human bone graft of the SCID-hu model is completely resorbed by the injected MM cells, there are minimal, if any, actual consequences to the rodent host in its quality of life. Barring systemic growth of cells metastasizing from the bone graft to other organs of the mouse, therefore, the life expectancy of mice in the SCID-hu model may not be radically different from mice bearing subcutaneous plasmacytomas. These aspects confound the interpretation of overall survival data obtained with use of the SCID-hu MM mice and limit the usefulness of this endpoint for evaluation of anti-MM activity by candidate investigational agents.

Furthermore, the SCID-hu model involves some technically and logistically demanding steps, including the acquisition of human bone grafts and their implantation in SCID mice. In principle, this model should be amenable to use of adult human bone grafts, but there are currently no detailed studies formally addressing the feasibility of using fetal versus adult human bone grafts in the SCID-hu MM model. In view of concerns related to research involving human fetal tissues, such comparative studies may become important. In part because of these considerations, the group of Yaccoby and colleagues [39] has proposed a variation of the original SCID-hu MM model, termed SCID-rab model. Instead of subcutaneously implanting fetal human bone grafts in SCID mice, Yaccoby and colleagues [39] implanted rabbit bone fragments in these mice, and then directly injected them with primary human MM cells. Tumor cells successfully engrafted in most patient samples (with unfractionated BM mononuclear cells or with injection of the CD138+ fraction), as evidenced by detection of the M-protein isotypes secreted by the respective patients and by osteolytic bone lesions in the rabbit bone graft. Similarly to the SCID-hu MM model, primary MM cells injected directly in one bone graft were able to metastasize into another bone graft at a remote site of the same mouse [39]. MM cells derived from patients who had extramedullary disease proliferated into contiguous soft tissues beyond the bone graft, consistent with the clinical behavior of the same cells in the human patients [39]. The SCID-rab model is therefore an approach that can potentially bypass some of the issues posed by the need for fetal bone grafts for the SCID-hu MM model. More experience with the SCD-rab model will be needed to ascertain whether the bone microenvironment of the rabbit provides a milieu that is as favorable to human MM cells as is the human bone milieu.

MODELS OF DIFFUSE MULTIPLE MYELOMA BONE LESIONS IN IMMUNOCOMPROMISED MICE

A key clinical feature of overt MM is the systemic and multifocal nature of its lesions. In the drug development process for MM, it would ideally be important to use in vivo models in which the MM lesions also exhibit a systemic and multifocal pattern of distribution in the skeleton, to better approximate the behavior of the disease in human patients. Subcutaneous plasmacytomas or the SCID-hu MM model involves injections of MM cells into specific singular locations of the body (ie, subcutaneous compartment and the implanted human bone graft, respectively). By default, therefore, they cannot recapitulate the multifocal and systemic nature of the disease [4]. To address this limitation, experimental animal models of MM require systemic injections of the MM cells (eg, intravenously or less frequently by way of the intracardiac route [40,41]). Several reports have shown that human MM cells injected intravenously in immunocompromised mice can indeed engraft in the BM and form MM bone lesions with features consistent with those of MM in human patients [3,4,42–51]. Some of the original studies of intravenous injection of MM cells into immunocompromised mice involved the ARH-77 cell line model, which did lead to development of osteolytic lesions [52–55]. Since then ARH-77 has been documented to be a lymphoblastoid EBV-positive cell line, instead of a bona fide MM line [56]. Nonetheless, the basic principle addressed by these early studies (ie, that human MM cells injected into the systemic circulation of immunocompromised mice can lead to multifocal MM bone lesions) has also been validated by several labs using many different bona fide human MM cell lines [3,4,42–51] and primary human MM cells [40,41,57]. Following the early studies with models of diffuse MM lesions, two caveats had been voiced: (1) the potential scenario that the murine BM microenvironment might not be fully compatible with the human MM cells and, thus, might not support them optimally, and (2) the difficulty of measuring the tumor burden, after the systemic injection of the MM cells in mice, and how it may change over time and with administration of treatment. These concerns have been addressed to a major extent.

The concern regarding the homing of human MM cells in a murine BM microenvironment relates to the notion that the tumor–microenvironment interaction in MM bone may depend on cytokine receptors and adhesion molecules that MM cells express and that do not optimally cross-react with their functional partners (eg, cytokines and counterpart adhesion molecules) from the murine milieu. Accumulating experience with the models of diffuse MM bone lesions indicates that a broad range of bone human bona fide

MM cell lines can lead to formation of bone lesions in immunocompromised mice. For example, the JJN-3 MM cell line and its subline JJN-3 T1 infiltrated the BM, produced radiologically identifiable osteolytic lesions, decreased osteoblast formation (as evidenced by histomorphometric studies), triggered mild hypercalcemia, and eventually caused paralysis of mice [3]. In studies in Japan, intravenous injection of KPMM2 cell line, which produces high levels of autocrine IL-6, led to formation of MM lesions predominantly localized in the BM, caused distinct osteolytic lesions at multiple skeletal sites, triggered diffuse decrease in bone reduction throughout the skeleton, led to increase in ionized plasma calcium levels, and ultimately caused hind-leg paralysis [42]. Tail vein injections of the RPMI-8226/S-GFP [4,47] and MM-1S-GFP/Luc [44] human MM cell lines also led to establishment of diffuse skeletal lesions that exhibited anatomic distribution and pathophysiologic manifestations consistent with the clinical course of MM in human patients. For instance, MM lesions identified in these models involved predominantly the axial skeleton (eg, spine, skull, and pelvis) and frequently caused hind-limb paralysis [4]. In contrast, tumor spread to the lungs, liver, spleen, or kidney was more infrequent. The results that were obtained with a luciferase-expressing MM-1S cell line model [44] were consistent with those obtained subsequently by Wu and colleagues [51] in a similar model of diffuse MM lesions.

Although the specific strain of immunocompromised mice used in these models may in theory affect, to a certain degree, the biologic behavior of the MM cells in these models, a common denominator of studies in different strains is the ability of MM cells to engraft in the BM and, depending on the cell line used, form occasional lesions in other sites. Miyakawa and colleagues [43] injected the human MM cell line U266 intravenously in NOD/SCID/γc null (NOG) mice: the MM cells caused hind-leg paralysis in all 20 mice tested; infiltrated only the BM, without any detectable presence in other organs; and caused lytic lesions in cortical bones and loss of density in trabecular bones. Intravenous injection of the same NOG mouse model with the KMM-1 cells led to BM infiltration, but also infiltration of the spleen, lung, and liver [45]. Wu and colleagues [46] reported that intravenous injection of the CAG human MM cell line in SCID/NOD mice led to establishment of multifocal lesions with anatomic distribution and pathophysiologic manifestations, consistent with the clinical course of MM in human patients, including: major involvement of the axial skeleton; osteolytic bone lesions captured by pathology and radiograph examinations (eg, spine, skull, and pelvis); frequent development of hind-limb paralysis secondary to spinal lesions; and no significant tumor spread to lungs, liver, spleen, or kidney. These findings were also confirmed in a subsequent study [50]. Xin and colleagues [48] injected female SCID-beige mice intravenously with KMS-11-luc human MM cells, which exhibited a typical diffuse pattern of multiple skeletal lesions in most mice, with prominent involvement of the skull, pelvis, and spine. Carlo-Stella and colleagues [49] also confirmed that intravenous injection of the KMS-11 cell line led to progressive BM infiltration and hind-leg paralysis.

In some of these studies, MM cells (particularly those that were originally derived from patients who were at advanced stages of their MM) did establish lesions in extraskeletal sites (eg, JJN3 cells formed lesions in the meninges, liver, and adipose tissue [3]; KPMM2 cells infiltrated the lymph nodes [42]; RPMI-8226/S-GFP [4] or MM-1S-GFP/Luc [44] led to infiltration of soft tissues in late stages of the disease; and KMM-1 cells can also infiltrate the spleen, lung, and liver of mice [45]). In all these studies, however, the predominant site of MM cell involvement was the BM. The capability of some human MM cell lines to grow not only in the BM but also at extramedullary sites does not minimize the biologic and clinical relevance of these cells lines or their use as in vivo models of diffuse MM lesions. In fact, even though MM cells have an osteo-tropic behavior and are clearly homing almost exclusively to the bone at the early stages of the natural history of this disease, patients who have advanced MM frequently present with extramedullary involvement [1,58]. That at least some of these models of diffuse MM lesions can include extramedullary compo-nents may provide a useful testing ground beneficial for the development of new anti-MM therapies for patients who have advanced MM.

So far, these models of diffuse MM lesions in immunocompromised mice have provided valuable insights in the preclinical, and eventually clinical, devel-opment of a series of investigational anti-MM therapies, including: humanized anti–IL-6 receptor antibody (hPM1) [42], small molecule inhibitors [44] or monoclonal antibodies [51] against IGF-1R, hsp90 inhibitors [47], FGF-R3 kinase inhibitors [48], synthetic epothilone analogs [46], antibodies against CD52 [49], and inhibitor against cyclin-dependent kinase 4/6 [50].

A second initial concern regarding the models of diffuse lesions of MM cells was that it would be difficult to monitor the anatomic localization, spatiotempo-ral progression, and total burden of the MM tumor lesions because these tu-mors would be located in internal organs and would not be as easily accessible and measurable. In the earlier versions of the models of diffuse MM lesions, radiographs were applied to estimate the degree of bone resorp-tion at sites of MM involvement [54]. Serial measurements of circulating levels of human monoclonal immunoglobulin in mouse serum samples were also oc-casionally applied (eg, in [42]), with the intent to provide an estimate of how the tumor burden changes over time and how it is affected (or not) by treatment. Radiographs cannot provide quantitative assessment of tumor burden, how-ever, and do not have high sensitivity for detection of MM bone involvement unless the associated bone resorption is advanced and has severely compro-mised the bone density. Some MM cells (particularly those originally derived from patients who had very advanced MM disease) exhibit a propensity to not only infiltrate the BM (even though this is still their predominant homing target) but also form extramedullary lesions that are not readily assessed with conventional radiographs. CT and MRI are potential alternatives to address these issues; however, their cost for preclinical studies is still prohibitive. Given the limitations of conventional imaging modalities, we adapted the model of dif-fuse MM bone lesions to include intravenous injections of human MM cell lines that stably express constructs for markers that can be detected in vivo by whole-body fluorescence or bioluminescence imaging. For instance, MM cell lines expressing green fluorescent protein (GFP) or its GFP/Luc fusion construct with luciferase (Luc) can be visualized by whole-body fluorescence imaging: MM-bearing mice are visualized by near-infrared light, because the small size of these animals causes less pronounced attenuation of the light emitted by the tumor lesions. With the use of sensitive digital cameras, the light signal is captured [4,44]. In addition, MM cell lines expressing Luc or a GFP/Luc fusion construct can be visualized by whole-body bioluminescence imaging: mice bearing lesions of luciferase-expressing MM cells are anesthetized and injected intraperitoneally with the substrate of luciferase, luciferin. The latter is then distributed through the systemic circulation to the various sites of the body where Luc-expressing tumor cells produce bioluminescence because of the interaction of Luc with its substrate. Similarly to the whole-body fluorescence studies, bioluminescence emitted by the tumor can penetrate modest lengths of solid tissues. Coupled with the small size of these experimental animals and the use of sensitive charged-couple device cameras, this allows for acquisition of whole-body images that reveal the sites of luciferase-expressing tumor involvement and sensitive quantification of tumor burden [4,44]. Both these modalities are noninvasive; can be used safely for the animals; do not require exposure to radiation or additional contrast agents; and can be used even in the case of cell lines that produce low levels of monoclonal immunoglobulin, free light chains, or other serum markers conventionally used for serial monitoring of tumor burden in other models. Since the first studies that applied fluorescence [4] and bioluminescence imaging [44] in mouse models of MM, several other studies in diverse experimental settings have used these approaches in the MM field and confirmed their feasibility and usefulness [35,46,48,50,51,59,60].

An important research field that has benefited from these models is the study of clonotypic B cells in patients who have MM [40,41,57] and the related study of proposed "myeloma stem cell." Pilarski and colleagues [40] reported that NOD/SCID mice can develop MM lesions not only after direct intraosseous injection of human MM cells but also after intracardiac injection with peripheral blood mononuclear cells from patients who have aggressive MM. Indeed, intracardiac injection of NOD/SCID mice with peripheral blood mononuclear cells from patients who have aggressive MM led to lytic bone lesions; detection of human Ig in mouse serum; detection of human plasma cells in the murine blood, BM, and spleen; and detection of clonotypic cells in the murine BM. In addition, human clonotypic B cells were detected in the femoral BM even after direct intraosseous injection of human MM cells in the sternum of the mice [40]. These observations were interpreted by the authors to suggest that MM cell can spread from a primary injection site to other distant locations in the murine BM [40].

THE MULTIPLE MYELOMA MODELS OF THE 5T SERIES

The MM models of the 5T series have been at the center of one of the most prolific lines of in vivo research studies in the MM field over the last 2 decades

[60–95]. The 5T models are actually not xenografts, because they involve injection of mice with syngeneic murine MM cells, in sharp contrast to the immunocompromised nature of the mice models in which human MM cells are injected. The 5T models involve serial transplantations of syngeneic recipients with murine MM cells spontaneously arising in C57BL/KaLwRij mice. This approach can address some notable limitations of bona fide MM xenograft models and has provided meaningful insight into the pathophysiology of MM and the preclinical development of novel agents for this disease.

The development of the 5T series was based on the initial observation of Radl and colleagues [96] that C57BL mice reaching an advanced age frequently develop an idiopathic paraproteinemia that is reminiscent in its features and natural history of human monoclonal gammopathy of undetermined significance (MGUS) and, eventually, human MM. This phenomenon was observed in various strains of C57BL mice, but the C57BL/KaLwRij strain exhibited the highest frequency of idiopathic paraproteinemia [96]. Radl and his group [5] then observed that the cells responsible for this idiopathic paraproteinemia reside in the BM or spleen and could be successfully transplanted into young C57BL/KaLwRij recipients, both irradiated and nonirradiated hosts.

In the most recent applications of the 5T models, the two main versions that are studied are the 5T2MM and the 5T33MM models, which share some common features. For example, these models have similar patterns of expression of adhesion molecules, such as LFA-1, CD44, VLA-4, and VLA-5 [84], which likely reflects their common derivation. There are, however, some notable differences: 5T33 cells infiltrate the BM of recipient mice faster that 5T2MM (within 2 weeks compared with 9 weeks, respectively), the development of lytic bone lesions is more consistent with the 5T2MM model [78], 5T33MM cells have the tendency to not only grow in the BM but also to home to the spleen and liver, and finally 5T2MM MM cells are generally deemed to behave less aggressively in vivo than the 5T33 MM cells in these models [84].

Studies based on the 5T models have provided valuable insight into the role of osteoprotegerin and RANK/RANKL interactions in MM bone disease [61], the impact of bisphosphonates on MM bone disease [63,64,95], and the functional involvement of cell adhesion molecules in MM cell proliferation or homing to the BM [65,66,71,75,76]. Furthermore, 5T models have provided insight into several aspects of MM pathophysiology, including the influence of chemokines on MM cell homing in vivo [67,97,98], the process of MM-associated neoangiogenesis [68,69], the status of normoxia versus hypoxia in the BM of MM [99], and the role of matrix metalloproteinases in the pathophysiology of MM [69]. In addition, several investigational anti-MM therapeutic strategies have been studied in these models: erythropoietin [72], all-trans retinoic acid [73], glucolipid synthase inhibitor P4 [82], bisphosphonates [100], IGF-1R kinase inhibitor [101], and HMG-CoA reductase inhibitor [102].

A key advantage of the 5T models is the syngeneic nature of interaction between MM cells and the BM microenvironment of the host. In particular, unlike all aforementioned human MM xenograft models, mouse recipients in the

5T models are immunocompetent and therefore suitable for evaluation of immunotherapeutic strategies, which cannot be readily addressed in SCID-hu or other xenograft models in immunocompromised rodents.

Unlike the SCID-hu models, which provide some insight into the biologic behavior of human MM cells, 5T models have the understandable limitation that their results have to be carefully interpreted within the context of the potential differences in the biology of human MM versus murine plasma cell dyscrasias. Furthermore, only a few 5T cell lines are currently available that do not fully capture the diverse spectrum of genetic heterogeneity within the context of human MM [86,93]. These factors do not neutralize the usefulness of the 5T models. It is possible that this issue could be addressed in the future with the development of more 5T cell lines, either through generation of sublines from currently available 5T cells (eg, as in the study of Libouban and colleagues [103] who developed the 5THL cell line, a more aggressive derivative cell line generated by successive passaging of 5T2MM cells in C57BL/KaLwRij mice) or by de novo generation of new 5T cell lines through a process similar to the original establishment of the 5T2MM or 5T33MM cells by Radl and his colleagues.

LAGλ-1 MODELS

The LAGλ-1 model was recently described as a new approach in the development of mouse models of human MM tumors [104]. In the first description of LAGλ-1 model, fresh whole core BM biopsies were obtained from 33 patients who had MM and engrafted en bloc into hind-limb muscles of SCID mice. Subsequently, human immunoglobulin was detected in 28 of 33 mice. Three of the mice with MM cell growth grew palpable tumors that were morphologically and immunophenotypically consistent with human MM [104]. These cells were then passaged in mice by intramuscular injections, leading to development of plasmacytomas. One of these, termed LAGλ-1, derived from cells of an IgG-λ–producing patient who had MM, was selected for further evaluation and studies. The cells of this LAGλ-1 model could lead to establishment of MM lesions after intramuscular, subcutaneous, or intravenous injection, and were tested for their in vivo response to established anti-MM agents, including melphalan, doxorubicin, and bortezomib. LAGλ-1 cells were responsive in vivo to high doses of bortezomib and low doses of doxorubicin, but not to low-dose bortezomib or conventional doses of melphalan, consistent with the patient who had MM, from whom LAGλ-1 cells were derived, being melphalan-resistant [104].

GENETIC MODELS OF MULTIPLE MYELOMA

With regard to pathogenesis, MM cells show a high level of Ig VH gene somatic mutation, consistent with their cellular origin as antigen-driven B cells found in postgerminal centers. Like other human malignancies, MM is regarded as a multistep process, requiring numerous genetic and epigenetic events that endow potential cancer cells with requisite malignant capabilities. The molecular characterization of several frequent translocations in MM and its precursor MGUS has revealed a juxtaposition of Ig enhancer elements with several cancer-relevant loci, including cyclin D1, FGFR3+MMSET, and c-*maf*, which are believed to be important for disease pathogenesis. Subsequent tumor progression correlates highly with deletion of chromosome 13, mutation of Ras, and inactivation of tumor suppressor genes p16INK4a and PTEN. Secondary translocations that activate c-*myc* and mutations that inactivate p53 are believed to drive progression into advanced stages of disease [58]. With the exception of XBP-1 and Blimp-1, little is known about the transcriptional factors that control the transition from activated B cell to plasma cell. XBP-1 (X-box–binding protein-1) is a basic-region leucine zipper protein in the CREB/ATF family of transcription factors, which is required for the generation of plasma cells [105].

Several mouse models of human plasma cell neoplasms (PCNs) have been developed built on the genetic changes described earlier. Most of these models have the disadvantages of not having adequately recapitulated in mice the clinical characteristic of human MM or of having limited preclinical use because of late onset, low incidence, and a propensity to grow in lymphoid tissues other than bone marrow. Established genetic mouse models of PCNs include tumors that arose spontaneously in old C57BL/KaLwRij mice and resemble human MGUS and MM. Once these mice have reached 2 years of age, 50% develop MGUS and 0.5% develop MM [96]. Both tumors are localized predominantly in the bone marrow, with MM developing osteolytic lesions. Virtually nothing is known about the molecular pathogenesis of these tumors except that, like early human MM, they rarely have Ig translocations involving c-*myc* [106]. The other models include mouse plasmacytomas, which are tumors of mature end-stage B cells that can be induced in high frequency in genetically susceptible strains of mice, such as BALB/cAN and NZB/BINJ, by the intraperitoneal administration of plastics, paraffin oils, or pristane, and further accelerated by injections of mice with transforming retroviruses [107]. Loss of Ink4a/Arf function has been shown to accelerate plasmacytomagenesis in nonpermissive strains [108]. Pristane-induced plasmacytomas secrete Igs, predominantly of the IgA isotype, and greater than 95% of these neoplasms carry translocations between the *myc* oncogene on chromosome 15 and the Ig heavy chain locus on chromosome 12. As such, they represent a mouse model system for studying the pathogenesis of B-cell tumors, such as Burkitt's lymphoma in humans, but not MM.

Currently emerging mouse models of human PCN are based on transgenic expression in B cells of IL-6 [109] and fusion protein of nucleophosmin and anaplastic lymphoma kinase [110], insertion of c-Myc into the IgH loci, and targeted deregulation of c-Myc and Bcl-XL in the B cell compartment [111,112].

In another model reported by Sebag and colleagues [113], c-myc is activated in postgerminal B cells of C57Bl6/J mice by somatic hypermutation. These mice (Vk*myc) spontaneously develop monoclonal gammopathies and plasma cell expansion in the BM (but not secondary lymphoid organs) and exhibit monoclonal paraproteinemia, BM infiltration with plasma cells that have low proliferative index, anemia, and decreased bone mineral density. Interestingly, these mice are responsive to drugs commonly used to treat MM (melphalan, dexamethasone, and bortezomib).

More recently, the biologic actions of XBP-1, the differentiation and unfolded protein/ER stress response factor, have been examined in the lymphoid compartment of transgenic mice. On the basis of XBP-1s prominence in human MM and its potent transactivation potential, transgenic mice engineered to express the *xbp-1s* open reading frame under the control of the immunoglobulin V_H promoter and *Em* enhancer elements (Em) have been generated and characterized [114]. This pEμXBP-1s model is prone to development of MM. Indeed, by one year of age, a significant proportion of the pEμXBP-1s transgenic mice present with a clinical and histopathologic picture similar to human MM, including marked elevation of serum IgM and IgG in most transgenic mice, expansion of the plasma cell population in the BM, development of plasmacytic tumors resembling human MGUS or MM, and eventual development of bone lytic lesions. Despite the long latency and low penetrance of the transformed phenotype, this model would be of value in investigating the genetic lesions responsible for the progression from MGUS to MM.

FUTURE PERSPECTIVES

This article focused on the accumulating experience generated in the MM field with the use of some key mouse models used for preclinical drug development and pathophysiologic studies for this disease. Each model has different strengths and limitations. A common feature of the xenograft models and of the 5T series is that the biologic behavior of the resulting MM tumors is ultimately determined to a significant degree by the biologic features of the human (or murine, in the case of the 5T series of models) MM cells injected into the mouse host. Longstanding efforts to develop genetic mouse models for spontaneous establishment of MM or related plasma cell dyscrasias [109–112] have mostly led to models of B-cell neoplasias with features compatible with earlier stages of the B-cell lineages, rather than typical MM. This void in the MM field is currently being addressed by recent advances that include the Vk*myc [113] and the pEμXBP-1s transgenic mouse model [114]. These novel models may provide useful insights in the pathophysiology of MM and function as useful tools for the evaluation of novel therapeutics for this disease, in a mutually complementary fashion with existing xenograft models, building on their respective strengths and addressing some of their limitations.

References
   [1] Mitsiades CS, Mitsiades N, Munshi NC, et al. Focus on multiple myeloma. Cancer Cell 2004;6(5):439–44.
   [2] Urashima M, Chen BP, Chen S, et al. The development of a model for the homing of multiple myeloma cells to human bone marrow. Blood 1997;90(2):754–65.
   [3] Hjorth-Hansen H, Seifert MF, Borset M, et al. Marked osteoblastopenia and reduced bone formation in a model of multiple myeloma bone disease in severe combined immunodeficiency mice. J Bone Miner Res 1999;14(2):256–63.

[4] Mitsiades CS, Mitsiades NS, Bronson RT, et al. Fluorescence imaging of multiple myeloma cells in a clinically relevant SCID/NOD in vivo model: biologic and clinical implications. Cancer Res 2003;63(20):6689–96.

[5] Radl J, De Glopper ED, Schuit HR, et al. Idiopathic paraproteinemia. II. Transplantation of the paraprotein-producing clone from old to young C57BL/KaLwRij mice. J Immunol 1979;122(2):609–13.

[6] Tong AW, Huang YW, Zhang BQ, et al. Heterotransplantation of human multiple myeloma cell lines in severe combined immunodeficiency (SCID) mice. Anticancer Res 1993;13(3): 593–7.

[7] LeBlanc R, Catley LP, Hideshima T, et al. Proteasome inhibitor PS-341 inhibits human myeloma cell growth in vivo and prolongs survival in a murine model. Cancer Res 2002;62(17):4996–5000.

[8] Chauhan D, Hideshima T, Anderson KC. A novel proteasome inhibitor NPI-0052 as an anticancer therapy. Br J Cancer 2006;95(8):961–5.

[9] Lentzsch S, Rogers MS, LeBlanc R, et al. S-3-Amino-phthalimido-glutarimide inhibits angiogenesis and growth of B-cell neoplasias in mice. Cancer Res 2002;62(8):2300–5.

[10] Sydor JR, Normant E, Pien CS, et al. Development of 17-allylamino-17-demethoxygeldanamycin hydroquinone hydrochloride (IPI-504), an anti-cancer agent directed against Hsp90. Proc Natl Acad Sci U S A 2006;103(46):17408–13.

[11] Hideshima T, Catley L, Yasui H, et al. Perifosine, an oral bioactive novel alkylphospholipid, inhibits Akt and induces in vitro and in vivo cytotoxicity in human multiple myeloma cells. Blood 2006;107(10):4053–62.

[12] Trudel S, Stewart AK, Rom E, et al. The inhibitory anti-FGFR3 antibody, PRO-001, is cytotoxic to t(4;14) multiple myeloma cells. Blood 2006;107(10):4039–46.

[13] Trudel S, Ely S, Farooqi Y, et al. Inhibition of fibroblast growth factor receptor 3 induces differentiation and apoptosis in t(4;14) myeloma. Blood 2004;103(9):3521–8.

[14] Trudel S, Li ZH, Wei E, et al. CHIR-258, a novel, multitargeted tyrosine kinase inhibitor for the potential treatment of t(4;14) multiple myeloma. Blood 2005;105(7):2941–8.

[15] Mitsiades CS, Treon SP, Mitsiades N, et al. TRAIL/Apo2L ligand selectively induces apoptosis and overcomes drug resistance in multiple myeloma: therapeutic applications. Blood 2001;98(3):795–804.

[16] Trudel S, Stewart AK, Li Z, et al. The Bcl-2 family protein inhibitor, ABT-737, has substantial antimyeloma activity and shows synergistic effect with dexamethasone and melphalan. Clin Cancer Res 2007;13(2 Pt 1):621–9.

[17] Podar K, Tonon G, Sattler M, et al. The small-molecule VEGF receptor inhibitor pazopanib (GW786034B) targets both tumor and endothelial cells in multiple myeloma. Proc Natl Acad Sci U S A 2006;103(51):19478–83.

[18] Navas TA, Nguyen AN, Hideshima T, et al. Inhibition of p38alpha MAPK enhances proteasome inhibitor-induced apoptosis of myeloma cells by modulating Hsp27, Bcl-X(L), Mcl-1 and p53 levels in vitro and inhibits tumor growth in vivo. Leukemia 2006;20(6): 1017–27.

[19] Lin B, Catley L, LeBlanc R, et al. Patupilone (epothilone B) inhibits growth and survival of multiple myeloma cells in vitro and in vivo. Blood 2005;105(1):350–7.

[20] Yan H, Frost P, Shi Y, et al. Mechanism by which mammalian target of rapamycin inhibitors sensitize multiple myeloma cells to dexamethasone-induced apoptosis. Cancer Res 2006;66(4):2305–13.

[21] Suzuki H, Yasukawa K, Saito T, et al. Anti-human interleukin-6 receptor antibody inhibits human myeloma growth in vivo. Eur J Immunol 1992;22(8):1989–93.

[22] Ozaki S, Kosaka M, Harada M, et al. Radioimmunodetection of human myeloma xenografts with a monoclonal antibody directed against a plasma cell specific antigen, HM1.24. Cancer 1998;82(11):2184–90.

[23] Hideshima T, Bergsagel PL, Kuehl WM, et al. Advances in biology of multiple myeloma: clinical applications. Blood 2004;104(3):607–18.

[24] Namikawa R, Kaneshima H, Lieberman M, et al. Infection of the SCID-hu mouse by HIV-1. Science 1988;242(4886):1684–6.

[25] McCune JM, Namikawa R, Kaneshima H, et al. The SCID-hu mouse: murine model for the analysis of human hematolymphoid differentiation and function. Science 1988;241(4873): 1632–9.

[26] Yaccoby S, Barlogie B, Epstein J. Primary myeloma cells growing in SCID-hu mice: a model for studying the biology and treatment of myeloma and its manifestations. Blood 1998;92(8):2908–13.

[27] Epstein J, Yaccoby S. The SCID-hu myeloma model. Methods Mol Med 2005;113: 183–90.

[28] Yaccoby S, Epstein J. The proliferative potential of myeloma plasma cells manifest in the SCID-hu host. Blood 1999;94(10):3576–82.

[29] Yaccoby S, Johnson CL, Mahaffey SC, et al. Antimyeloma efficacy of thalidomide in the SCID-hu model. Blood 2002;100(12):4162–8.

[30] Pearse RN, Sordillo EM, Yaccoby S, et al. Multiple myeloma disrupts the TRANCE/osteo-protegerin cytokine axis to trigger bone destruction and promote tumor progression. Proc Natl Acad Sci U S A 2001;98(20):11581–6.

[31] Yaccoby S, Pearse RN, Johnson CL, et al. Myeloma interacts with the bone marrow micro-environment to induce osteoclastogenesis and is dependent on osteoclast activity. Br J Hae-matol 2002;116(2):278–90.

[32] Sordillo EM, Pearse RN. RANK-Fc: a therapeutic antagonist for RANK-L in myeloma. Can-cer 2003;97(3 Suppl):802–12.

[33] Hideshima T, Neri P, Tassone P, et al. MLN120B, a novel IkappaB kinase beta inhibitor, blocks multiple myeloma cell growth in vitro and in vivo. Clin Cancer Res 2006;12(19): 5887–94.

[34] Zhu K, Gerbino E, Beaupre DM, et al. Farnesyltransferase inhibitor R115777 (Zarnestra, Tipifarnib) synergizes with paclitaxel to induce apoptosis and mitotic arrest and to inhibit tumor growth of multiple myeloma cells. Blood 2005;105(12):4759–66.

[35] Tassone P, Goldmacher VS, Neri P, et al. Cytotoxic activity of the maytansinoid immunocon-jugate B-B4-DM1 against CD138+ multiple myeloma cells. Blood 2004;104(12): 3688–96.

[36] Araki K, Sangai T, Miyamoto S, et al. Inhibition of bone-derived insulin-like growth fac-tors by a ligand-specific antibody suppresses the growth of human multiple myeloma in the human adult bone explanted in NOD/SCID mouse. Int J Cancer 2006;118(10): 2602–8.

[37] Tassone P, Neri P, Burger R, et al. Combination therapy with interleukin-6 receptor super-antagonist Sant7 and dexamethasone induces antitumor effects in a novel SCID-hu In vivo model of human multiple myeloma. Clin Cancer Res 2005;11(11):4251–8.

[38] Tassone P, Gozzini A, Goldmacher V, et al. In vitro and in vivo activity of the maytansinoid immunoconjugate huN901-N2'-deacetyl-N2'-(3-mercapto-1-oxopropyl)-maytansine against CD56+ multiple myeloma cells. Cancer Res 2004;64(13):4629–36.

[39] Yata K, Yaccoby S. The SCID-rab model: a novel in vivo system for primary human mye-loma demonstrating growth of CD138-expressing malignant cells. Leukemia 2004; 18(11):1891–7.

[40] Pilarski LM, Hipperson G, Seeberger K, et al. Myeloma progenitors in the blood of patients with aggressive or minimal disease: engraftment and self-renewal of primary human mye-loma in the bone marrow of NOD SCID mice. Blood 2000;95(3):1056–65.

[41] Pilarski LM, Seeberger K, Coupland RW, et al. Leukemic B cells clonally identical to mye-loma plasma cells are myelomagenic in NOD/SCID mice. Exp Hematol 2002;30(3): 221–8.

[42] Tsunenari T, Koishihara Y, Nakamura A, et al. New xenograft model of multiple myeloma and efficacy of a humanized antibody against human interleukin-6 receptor. Blood 1997;90(6):2437–44.

[43] Miyakawa Y, Ohnishi Y, Tomisawa M, et al. Establishment of a new model of human multiple myeloma using NOD/SCID/gammac(null) (NOG) mice. Biochem Biophys Res Commun 2004;313(2):258–62.

[44] Mitsiades CS, Mitsiades NS, McMullan CJ, et al. Inhibition of the insulin-like growth factor receptor-1 tyrosine kinase activity as a therapeutic strategy for multiple myeloma, other hematologic malignancies, and solid tumors. Cancer Cell 2004;5(3):221–30.

[45] Dewan MZ, Watanabe M, Terashima K, et al. Prompt tumor formation and maintenance of constitutive NF-kappaB activity of multiple myeloma cells in NOD/SCID/gammacnull mice. Cancer Sci 2004;95(7):564–8.

[46] Wu KD, Cho YS, Katz J, et al. Investigation of antitumor effects of synthetic epothilone analogs in human myeloma models in vitro and in vivo. Proc Natl Acad Sci U S A 2005;102(30):10640–5.

[47] Mitsiades CS, Mitsiades NS, McMullan CJ, et al. Antimyeloma activity of heat shock protein-90 inhibition. Blood 2006;107(3):1092–100.

[48] Xin X, Abrams TJ, Hollenbach PW, et al. CHIR-258 is efficacious in a newly developed fibroblast growth factor receptor 3-expressing orthotopic multiple myeloma model in mice. Clin Cancer Res 2006;12(16):4908–15.

[49] Carlo-Stella C, Guidetti A, Di Nicola M, et al. CD52 antigen expressed by malignant plasma cells can be targeted by alemtuzumab in vivo in NOD/SCID mice. Exp Hematol 2006;34(6):721–7.

[50] Baughn LB, Di Liberto M, Wu K, et al. A novel orally active small molecule potently induces G1 arrest in primary myeloma cells and prevents tumor growth by specific inhibition of cyclin-dependent kinase 4/6. Cancer Res 2006;66(15):7661–7.

[51] Wu KD, Zhou L, Burtrum D, et al. Antibody targeting of the insulin-like growth factor I receptor enhances the anti-tumor response of multiple myeloma to chemotherapy through inhibition of tumor proliferation and angiogenesis. Cancer Immunol Immunother 2007;56(3): 343–57.

[52] Huang YW, Richardson JA, Tong AW, et al. Disseminated growth of a human multiple myeloma cell line in mice with severe combined immunodeficiency disease. Cancer Res 1993;53(6):1392–6.

[53] Alsina M, Boyce BF, Mundy GR, et al. An in vivo model of human multiple myeloma bone disease. Stem Cells 1995;13(Suppl 2):48–50.

[54] Alsina M, Boyce B, Devlin RD, et al. Development of an in vivo model of human multiple myeloma bone disease. Blood 1996;87(4):1495–501.

[55] Bellamy WT, Mendibles P, Bontje P, et al. Development of an orthotopic SCID mouse-human tumor xenograft model displaying the multidrug-resistant phenotype. Cancer Chemother Pharmacol 1996;37(4):305–16.

[56] Drexler HG, Matsuo Y, MacLeod RA. Persistent use of false myeloma cell lines. Hum Cell 2003;16(3):101–5.

[57] Pilarski LM, Belch AR. Clonotypic myeloma cells able to xenograft myeloma to nonobese diabetic severe combined immunodeficient mice copurify with CD34 (+) hematopoietic progenitors. Clin Cancer Res 2002;8(10):3198–204.

[58] Kuehl WM, Bergsagel PL. Multiple myeloma: evolving genetic events and host interactions. Nat Rev Cancer 2002;2(3):175–87.

[59] Tassone P, Neri P, Carrasco DR, et al. A clinically relevant SCID-hu in vivo model of human multiple myeloma. Blood 2005;106(2):713–6.

[60] Alici E, Konstantinidis KV, Aints A, et al. Visualization of 5T33 myeloma cells in the C57BL/KaLwRij mouse: establishment of a new syngeneic murine model of multiple myeloma. Exp Hematol 2004;32(11):1064–72.

[61] Heath DJ, Vanderkerken K, Cheng X, et al. An osteoprotegerin-like peptidomimetic inhibits osteoclastic bone resorption and osteolytic bone disease in myeloma. Cancer Res 2007;67(1):202–8.

[62] Potter M. Neoplastic development in plasma cells. Immunol Rev 2003;194:177–95.

[63] Libouban H, Moreau MF, Basle MF, et al. Increased bone remodeling due to ovariectomy dramatically increases tumoral growth in the 5T2 multiple myeloma mouse model. Bone 2003;33(3):283–92.

[64] Croucher PI, Shipman CM, Van Camp B, et al. Bisphosphonates and osteoprotegerin as inhibitors of myeloma bone disease. Cancer 2003;97(3 Suppl):818–24.

[65] Asosingh K, Vankerkhove V, Van Riet I, et al. Selective in vivo growth of lymphocyte function- associated antigen-1-positive murine myeloma cells. Involvement of function-associated antigen-1-mediated homotypic cell-cell adhesion. Exp Hematol 2003;31(1): 48–55.

[66] Asosingh K. Migration, adhesion and differentiation of malignant plasma cells in the 5T murine model of myeloma. Verh K Acad Geneeskd Belg 2003;65(2):127–34.

[67] Vanderkerken K, Vande Broek I, Eizirik DL, et al. Monocyte chemoattractant protein-1 (MCP-1), secreted by bone marrow endothelial cells, induces chemoattraction of 5T multiple myeloma cells. Clin Exp Metastasis 2002;19(1):87–90.

[68] Van Valckenborgh E, De Raeve H, Devy L, et al. Murine 5T multiple myeloma cells induce angiogenesis in vitro and in vivo. Br J Cancer 2002;86(5):796–802.

[69] Van Valckenborgh E, Bakkus M, Munaut C, et al. Upregulation of matrix metalloproteinase-9 in murine 5T33 multiple myeloma cells by interaction with bone marrow endothelial cells. Int J Cancer 2002;101(6):512–8.

[70] Menu E, Braet F, Timmers M, et al. The F-actin content of multiple myeloma cells as a measure of their migration. Ann N Y Acad Sci 2002;973:124–36.

[71] Asosingh K, Menu E, Van Valckenborgh E, et al. Mechanisms involved in the differential bone marrow homing of CD45 subsets in 5T murine models of myeloma. Clin Exp Metastasis 2002;19(7):583–91.

[72] Mittelman M, Neumann D, Peled A, et al. Erythropoietin induces tumor regression and antitumor immune responses in murine myeloma models. Proc Natl Acad Sci U S A 2001;98(9):5181–6.

[73] Henry JM, Morley AA, Sykes PJ. Purging of myeloma cells using all-trans retinoic acid in a mouse model. Exp Hematol 2001;29(3):315–21.

[74] Bakkus MH, Asosingh K, Vanderkerken K, et al. Myeloma isotype-switch variants in the murine 5T myeloma model: evidence that myeloma IgM and IgA expressing subclones can originate from the IgG expressing tumour. Leukemia 2001;15(7):1127–32.

[75] Asosingh K, Gunthert U, De Raeve H, et al. A unique pathway in the homing of murine multiple myeloma cells: CD44v10 mediates binding to bone marrow endothelium. Cancer Res 2001;61(7):2862–5.

[76] Asosingh K, De Raeve H, Croucher P, et al. In vivo homing and differentiation characteristics of mature (CD45-) and immature (CD45+) 5T multiple myeloma cells. Exp Hematol 2001;29(1):77–84.

[77] Vanderkerken K, Van Camp B, De Greef C, et al. Homing of the myeloma cell clone. Acta Oncol 2000;39(7):771–6.

[78] Vanderkerken K, De Greef C, Asosingh K, et al. Selective initial in vivo homing pattern of 5T2 multiple myeloma cells in the C57BL/KalwRij mouse. Br J Cancer 2000;82(4):953–9.

[79] Oyajobi BO, Deng JH, Dallas SL, et al. Absence of herpesvirus DNA sequences in the 5T murine model of human multiple myeloma. Br J Haematol 2000;109(2):413–9.

[80] Asosingh K, Radl J, Van Riet I, et al. The 5TMM series: a useful in vivo mouse model of human multiple myeloma. Hematol J 2000;1(5):351–6.

[81] Vanderkerken K, Asosingh K, Braet F, et al. Insulin-like growth factor-1 acts as a chemoattractant factor for 5T2 multiple myeloma cells. Blood 1999;93(1):235–41.

[82] Manning LS, Radin NS. Effects of the glucolipid synthase inhibitor, P4, on functional and phenotypic parameters of murine myeloma cells. Br J Cancer 1999;81(6):952–8.

[83] Zhu D, van Arkel C, King CA, et al. Immunoglobulin VH gene sequence analysis of spontaneous murine immunoglobulin-secreting B-cell tumours with clinical features of human disease. Immunology 1998;93(2):162–70.

[84] Vanderkerken K, De Raeve H, Goes E, et al. Organ involvement and phenotypic adhesion profile of 5T2 and 5T33 myeloma cells in the C57BL/KaLwRij mouse. Br J Cancer 1997;76(4):451–60.

[85] Vanderkerken K, Goes E, De Raeve H, et al. Follow-up of bone lesions in an experimental multiple myeloma mouse model: description of an in vivo technique using radiography dedicated for mammography. Br J Cancer 1996;73(12):1463–5.

[86] van den Akker TW, Radl J, Franken-Postma E, et al. Cytogenetic findings in mouse multiple myeloma and Waldenstrom's macroglobulinemia. Cancer Genet Cytogenet 1996;86(2): 156–61.

[87] Bradley TR, Kriegler AB, Verschoor SM, et al. Interaction between a murine myeloma cell line and bone marrow stromal cells. Exp Hematol 1996;24(2):307–9.

[88] Manning LS, Chamberlain NL, Leahy MF, et al. Assessment of the therapeutic potential of cytokines, cytotoxic drugs and effector cell populations for the treatment of multiple myeloma using the 5T33 murine myeloma model. Immunol Cell Biol 1995;73(4):326–32.

[89] Turner JH, Claringbold PG, Manning LS, et al. Radiopharmaceutical therapy of 5T33 murine myeloma by sequential treatment with samarium-153 ethylenediaminetetramethylene phosphonate, melphalan, and bone marrow transplantation. J Natl Cancer Inst 1993;85(18):1508–13.

[90] Manning LS, Berger JD, O'Donoghue HL, et al. A model of multiple myeloma: culture of 5T33 murine myeloma cells and evaluation of tumorigenicity in the C57BL/KaLwRij mouse. Br J Cancer 1992;66(6):1088–93.

[91] Croese JW, Vissinga CS, Boersma WJ, et al. Immune regulation of mouse 5T2 multiple myeloma. I. Immune response to 5T2 MM idiotype. Neoplasma 1991;38(5):457–66.

[92] Croese JW, Van den Enden-Vieveen MH, Radl J. Immune regulation of 5T2 mouse multiple myeloma. II. Immunological treatment of 5T2 MM residual disease. Neoplasma 1991;38(5):467–74.

[93] Radl J, Punt YA, van den Enden-Vieveen MH, et al. The 5T mouse multiple myeloma model: absence of c-myc oncogene rearrangement in early transplant generations. Br J Cancer 1990;61(2):276–8.

[94] Croese JW, Vas Nunes CM, Radl J, et al. The 5T2 mouse multiple myeloma model: characterization of 5T2 cells within the bone marrow. Br J Cancer 1987;56(5):555–60.

[95] Radl J, Croese JW, Zurcher C, et al. Influence of treatment with APD-bisphosphonate on the bone lesions in the mouse 5T2 multiple myeloma. Cancer 1985;55(5):1030–40.

[96] Radl J, Hollander CF, van den Berg P, et al. Idiopathic paraproteinaemia. I. Studies in an animal model–the ageing C57BL/KaLwRij mouse. Clin Exp Immunol 1978;33(3): 395–402.

[97] Menu E, De Leenheer E, De Raeve H, et al. Role of CCR1 and CCR5 in homing and growth of multiple myeloma and in the development of osteolytic lesions: a study in the 5TMM model. Clin Exp Metastasis 2006;23(5–6):291–300.

[98] Menu E, Asosingh K, Indraccolo S, et al. The involvement of stromal derived factor 1alpha in homing and progression of multiple myeloma in the 5TMM model. Haematologica 2006;91(5):605–12.

[99] Asosingh K, De Raeve H, de Ridder M, et al. Role of the hypoxic bone marrow microenvironment in 5T2MM murine myeloma tumor progression. Haematologica 2005;90(6): 810–7.

[100] Croucher PI, De Hendrik R, Perry MJ, et al. Zoledronic acid treatment of 5T2MM-bearing mice inhibits the development of myeloma bone disease: evidence for decreased osteolysis, tumor burden and angiogenesis, and increased survival. J Bone Miner Res 2003; 18(3):482–92.

[101] Menu E, Jernberg-Wiklund H, Stromberg T, et al. Inhibiting the IGF-1 receptor tyrosine kinase with the cyclolignan PPP: an in vitro and in vivo study in the 5T33MM mouse model. Blood 2006;107(2):655–60.

[102] Edwards CM, Mueller G, Roelofs AJ, et al. Apominetrade mark, an inhibitor of HMG-CoA-reductase, promotes apoptosis of myeloma cells in vitro and is associated with a modulation of myeloma in vivo. Int J Cancer 2007;120(8):1657–63.

[103] Libouban H, Moreau MF, Basle MF, et al. Selection of a highly aggressive myeloma cell line by an altered bone microenvironment in the C57BL/KaLwRij mouse. Biochem Biophys Res Commun 2004;316(3):859–66.

[104] Campbell RA, Manyak SJ, Yang HH, et al. LAGlambda-1: a clinically relevant drug resistant human multiple myeloma tumor murine model that enables rapid evaluation of treatments for multiple myeloma. Int J Oncol 2006;28(6):1409–17.

[105] Iwakoshi NN, Lee AH, Glimcher LH. The X-box binding protein-1 transcription factor is required for plasma cell differentiation and the unfolded protein response. Immunol Rev 2003;194:29–38.

[106] Radl J. Multiple myeloma and related disorders. Lessons from an animal model. Pathol Biol (Paris) 1999;47(2):109–14.

[107] Potter M. Experimental plasmacytomagenesis in mice. Hematol Oncol Clin North Am 1997;11(2):323–47.

[108] Zhang SL, DuBois W, Ramsay ES, et al. Efficiency alleles of the Pctr1 modifier locus for plasmacytoma susceptibility. Mol Cell Biol 2001;21(1):310–8.

[109] Kovalchuk AL, Kim JS, Park SS, et al. IL-6 transgenic mouse model for extraosseous plasmacytoma. Proc Natl Acad Sci U S A 2002;99(3):1509–14.

[110] Chiarle R, Gong JZ, Guasparri I, et al. NPM-ALK transgenic mice spontaneously develop T-cell lymphomas and plasma cell tumors. Blood 2003;101(5):1919–27.

[111] Cheung WC, Kim JS, Linden M, et al. Novel targeted deregulation of c-Myc cooperates with Bcl-X(L) to cause plasma cell neoplasms in mice. J Clin Invest 2004;113(12):1763–73.

[112] Kim JS, Han SS, Park SS, et al. Plasma cell tumour progression in iMycEmu gene-insertion mice. J Pathol 2006;209(1):44–55.

[113] Sebag M, Stewart K, Palmer S, et al. A novel transgenic mouse model of multiple myeloma reliably predicts drug response. Blood 2006;108(11):75a.

[114] Carrasco DR, Sukhdeo K, Protopopova M, et al. The differentiation and stress response factor XBP-1 drives multiple myeloma pathogenesis. Cancer Cell 2007;11(4):349–60.

Hematol Oncol Clin N Am 21 (2007) 1071–1091

HEMATOLOGY/ONCOLOGY CLINICS
OF NORTH AMERICA

Preclinical Studies of Novel Targeted Therapies

Teru Hideshima, MD, PhD[a],*, Kenneth C. Anderson, MD[a]

[a]Jerome Lipper Multiple Myeloma Center, Department of Medical Oncology,
Dana-Farber Cancer Institute, Harvard Medical School, 44 Binney Street, Boston, MA 02115, USA

Despite advances in systemic and supportive therapies, MM remains incurable because of intrinsic or acquired chemotherapeutic resistance. High-dose chemotherapy with stem cell transplantation has significantly extended progression-free and overall survival, but cures few, if any, patients. Novel therapeutic approaches overcoming drug resistance are therefore urgently needed in MM. The interaction of MM cells with extracellular matrix (ECM) proteins and BM stromal cells (BMSCs), along with other components in the BM milieu (ie, osteoblast, osteoclast, vascular endothelial cells), plays a crucial role in MM cell pathogenesis and drug resistance. Importantly, novel biologically based treatments that target not only the MM cell but also the MM cell interaction with other accessory cells and cytokines/growth factors in the BM milieu can overcome resistance to conventional therapies in preclinical and clinical studies and has great promise to improve patient outcome in MM.

THE ROLE OF THE BONE MARROW MICROENVIRONMENT IN MULTIPLE MYELOMA

The BM microenvironment promotes MM cell growth, survival, migration, and drug resistance. It is composed of different types of cellular components, including hematopoietic stem cells, progenitor and precursor cells, immune cells, erythrocytes, BMSCs, BM endothelial cells (ECs), and osteoclasts and osteoblasts. These cells not only physically interact with MM cells but also secrete growth or antiapoptotic factors, such as interleukin (IL)–6, insulinlike growth factor (IGF)–1, vascular endothelial growth factor (VEGF), tumor necrosis factor (TNF)–α, stromal cell–derived factor (SDF)1α, and B-cell activating factor (BAFF). The interaction with these cellular components and growth/antiapoptotic factors triggers, several proliferative/antiapoptotic signaling cascades in MM cells: phosphatidylinositol-3 kinase (PI3K)/Akt; Ras/Raf/mitogen-activated

*Corresponding author. Jerome Lipper Multiple Myeloma Center, Dana-Farber Cancer Institute, Harvard Medical School, 44 Binney Street, Boston, MA 02115. E-mail address: teru_hideshima@dfci.harvard.edu (T. Hideshima).

0889-8588/07/$ – see front matter
doi:10.1016/j.hoc.2007.08.013

protein kinase (MAPK) kinase (MEK)/extracellular signal-related kinase (ERK); Janus kinase (JAK) 2/signal transducers and activators of transcription (STAT)3; and nuclear factor (NF)–κB. These signaling cascades further activate downstream target kinases or transcription factors that regulate MM cell cycle progression, proliferation, and antiapoptosis. Importantly, cytokines secreted from MM cells and BMSCs in turn further augment these signaling pathways [1–3]. Cytokines, their receptors, transcription factors, and protein kinases therefore represent potential targets for novel therapies (Fig. 1).

TARGETING GROWTH FACTORS AND THEIR RECEPTORS
Interleukin-6
IL-6 mediates autocrine and paracrine growth of MM cells within the BM milieu (see Fig. 1). Specifically, some MM cells spontaneously secrete IL-6, which can be enhanced by CD 40 activation of tumor cells [4] or by cytokines (TNFα, VEGF, IL-1) within the BM microenvironment [5,6]. Most IL-6 in the BM milieu is secreted by BMSCs; importantly, transcription and secretion of

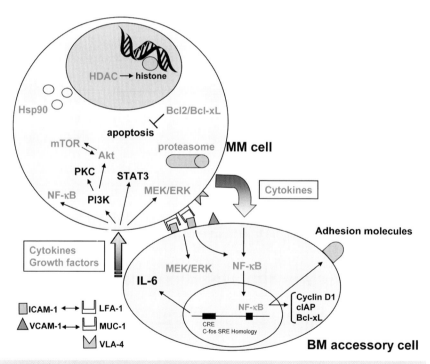

Fig. 1. Cell surface and intracellular targets of novel therapeutic agents. Novel agents block signaling cascade triggered by MM cell–BM accessory cell interaction and induce growth inhibition in the BM microenvironment. Novel agents inhibit interaction of cytokines/growth factors and their receptors expressed on MM cells; inhibit intracellular molecules (kinases, anti-apoptotic proteins, molecular chaperons, and transcription factors).

IL-6 in BMSCs is up-regulated by binding of MM cells to BMSCs [7,8] and by secretion of cytokines (VEGF, TGF-β, TNFα) from MM cells [9–11]. IL-6–induced proliferation is associated with activation of Ras/Raf/MEK/ERK signaling cascade [12,13], and can be abrogated by either MAPK antisense oligonucleotide or by the ERK or MEK inhibitor [14]. Survival of MM cells triggered by IL-6 is conferred by way of JAK2/STAT3 signaling and downstream induction of Bcl-xL [15] and Mcl-1 expression [16,17]. IL-6–triggered drug (dexamethasone [Dex]) resistance is mediated by way of PI3-K/Akt signaling cascade, which can be neutralized by PI3K inhibitors (ie, wartmannin or LY294002). Specifically, Dex-mediated MM apoptosis is not associated with mitochondrial cytochrome c release [18], but is mediated by Second mitochondria activator of caspase (Smac) release from mitochondria [19]; cytosolic Smac disrupts the inhibitor of apoptosis XIAP/caspase-9 complex, thereby allowing activation of caspase-9, caspase-3 cleavage, and apoptosis [20]. We have used gene microarray profiling to further delineate these cytokine-induced growth and antiapoptotic pathways and to derive targeted therapeutic strategies to overcome drug resistance based on interrupting growth or triggering apoptotic signaling cascades [21]. For example, these studies have demonstrated that IL-6 induces the XBP-1 transcription factor [22], which is implicated in differentiation of normal B cells to plasma cells [23,24] and is markedly up-regulated in freshly isolated MM patient tumor cells.

Clinically, serum IL-6 and IL-6 receptors are prognostic factors that reflect the proliferative fraction of MM cells [25–27]. IL-6 or CRP, either alone or coupled with serum β2 microglobulin (β2 m) as a measure of MM cell mass [28], provide one example of a biologically based staging system in MM. Attempts to target IL-6 in treatment strategies to date have included antibodies to IL-6 and IL-6 receptor along with IL-6 superantagonists (ie, Sant7) [29,30] that bind to IL-6R but do not trigger downstream signaling; although in vivo anti-MM activities have been observed, to date responses have only been limited and transient.

Insulinlike Growth Factor-1

IGF-1 is a multifunctional peptide that regulates cell proliferation, differentiation, and apoptosis [31,32]. In the circulation, IGF-1 binds mainly to the main IGF binding protein (IGFBP-3). Several studies suggest that high concentrations of circulating IGF-1 are associated with an increased risk for prostate, breast, lung, and colorectal cancer, whereas high IGFBP-3 concentrations are associated with a decreased risk [32]. The direct relationship of serum IGF-1 level and prognosis in MM has not yet been clarified, however. Standal and colleagues [33] reported that the mean IGF-1 level did not differ between MM patients and controls. IGF-1 was a strong indicator of prognosis: median survival of patients who had low levels (<13 nmol/L) of serum IGF-1 had not been reached at 80 months. Previous studies have delineated the biologic sequelae of IGF-1 in MM cells. Specifically, IGF-1 augments the proliferative and antiapoptotic effects of IL-6 [34]. In contrast to IL-6, IGF-1 activates

Ras/Raf/MAPK kinase/ERK and PI3K/Akt, but not JAK2/STAT3 pathways, by way of type 1 IGF receptor (IGF1R) [35].

IGF-1 stimulates sustained activation of PI3 K/Akt and NFκB; induces phosphorylation of FKHR (forkhead) transcription factor; up-regulates a series of intracellular antiapoptotic proteins, including FLIP, survivin, cIAP-2, A1/Bfl-1, and XIAP; and decreases drug sensitivity of MM cells [36]. IGF-1 primes MM cell responsiveness to IL-6 and stimulates production of angiogenic cytokines [37]. Importantly, it is more potent than IL-6 in mediating these effects, setting the stage for novel MM treatments targeting IGF-1. IGF-1 also mediates MM cell migration by activation of PI3 K/Akt signaling cascade [38]. The antiapoptotic effect of IGF-1 has also been studied using an in vitro model system of MM cells in the BM milieu. Specifically, IGF-1 inhibits Dex-induced apoptosis in MM cell lines without altering Bcl-2 or Bcl-XL proteins associated with activation of ERK and PI3 K/Akt signaling pathways [36]. IGF-1 mediates MM cell growth and survival in MM cells in vitro [34] and in vivo [31]. Recently we showed that caveolin-1, which is usually absent in blood cells, is expressed in MM cells and plays a crucial role in IL-6– and IGF-1–mediated signaling cascades [39]. Preclinical studies of IGF1R targeted strategies have shown efficacy comparable with that of other antineoplastic strategies (ie, proteasome inhibitors and immunomoduratory derivatives of thalidomide (IMiDs) that have proven to be clinically useful [32]. Small-molecule IGF1R kinase inhibitor NVP-ADW742 [31], anti-IGF1R antibodies, or anti-IGF-1 ligand antibodies, will be evaluated in clinical trials in several cancers, including MM [40].

Vascular Endothelial Growth Factor

VEGF is a known angiogenic factor in solid tumors and hematologic malignancies [41]. In MM, VEGF is produced by MM cells and BMSCs and may account, at least in part, for the increased angiogenesis the BM of patients who have MM. Our recent studies show that VEGF triggers ERK activation, proliferation, and migration of MM cells [42,43], which can be neutralized by VEGF receptor tyrosine kinase inhibitors PTK787 [44] and GW654652 [45]. VEGF also triggers Src-dependent phosphorylation of caveolin-1, which is required for p130Cas phosphorylation and MM cell migration [46]. Recently, we have shown that VEGF up-regulates Mcl-1 expression in MM cell lines and MM patient cells; conversely, pan-VEGF inhibitor GW654652 inhibits VEGF-induced up-regulation of Mcl-1, associated with decreased proliferation and induction of apoptosis [47].

We have also shown that a VEGF receptor inhibitor pazopanib (GW786034B) inhibits VEGF-triggered signaling pathways in tumor and endothelial cells [48]. Humanized monoclonal antibody against VEGF bevacizumab (Avastin) was recently approved by the United States Food and Drug Administration for the therapy of metastatic colorectal cancer, and ongoing studies in MM are evaluating the efficacy of bevacizumab, with or without thalidomide, in patients who have relapsed or refractory MM [41].

Fibroblast Growth Factor

MM cells express and secrete bFGF, which contributes to the increased angiogenic potential of BM plasma cells in progressive MM [49]. BMSCs from patients who have MM and control subjects express high-affinity FGF receptors R1–R4. Importantly, stimulation of BMSCs with bFGF induces a time- and dose-dependent increase in IL-6 secretion; conversely, stimulation with IL-6 enhances bFGF expression and secretion by MM cell lines and tumor cells from patients who have MM [50]. In MM, dysregulation of fibroblast growth factor receptor 3 (FGFR3) by the t(4;14) translocation is a primary event in 10% to 20% of MM patients and confers poor prognosis [51–54]. As a surface receptor, FGFR3 can be targeted by monoclonal antibodies [55,56] or be inhibited by selective tyrosine kinase inhibitors (SU5402, SU10991, PD173074, or PKC412) [57,58]. Preclinical studies have validated FGFR3 as a therapeutic target in t(4;14) MM, and FGFR3 inhibitors are currently under clinical evaluation to improve prognosis of this patient subgroup.

B-Cell Activating Factor

B-lymphocyte stimulating factor (Blys) is a TNF family member that plays a critical role for maintenance of normal B-cell development and homeostasis. BAFF and a proliferation-inducing ligand (APRIL), another TNF family member sharing significant homology, are expressed on MM cells [59,60]. Three receptors for BAFF have been identified: B-cell maturation antigen (BCMA), transmembrane activator and calcium-modulating cyclophilin ligand interactor (TACI), and BAFF receptor (BAFF-R). TACI and BCMA can also bind to APRIL, whereas BAFF-R is specific for BAFF. It has been shown that the serum levels of BAFF and APRIL are increased in patients who have MM [61]. BAFF and APRIL promote MM cell growth and activate NF-κB, PI3 K/Akt, and Ras/Raf/MAPK pathways with up-regulation of Mcl-1 and Bcl- 2 antiapoptotic proteins, leading to protection of MM cells against Dex-induced apoptosis [59]. Blockade of BAFF/BAFR axis therefore represents a potential therapeutic target.

Wingless-Type Mouse Mammary Tumor Virus Integration-Site Family

Wnt signaling regulates various developmental processes and can lead to malignant transformation. Wnts are a family of secreted cysteine-rich glycoproteins that act as short-range ligands locally and bind to frizzled transmembrane receptors. Intracellularly, a canonical Wnt/β-catenin signaling cascade inhibits GSK-3β activity, thereby blocking β-catenin phosphorylation and degradation by proteasomes. In MM, Wnt/β-catenin pathway is activated following treatment with Wnt-3a. MM cells highly express β-catenin, which is consistent with active β-catenin/T-cell factor (TCF)-mediated transcription [62]. Further accumulation and nuclear localization of β-catenin, or increased cell proliferation, is achieved by stimulation of Wnt signaling with either the Wnt-3a or the constitutively active mutant of β-catenin [62]. Recent studies have shown that inhibition of β-catenin and TCF-4 interaction by PKF115-584 induces cytotoxicity in MM patient tumor cells and MM cell lines and inhibits tumor growth in mouse xenograft models of human MM [63].

In the BM microenvironment, Wnt signaling is involved in osteoblastogenesis. MM cells in patient BM biopsy specimens express dickkopf 1 (DKK1), a negative regulator of the Wnt/β-catenin signaling cascade [64]. Moreover, elevated DKK1 levels in BM plasma and peripheral blood from patients who have MM correlate with DKK1 gene expression patterns and were associated with focal bone lytic lesions [65]. Importantly, recent studies have shown that anti-DKK1 neutralizing Ab increases numbers of osteocalcin-expressing osteoblasts and bone mineral density of implanted bone in SCID mice [66].

CD40

CD40 is a TNFα superfamily member. CD40 ligand (CD40-L) triggers p53-dependent MM cell proliferation and PI3 K/Akt/NFκB-dependent migration in MM cells [67,68]. In BMSCs, CD40 triggers secretion of IL-6 and VEGF, which further promotes MM cell growth in the BM milieu. Inhibition of CD40–CD40L interaction therefore is a possible therapeutic strategy in MM. Indeed, anti-CD40 antibodies (SGN-40, CHIR-12.12) modestly inhibit MM cell proliferation [69]. Importantly, these antibodies can induce antibody-dependent cell-mediated cytotoxicity (ADCC) against CD40-positive MM cells, which can be further enhanced by lenalidomide [70,71].

Others

Serotherapy directed against CD20 targets only a minority of MM patient tumor cells, because CD20 expression is not common in MM (20% CD20+). The anti-CD20 monoclonal antibody (Rituximab) achieved response in 32% of previously treated patients who had MM, all of whom had CD20+ tumor cells [72]. CS1 (CD2 subset 1) is a member of the CD2 family of cell surface glycoproteins and highly expresses on myeloma cells. Recent studies have shown that a novel humanized anti-CS1 mAb, HuLuc63, induces significant ADCC against MM cells including drug-resistant cells, and inhibited their interaction with BMSCs [73].

TARGETING INTRACELLULAR MOLECULES

Proteasome

Ubiquitin-proteasome pathway is a protein degradation system that maintains intracellular protein homeostasis. It plays a central role in the targeted degradation of cellular proteins, including cell cycle regulatory proteins and apoptosis-associated proteins. Ubiquitin is a small protein (76 amino acids). The C-terminus of ubiquitin forms an isopeptide bond with the amino group of a lysine side chain in a target protein. After attaching multiple copies of ubiquitin to target proteins, the protein is degraded by 26S proteasome, which consists of a proteolytic core, the 20S proteasome, sandwiched between two 19S regulatory complexes. The 20S proteasome has multiple active sites, including caspase-like, trypsin-like, and chymotrypsin-like sites. Because the ubiquitin–proteasome pathway is crucial for survival of cancer cells, its inhibition represents a novel therapeutic strategy in cancer. The proteasome inhibitors are classified as reversible and irreversible according to their inhibition of chymotrypsin-like, trypsin-like, or caspase-like activities. Bortezomib is a reversible inhibitor of chymotrypsin-like activity and has demonstrated significant antitumor activity in preclinical and clinical studies in MM.

Bortezomib (Velcade)

Bortezomib (N-pyrazinecarbonyl-L-phenylalanine-L-leucine boronic acid) is a boronic acid dipeptide that inhibits β1, β1i, and β5 subunits of the 20S proteasome core in the 26S proteasome complex [74]. The initial rationale to use bortezomib in MM is its inhibitory effect of NF-κB, which plays a crucial role in the pathogenesis in cancer cells, including MM. The NF-κB complex is a dimer of different combinations of Rel family proteins, including p65 (RelA), RelB, c-Rel, p50 (NF-κB1), and p52 (NF-κB2). Recent studies have revealed that NF-κB activity is mediated by way of two distinct pathways. In the canonical pathway, NF-κB is typically a heterodimer composed of p50 and p65 subunits [75], and its activity is regulated by association with IκB family proteins [76]. Following stimulation by various factor, including cytokines (ie, TNFα, IL-1β, IGF-1), IκB protein is phosphorylated by IκB kinase (IKK), typically IKKβ. Phosphorylated IκB is subsequently polyubiquitinated and degraded by the 26S proteasome [77,78], which allows p50/p65 NF-κB nuclear translocation. Bortezomib inhibits degradation of IκB thereby blocking NF-κB activity.

Although NF-κB is a major target of bortezomib, it also has other target molecules. First, it directly induces apoptosis of human MM cell lines and freshly isolated patient MM cells despite induction of p53-independent p21^{Cip1} and p27^{Kip1}. Second, it triggers apoptosis even in drug-resistant cells and adds to the anti-MM activity of Dex. Importantly, IL-6 and other growth factors do not overcome bortezomib-induced apoptosis, which is triggered by activation of caspase-3 via caspase-8/9 [79,80]. Third, bortezomib cleaves DNA repair enzymes (DNA-PKcs, ATM) [81,82] and enhances sensitivity of MM cells to conventional chemotherapeutic agents, especially to DNA-damaging agents (ie, doxorubicin, melphalan) [81]. Fourth, previous studies have also shown that normal plasma cells, along with MM cells, produce and secrete abundant immunoglobulins, which require a highly developed endoplasmic reticulum (ER) and chaperone proteins (ie, heat shock proteins [Hsps]) that effect proper translation and folding. The unfolded protein response ensures that the plasma cells can catabolize immunoglobulins; therefore proteasome inhibition is an ideal novel therapeutic strategy for MM [83]. Fifth, bortezomib induces a stress response in MM cells. For example, bortezomib up-regulates Hsps and c-Jun NH$_2$-terminal kinase (JNK), which mediate apoptosis triggered by unfolded proteins. Although bortezomib directly induces caspase-dependent apoptosis, it also targets the BM microenvironment. Specifically, in MM cells, it triggers down-regulation of gp130 [84], which is phosphorylated after IL-6 binding to its receptor, thereby inhibiting phosphorylation of ERK, STAT3, and Akt induced by either IL-6 or by binding of MM cells to BMSCs. Sixth, bortezomib also inhibits VEGF-triggered caveolin-1 phosphorylation and markedly decreases caveolin-1 expression, thereby inhibiting VEGF-induced MM cell migration [46]. Seventh, expression of adhesion molecules (ie, ICAM-1, VCAM-1) on MM cells and BMSCs is also regulated by NF-κB; inhibition of NF-κB by bortezomib decreases adhesion and thereby enhances susceptibility of MM cells to therapeutic agents (Fig. 2) [85,86]. Importantly, bortezomib also inhibits the paracrine growth of human MM cells in the BM milieu by decreasing their adherence to BMSCs and related NF-κB–dependent induction of IL-6 secretion in BMSCs (see Fig. 1).

Most recently, the effects of bortezomib in bone remodeling, specifically on osteoblasts and osteoclasts, have been reported [87,88]. Bortezomib significantly induced a stimulatory effect on osteoblast markers in human mesenchymal cells without affecting the number of osteoblast progenitors in bone marrow cultures or the viability of mature osteoblasts associated with up-regulated Runx2/Cbfa1 activity in human osteoblast progenitors and osteoblasts. Importantly, numbers of osteoblastic cells were significantly increased by bortezomib. Specifically, Runx2/Cbfa1-positive osteoblastic cells were observed in patients who had MM responding to bortezomib treatment [88]. Moreover, bortezomib inhibited osteoclast differentiation and bone resorption activity. The mechanisms of action targeting early osteoclast differentiation were related to the inhibition of p38 MAPK pathways, whereas targeting the later phase of

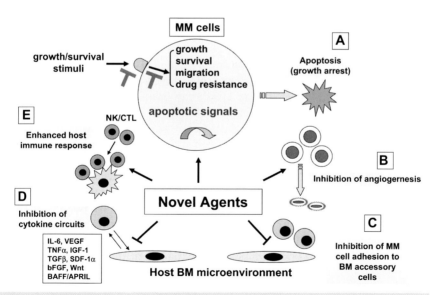

Fig. 2. Novel biologically based therapies targeting MM cells and the BM microenvironment. Novel agents (A) directly inhibit MM cell growth, (B) inhibit angiogenesis, (C) inhibit MM cell adhesion to BM accessory cells, (D) decrease cytokine production and sequelae in the BM microenvironment, and (E) enhance host anti-MM immunity.

differentiation and activation was attributable to inhibition of p38 MAPK, AP-1 and NF-κB activation [89].

Other proteasome inhibitors

NPI-0052 is a novel proteasome inhibitor from Salinospora tropica, a marine actinomycete. Although bortezomib only blocks chymotryptic activity, NPI-0052 inhibits chymotryptic, trypsin-like, and caspase-like activities. NPI-0052–induced cytotoxicity is predominantly triggered by caspase-dependent apoptosis. It induces cytotoxicity in MM cells resistant to conventional agents. Importantly, it is also able to overcome bortezomib resistance in vitro [90]. NPI-0052 triggers reactive oxygen species/caspase-8–dependent apoptosis, which can be enhanced by histone deacetylase inhibitor in acute lymphocytic leukemia cells [91].

PR-171 is another novel epoxyketone-based irreversible proteasome inhibitor, which primarily inhibits chymotryptic activity of 20S proteasome. It triggers JNK/caspase-dependent apoptosis. Compared with bortezomib, PR-171 exhibits equal potency but greater selectivity for the chymotrypsin-like activity of the proteasome. In vitro studies, PR-171 is more cytotoxic than bortezomib following brief treatments that mimic the in vivo pharmacokinetics of both molecules [92]. Multicenter phase I studies to evaluate the safety, tolerability, and clinical response to intensive dosing with PR-171 in patients who have relapsed or refractory hematologic malignancies has already been reported. In this study, 51 patients are enrolled, and 17 of 21 patients who had myeloma were previously treated with bortezomib; importantly, 4 patients who had myeloma responded to PR-171 treatment (partial response, 19%) [93].

Lenalidomide (Revlimid)

Lenalidomide, an immunomodulatory derivative of thalidomide (IMiDs), has multiple mechanisms of anti-MM activities, including directly inducing G1 growth arrest or apoptosis; inhibiting MM cell adherence to BMSCs; decreasing production of cytokines; inhibiting BM angiogenesis, which is increased in patients who have MM; and enhancing anti-MM immunity with stimulation of T-cell and natural killer cell responses. We and others have studied the mechanism of anti-MM activity of IMiDs, which have significantly higher potency at inducing apoptosis or growth arrest in MM cells resistant to melphalan, doxorubicin, and dexamethasone [94]. The IMiDs reduce the secretion of IL-6 and VEGF triggered by the binding of MM cells to BMSCs and inhibit angiogenesis [11]. We and others demonstrated that the IMiDs stimulated T-cell proliferation by way of T-cell costimulatory mechanism. Specifically, IMiDs trigger tyrosine phosphorylation of CD28 on T cells, followed by activation of nuclear factor of activated T cell 2 (NFAT2) and production of IL-2 [70,95]. Moreover, IMiDs induce NK cell cytotoxicity, because NK cell proliferation and ADCC activity were enhanced by IL-2 production from T cells (see Fig. 2) [70,71,96]. These data provide the cellular and molecular basis for use of IMiDs as an adjuvant in immunotherapeutic treatment strategies for MM.

Histone Deacetylase

Histone deacetylase (HDAC) inhibitors are members of a novel class of anti-tumor agents for malignancies, and a large number of structurally diverse HDAC inhibitors have been purified from natural sources or synthetically developed. HDAC inhibitors can be divided into six classes based on their chemical structure. These classes are short-chain fatty acid, hydroxamate, benzamide, cyclic tetrapeptide, electrophilic ketone, and others [97]. Accumulated histone acetylation by HDAC inhibitors attenuates their electrostatic interaction with the negatively charged DNA backbone, promoting the unfolding of histone–DNA complex, thereby modulating access of transcription factors to their binding sites of action and transcription of their target genes (see Fig. 1) [98–100]. Previous studies have shown that deletions or inactivating mutations of histone acetyltransferases (HATs) that decrease histone acetylation are involved in development of human neoplasms [101,102]. In contrast, inhibition of HDAC activity triggers growth arrest or apoptosis of tumor cells. Possible mechanisms of antitumor activities of HDAC inhibitors have recently been comprehensively described [97]; however, their mechanisms of growth inhibitory effects in MM cells have not yet been fully characterized.

Suberoylanilide hydroxamic acid

Suberoylanilide hydroxamic acid (SAHA) is prototype class I, II HDAC inhibitor that directly interacts with the catalytic site of HDAC-like protein and inhibits its enzymatic activity. Inhibition of HDAC activity by SAHA therefore results in alteration of gene expression in various cell types, including MM [103]. Like other HDAC inhibitors, SAHA up-regulates $p21^{WAF1}$ expression [104,105], thereby inhibiting tumor cell growth. In MM, SAHA modulates expression of many genes and inhibits tumor cell growth [103,106], associated with up-regulation of $p21^{WAF1}$, up-regulates p53 protein expression, and de-phosphorylates Rb, followed by apoptosis. Importantly, up-regulation of $p21^{WAF1}$ occurs before p53 induction, suggesting that $p21^{WAF1}$ up-regulation is independent of p53 activity [103]. SAHA-induced apoptosis in MM cells is also associated with Bcl-2 interacting protein Bid; conversely, overexpression of Bcl-2 blocks SAHA-induced apoptosis, suggesting that Bcl-2 plays a crucial role regulating SAHA-induced apoptosis in MM cells. Interestingly, SAHA does not trigger caspase activation, and the caspase inhibitor does not protect against SAHA-induced cytotoxicity. Poly (ADP) ribose polymerase (PARP) is significantly cleaved by SAHA, suggesting that SAHA triggers atypical PARP cleavage in MM cells [103]. Importantly, SAHA suppresses expression and activity of the proteasome and its subunits, providing the rationale for its use in combination with bortezomib to enhance its cytotoxicity [106]. It has also shown that SAHA enhances tumor necrosis factor-related apoptosis-inducing ligand (TRAIL)–induced cytotoxicity, associated with up-regulation of the proapoptotic proteins (Bim, Bak, Bax, Noxa, and PUMA) and down-regulation of anti-apoptotic proteins (Bcl-2 and Bcl-xL) [107].

MVP-LAQ824 (LAQ824)

LAQ824 is a member of hydroxamate HDAC inhibitor that blocks class I and II HDAC activity. LAQ824 inhibits proliferation of cancer cell lines with IC50s of 10- to 150-nM ranges in vitro, indicating that antiproliferative potency of LAQ824 is up to 200-fold higher than that of SAHA [108,109]. Antitumor activity of LAQ824 has been extensively studied in leukemia cells [110–114]. In MM, LAQ824 induces apoptosis at IC50 of 100 nM at 24 hours in most MM cell lines and patient tumor cells. Importantly, LAQ824 is effective in cells that are resistant to conventional therapies (dexamethasone, doxorubicin, melphalan). Moreover, LAQ824 inhibits cell growth in vivo in a preclinical murine myeloma model. Unlike SAHA, LAQ824-induced apoptosis is associated with caspase activation [115].

LBH589

LBH589 is a hydroxamic acid analog that blocks class I and II HDAC activity. LBH589 has been studied in many malignancies as a single agent and combined with other anticancer agents [116–119]. LBH589 has also been shown to inhibit angiogenesis in vitro [120]. In MM, LBH589 blocks cell cycle progression, associated with up-regulation of $p21^{WAF1}$, p53, and p57, and induces cytotoxicity through an increase in mitochondrial outer membrane permeability [121]. The IC50 of LBH589 is 40 to 80 nM in most MM cell lines [121,122]. LBH589-induced cytotoxicity is associated with caspase/PARP cleavage; however, interestingly, LBH589 also triggers a caspase-independent apoptotic pathway through the release of apoptosis-inducing factor (AIF) from mitochondria [121]. Synergistic cytotoxicity against MM cells is observed with LBH589 in combination with bortezomib [122]. Phase II clinical trials of LBH589 are ongoing in MM, and a clinical trial of bortezomib with LBH589 to block proteasomal and aggresomal breakdown of protein, respectively, is soon to begin.

Other histone deacetylase inhibitors

Tubacin is a hydroxamic acid HDAC inhibitor and inhibits only HDAC6 activity [123]. Previous studies have characterized the aggresome as an alternative system to the proteasome for degradation of polyubiquitinated proteins. The aggresome pathway therefore likely provides a novel system for delivery of aggregated proteins from the cytoplasm to lysosomes for degradation [124]. In this aggresomal protein degradation pathway, HDAC6 has an essential role, because it can bind polyubiquitinated proteins and dynein motors, thereby acting to recruit protein cargo to dynein motors for transport to aggresomes [125]. We have demonstrated that blockade of proteasomal and aggresomal protein degradation by bortezomib and tubacin, respectively, synergistically enhances cytotoxicity in MM cells in vitro [126]. Depsipeptide (FR901228, FK228) is a class of cyclic tetrapeptide and inhibits only class I HDAC activity [127]. Depsipeptide induces apoptosis in MM cell lines and in primary patient tumor cells, associated with down-regulation of Bcl-2, BCL-xL, and Mcl-1 expression [128]. PXD101 is a hydroxamate class HDAC inhibitor [129] that has antiproliferative activity in MM cell lines and shows additive or synergistic effects with conventional agents used in MM. MS-275 belongs to the benzamide class and inhibits class I and II HDACs. KD5170 is non-hydroxamate, orally bioavailable HDAC inhibitor that significantly inhibits osteoclast formation at lower μM range and triggers apoptosis in MM cells [130].

Heat Shock Protein 90

Hsp90 is a molecular chaperone that facilitates intracellular protein trafficking, conformational maturation, and three-dimensional folding required for protein function. Intracellular overexpression of Hsp90 proteins is observed in most MM tumor cells, but not in monoclonal gammopathy of undetermined significance (MGUS) or in normal plasma cells [131]. The ansamycin antibiotic geldanamycin (GA) and its analogs bind to the critical ATP-binding site of Hsp90, thereby abrogating its chaperoning activity, decreasing IGF-1R and IL-6R expression on MM cells, depleting growth kinases (eg, Akt, IKK, Raf) and antiapoptotic proteins (FLIP, XIAP, cIAP, telomerase), and inhibiting constitutive and cytokine-induced activation of NF-κB and telomerase (hTERT) in the BM milieu [132]. GA and other Hsp90 inhibitors induce apoptosis of MM cell lines and patient cells that are resistant to Dex, anthracyclines, Thal or IMiDs, TRAIL/Apo2L, and bortezomib. Moreover, a GA analog 17-AAG suppresses the expression or function of multiple levels of IGF receptor (IGF-1R) and IL-6 receptor (IL-6R) signaling (eg, IKK/NF-κB, PI-3 K/Akt, and Raf/MAPK) and downstream effectors (eg, proteasome, telomerase, and HIF-1α activities) in MM cells [132]. Most recently, Hsp90 inhibitors have been reported to induce myeloma cell death, at least in part, by way of ER stress and the unfolded protein response death pathway [133].

IPI-504 is a hydroquinone hydrochloride derivative of 17-AAG. In MM, IPI-504 inhibits MM cell growth in vitro and in mouse models. Like other Hsp90 inhibitors, IPI-504 synergistically enhances cytotoxicity of bortezomib [134]. The water-soluble novel Hsp90 inhibitor 17-dimethylaminoethylamino-17-demethoxygeldanamycin hydrochloride (17-DMAG) attenuates the levels of STAT3 and phospho-ERK and decreases the viability of MM cells [131].

Akt (Protein Kinase B)

Akt signaling mediates MM cell resistance to conventional therapeutics [20,36,135]; therefore, biologically based treatments targeting Akt are a promising therapeutic strategy in MM. Perifosine is a synthetic novel alkylphospholipid that inhibits Akt activation. In MM cells, we have shown that perifosine inhibits baseline and cytokine (IL-6, IGF-1)–triggered Akt activation. Importantly, perifosine triggers significant cytotoxicity even of MM cells adherent to BM stromal cells (SCs) and therefore overcomes cell adhesion-mediated drug resistance (CAM-DR). Furthermore, perifosine augments conventional agent- and bortezomib-induced MM cell cytotoxicity. Importantly, we have also demonstrated in vivo anti-MM activity of perifosine in a human plasmacytoma mouse model, associated with down-regulation of Akt phosphorylation in tumor cells [136]. Perifosine has been shown to induce selective apoptosis in MM cells by recruitment of death receptors, such as TNF-related apoptosis-inducing ligand (TRAIL)-R1/DR4 and TRAIL-R2/DR5 [137]. Most recently, we have shown that perifosine-induced cytotoxicity is strongly associated with down-regulation of survivin [138].

Mammalian Target of Rapamycin

Mammalian target of rapamycin (mTOR) is a serine/threonine protein kinase that regulates transcription, cell proliferation, and survival. Inhibition of mTOR by its inhibitors therefore induces potent cytotoxicity in MM cells [139,140]. Specifically, rapamycin induced G0/G1 arrest associated with an increase of the cyclin-dependent kinase inhibitor p27 and a decrease of cyclins D2 and D3 in MM cells [141]. Interestingly, PTEN-negative myeloma cells are more sensitive to mTOR inhibition than PTEN-positive cells [142]. Rapamycin shows synergistic cytotoxicity in combination with dexamethasone [141] and lenalidomide [143]. CCI-779 is a rapamycin analog that demonstrates inhibition of proliferation and induction of apoptosis, associated with cyclin D1 and c-myc down-regulation and up-regulation of p27^{Kip1} in OPM-2 cells [144]. Moreover, CCI-779 down-regulates VEGF translation, and ultimately blocks angiogenesis [145].

MAPK Kinase

MEK/ERK pathway is one of the major signaling cascades that can be activated by many cytokines (ie, IL-6, IGF-1, SDF1α, BAFF) in MM cells. We have shown that inhibition of ERK by antisense oligonucleotide blocks MM cell proliferation [12,13]. Inhibition of MEK/ERK signaling is therefore a promising therapeutic strategy.

Recent studies have shown that clinical grade novel MEK1/2 inhibitor AZD6244 (ARRY-142886) induces apoptosis in MM cell lines and patient MM cells, associated with caspase-3 activation. Importantly, AZD6244 down-regulates the expression/secretion of osteoclast (OC)-activating factors from MM cells and inhibits in vitro differentiation of MM patient PBMCs to OCs [14].

Bcl2 and Bcl-xL

Bcl2 family members have a crucial role in protecting cells from apoptotic stimuli. In MM, Bcl-2 antisense oligonucleotide (G3139) [146,147] and Bcl2/Bcl-XL inhibitor (ABT-737) [148,149] induce strong anti-MM activities as single agents and in combination with Dex [150].

FUTURE DIRECTIONS

Although each novel agent demonstrates significant preclinical anti-MM activity in vitro and in vivo mouse model of human MM, treatment with single agents may not achieve sufficient clinical efficacy. Treatments combining novel agents with conventional or novel agents to overcome clinical drug resistance are therefore required. Among these combination therapies, thalidomide with dexamethasone, bortezomib with dexamethasone, and bortezomib with doxorubicin have shown promising results in clinical studies based on our preclinical studies. Our recent preclinical studies further indicate that other novel agents enhance cytotoxicity induced by conventional agents. For example, bortezomib induces stress response–related proteins, such as Hsp27, Hsp70, and Hsp90. Blockade of Hsp90 or Hsp27 by their inhibitors restores sensitivity to bortezomib. Recent studies have demonstrated that unfolded and ubiquitinated proteins are degraded not only by proteasomes but also by aggresomes dependent on HDAC6 activity. Inhibition of proteasome and aggresome mechanisms using bortezomib and HDAC6-specific inhibitor tubacin induces accumulation of ubiquitinated proteins, followed by significant cell stress and cytotoxicity in MM cells. Most recently, we also demonstrated that the potent Akt inhibitor perifosine augments bortezomib-induced cytotoxicity in MM. These preclinical studies of combination therapies of bortezomib with novel agents provide the rational framework for clinical evaluation of these treatment options.

References

[1] Hideshima T, Anderson KC. Molecular mechanisms of novel therapeutic approaches for multiple myeloma. Nat Rev Cancer 2002;2:927–37.

[2] Hideshima T, Bergsagel PL, Kuehl WM, et al. Advances in biology of multiple myeloma: clinical applications. Blood 2004;104:607–18.

[3] Hideshima T, Mitsiades C, Tonon G, et al. Understanding multiple myeloma pathogenesis in the bone marrow to identify new therapeutic targets. Nat Rev Cancer 2007;7:585–98.

[4] Chauhan D, Kharbanda S, Ogata A, et al. Oncostatin M induces association of Grb2 with Janus kinase JAK2 in multiple myeloma cells. J Exp Med 1995;182:1801–6.

[5] Costes V, Portier M, Lu ZY, et al. Interleukin-1 in multiple myeloma: producer cells and their role in the control of IL-6 production. Br J Haematol 1998;103:1152–60.

[6] Lust JA, Donovan KA. The role of interleukin-1 beta in the pathogenesis of multiple myeloma. Hematol Oncol Clin North Am 1999;13:1117–25.

[7] Uchiyama H, Barut BA, Mohrbacher AF, et al. Adhesion of human myeloma-derived cell lines to bone marrow stromal cells stimulates IL-6 secretion. Blood 1993;82:3712–20.

[8] Chauhan D, Uchiyama H, Akbarali Y, et al. Multiple myeloma cell adhesion-induced interleukin-6 expression in bone marrow stromal cells involves activation of NF-kB. Blood 1996;87:1104–12.

[9] Urashima M, Ogata A, Chauhan D, et al. Transforming growth factor b1: Differential effects on multiple myeloma versus normal B cells. Blood 1996;87:1928–38.

[10] Dankbar B, Padro T, Leo R, et al. Vascular endothelial growth factor and interleukin-6 in paracrine tumor-stromal cell interactions in multiple myeloma. Blood 2000;95:2630–6.

[11] Gupta D, Treon SP, Shima Y, et al. Adherence of multiple myeloma cells to bone marrow stromal cells upregulates vascular endothelial growth factor secretion: therapeutic applications. Leukemia 2001;15:1950–61.

[12] Ogata A, Chauhan D, Teoh G, et al. Interleukin-6 triggers cell growth via the ras-dependent mitogen-activated protein kinase cascade. J Immunol 1997;159:2212–21.

[13] Ogata A, Chauhan D, Urashima M, et al. Blockade of mitogen-activated protein kinase cascade signaling in interleukin-6 independent multiple myeloma cells. Clin Cancer Res 1997;3:1017–22.

[14] Tai YT, Fulciniti M, Hideshima T, et al. Targeting MEK induces myeloma cell cytotoxicity and inhibits osteoclastogenesis. Blood 2007;110:1656–63.

[15] Catlett-Falcone R, Landowski TH, Oshiro MM, et al. Constitutive activation of STAT-3 signaling confers resistance to apoptosis in human U266 myeloma cells. Immunity 1999;10:105–15.

[16] Puthier D, Bataille R, Amiot M. IL-6 up-regulates mcl-1 in human myeloma cells through JAK/STAT rather than ras/MAP kinase pathway. Eur J Immunol 1999;29:3945–50.

[17] Epling-Burnette PK, Liu JH, Catlett-Falcone R, et al. Inhibition of STAT3 signaling leads to apoptosis of leukemic large granular lymphocytes and decreased Mcl-1 expression. J Clin Invest 2001;107:351–62.

[18] Chauhan D, Pandey P, Ogata A, et al. Cytochrome-c dependent and independent induction of apoptosis in multiple myeloma cells. J Biol Chem 1997;272:29995–7.

[19] Chauhan D, Hideshima T, Rosen S, et al. Apaf-1/cytochrome c independent and Smac dependent induction of apoptosis in multiple myeloma cells. J Biol Chem 2001;276: 24453–6.

[20] Hideshima T, Nakamura N, Chauhan D, et al. Biologic sequelae of interleukin-6 induced PI3-K/Akt signaling in multiple myeloma. Oncogene 2001;20:5991–6000.

[21] Chauhan D, Auclair D, Robinson EK, et al. Identification of genes regulated by dexamethasone in multiple myeloma cells using oligonucleotide arrays. Oncogene 2002;21: 1346–58.

[22] Chauhan D, Li G, Auclair D, et al. Identification of genes regulated by 2-methoxyestradiol (2ME2) in multiple myeloma cells using oligonucleotide arrays. Blood 2003;101: 3606–14.

[23] Iwakoshi NN, Lee AH, Vallabhajosyula P, et al. Plasma cell differentiation and the unfolded protein response intersect at the transcription factor XBP-1. Nat Immunol 2003; 4:321–9.

[24] Carrasco DR, Sukhdeo K, Protopopov M, et al. The differentiation and stress response factor XBP-1 drives multiple myeloma pathogenesis. Cancer Cell 2007;11:349–60.

[25] Pulkki K, Pelliniemi TT, Rajamaki A, et al. Soluble interleukin-6 receptor as a prognostic factor in multiple myeloma. Br J Haematol 1996;92:370–4.

[26] Kyrtsonis MC, Dedoussis G, Zervas C, et al. Soluble interleukin-6 receptor (sIL-6R), a new prognostic factor in multiple myeloma. Br J Haematol 1996;93:398–400.

[27] Stasi R, Brunetti M, Parma A, et al. The prognostic value of soluble interleukin-6 receptor in patients with multiple myeloma. Cancer 1998;82:1860–6.

[28] Tricot G, Spencer T, Sawyer J, et al. Predicting long-term ($\geq$ 5 years) event-free survival in multiple myeloma patients following planned tandem autotransplants. Br J Haematol 2002;116:211–7.

[29] Tassone P, Galea E, Forciniti S, et al. The IL-6 receptor super-antagonist Sant7 enhances antiproliferative and apoptotic effects induced by dexamethasone and zoledronic acid on multiple myeloma cells. Int J Oncol 2002;21:867–73.

[30] Tassone P, Neri P, Burger R, et al. Combination therapy with IL-6 receptor super-antagonist Sant7 and dexamethasone induces antitumor effects in a novel SCID-hu in vivo model of human multiple myeloma. Clin Cancer Res 2005;11:4251–8.

[31] Mitsiades CS, Mitsiades NS, McMullan CJ, et al. Inhibition of the insulin-like growth factor receptor-1 tyrosine kinase activity as a therapeutic strategy for multiple myeloma, other hematologic malignancies, and solid tumors. Cancer Cell 2004;5:221–30.

[32] Pollak MN. Insulin-like growth factors and neoplasia. Novartis Found Symp 2004;262: 84–98.

[33] Standal T, Borset M, Lenhoff S, et al. Serum insulinlike growth factor is not elevated in patients with multiple myeloma but is still a prognostic factor. Blood 2002;100:3925–9.

[34] Jelinek DF, Witzig TE, Arendt BK. A role for insulin-like growth factor in the regulation of IL-6-responsive human myeloma cell line growth. J Immunol 1997;159:487–96.

[35] Qiang YW, Kopantzev E, Rudikoff S. Insulinlike growth factor-I signaling in multiple myeloma: downstream elements, functional correlates, and pathway cross-talk. Blood 2002;99:4138–46.

[36] Mitsiades CS, Mitsiades N, Poulaki V, et al. Activation of NF-kB and upregulation of intracellular anti-apoptotic proteins via the IGF-1/Akt signaling in human multiple myeloma cells: therapeutic implications. Oncogene 2002;21:5673–83.

[37] Mitsiades CS, Mitsiades N, Kung AL, et al. The IGF/IGF-1R system is a major therapeutic target for multiple myeloma, other hematologic malignancies and solid tumors. Blood 2002;100:170a.

[38] Tai YT, Podar K, Catley L, et al. Insulin-like growth factor-1 induces adhesion and migration in human multiple myeloma cells via activation of beta1-integrin and phosphatidylinositol 3′-kinase/AKT signaling. Cancer Res 2003;63:5850–8.

[39] Podar K, Tai YT, Cole CE, et al. Essential role of caveolae in interleukin-6- and insulin-like growth factor I-triggered Akt-1-mediated survival of multiple myeloma cells. J Biol Chem 2003;278:5794–801.

[40] Mitsiades CS, Mitsiades N, Munshi NC, et al. Focus on multiple myeloma. Cancer Cell 2004;6:439–44.

[41] Podar K, Anderson KC. The pathophysiological role of VEGF in hematological malignancies: therapeutic implications. Blood 2005;105:1383–95.

[42] Podar K, Tai YT, Davies FE, et al. Vascular endothelial growth factor triggers signaling cascades mediating multiple myeloma cell growth and migration. Blood 2001;98: 428–35.

[43] Podar K, Tai YT, Lin BK, et al. Vascular endothelial growth factor-induced migration of multiple myeloma cells is associated with beta 1 integrin- and phosphatidylinositol 3-kinase-dependent PKC alpha activation. J Biol Chem 2002;277:7875–81.

[44] Lin B, Podar K, Gupta D, et al. The vascular endothelial growth factor receptor tyrosine kinase inhibitor PTK787/ZK222584 inhibits growth and migration of multiple myeloma cells in the bone marrow microenvironment. Cancer Res 2002;62: 5019–26.

[45] Podar K, Catley LP, Tai YT, et al. GW654652, the pan-inhibitor of VEGF receptors, blocks the growth and migration of multiple myeloma cells in the bone marrow microenvironment. Blood 2004;103:3474–9.

[46] Podar K, Shringarpure R, Tai YT, et al. Caveolin-1 is required for vascular endothelial growth factor-triggered multiple myeloma cell migration and is targeted by bortezomib. Cancer Res 2004;64:7500–6.

[47] Le Gouill S, Podar K, Amiot M, et al. VEGF induces MCL-1 upregulation and protects multiple myeloma cells against apoptosis. Blood 2004;104:2886–92.

[48] Podar K, Tonon G, Sattler M, et al. The small-molecule VEGF receptor inhibitor pazopanib (GW786034B) targets both tumor and endothelial cells in multiple myeloma. Proc Natl Acad Sci U S A 2006;103:19478–83.

[49] Vacca A, Ribatti D, Presta M, et al. Bone marrow neovascularization, plasma cell angiogenic potential, and matrix metalloproteinase-2 secretion parallel progression of human multiple myeloma. Blood 1999;93:3064–73.

[50] Bisping G, Leo R, Wenning D, et al. Paracrine interactions of basic fibroblast growth factor and interleukin-6 in multiple myeloma. Blood 2003;101:2775–83.

[51] Chesi M, Nardini E, Lim RSC, et al. The t(4;14) translocation in myeloma dysregulates both FGFR3 and a novel gene, MMSET, resulting in IgH/MMSET hybrid transcripts. Blood 1998;92:3025–34.

[52] Chesi M, Nardini E, Brents LA, et al. Frequent translocation t(4;14)(p16.3;q32.3) in multiple myeloma: association with increased expression and activating mutations of fibroblast growth factor receptor 3. Nat Genet 1997;16:260–4.

[53] Keats JJ, Reiman T, Maxwell CA, et al. In multiple myeloma, t(4;14)(p16;q32) is an adverse prognostic factor irrespective of FGFR3 expression. Blood 2003;101:1520–9.

[54] Chang H, Stewart AK, Qi XY, et al. Immunohistochemistry accurately predicts FGFR3 aberrant expression and t(4;14) in multiple myeloma. Blood 2005;106:353–5.

[55] Trudel S, Li ZH, Wei E, et al. CHIR-258, a novel, multitargeted tyrosine kinase inhibitor for the potential treatment of t(4;14) multiple myeloma. Blood 2005;105:2941–8.

[56] Trudel S, Stewart AK, Rom E, et al. The inhibitory anti-FGFR3 antibody, PRO-001, is cytotoxic to t(4;14) multiple myeloma cells. Blood 2006;107:4039–46.

[57] Trudel S, Ely S, Farooqi Y, et al. Inhibition of fibroblast growth factor receptor 3 induces differentiation and apoptosis in t(4;14) myeloma. Blood 2004;103:3521–8.

[58] Chen J, Lee BH, Williams IR, et al. FGFR3 as a therapeutic target of the small molecule inhibitor PKC412 in hematopoietic malignancies. Oncogene 2005;24:8259–67.

[59] Moreaux J, Legouffe E, Jourdan E, et al. BAFF and APRIL protect myeloma cells from apoptosis induced by interleukin 6 deprivation and dexamethasone. Blood 2004;103:3148–57.

[60] Novak AJ, Darce JR, Arendt BK, et al. Expression of BCMA, TACI, and BAFF-R in multiple myeloma: a mechanism for growth and survival. Blood 2004;103:689–94.

[61] Tai YT, Li XF, Breitkreutz I, et al. Role of B-cell-activating factor in adhesion and growth of human multiple myeloma cells in the bone marrow microenvironment. Cancer Res 2006;66:6675–82.

[62] Derksen PW, Tjin E, Meijer HP, et al. Illegitimate WNT signaling promotes proliferation of multiple myeloma cells. Proc Natl Acad Sci U S A 2004;101:6122–7.

[63] Sukhdeo K, Mani M, Zhang Y, et al. Targeting the beta-catenin/TCF transcriptional complex in the treatment of multiple myeloma. Proc Natl Acad Sci U S A 2007;104:7516–21.

[64] Niida A, Hiroko T, Kasai M, et al. DKK1, a negative regulator of Wnt signaling, is a target of the beta-catenin/TCF pathway. Oncogene 2004;23:8520–6.

[65] Tian E, Zhan F, Walker R, et al. The role of the Wnt-signaling antagonist DKK1 in the development of osteolytic lesions in multiple myeloma. N Engl J Med 2003;349:2483–94.

[66] Yaccoby S, Ling W, Zhan F, et al. Antibody-based inhibition of DKK1 suppresses tumor-induced bone resorption and multiple myeloma growth in vivo. Blood 2007;109:2106–11.

[67] Tai YT, Podar K, Gupta D, et al. CD40 activation induces p53-dependent vascular endothelial growth factor secretion in human multiple myeloma cells. Blood 2002;99:1419–27.

[68] Tai YT, Podar K, Mitsiades N, et al. CD40 induces human multiple myeloma cell migration via phosphatidylinositol 3-kinase/AKT/NF-kappa B signaling. Blood 2003;101:2762–9.

[69] Tai YT, Catley LP, Mitsiades CS, et al. Mechanisms by which SGN-40, a humanized anti-CD40 antibody, induces cytotoxicity in human multiple myeloma cells: clinical implications. Cancer Res 2004;64:2846–52.

[70] Hayashi T, Hideshima T, Akiyama M, et al. Molecular mechanisms whereby immunomodulatory drugs activate natural killer cells: clinical application. Br J Haematol 2005;128:192–203.

[71] Tai YT, Li XF, Catley L, et al. Immunomodulatory drug lenalidomide (CC-5013, IMiD3) augments anti-CD40 SGN-40-induced cytotoxicity in human multiple myeloma: clinical implications. Cancer Res 2005;65:11712–20.

[72] Treon SP, Pilarski LM, Belch AR, et al. CD20-directed serotherapy in patients with multiple myeloma: biologic considerations and therapeutic applications. J Immunother 2002;25:72–81.

[73] Tai Y-T, Song W, Li X-F, et al. Killing of drug-sensitive and resistant myeloma cells and disruption of their bone marrow stromal interaction by HuLuc63, a novel humanized anti-CS1 monoclonal antibody. Blood 2006;108:990a.

[74] Berkers CR, Verdoes M, Lichtman E, et al. Activity probe for in vivo profiling of the specificity of proteasome inhibitor bortezomib. Nat Methods 2005;2:357–62.

[75] Baldwin AS Jr. The NF-kB and I kB proteins: new discoveries and insights. Annu Rev Immunol 1996;14:649–83.

[76] Beg AA, Baldwin AS Jr. The IkB proteins: multifunctional regulators of Rel NF-kB transcription factors. Genes Dev 1993;7:2064–70.

[77] Zandi E, Chen Y, Karin M. Direct phosphorylation of IkappaB by IKKalpha and IKKbeta: discrimination between free and NF-kappaB-bound substrate. Science 1998;281:1360–3.

[78] Zandi E, Rothwarf DM, Delhase M, et al. The IkB kinase complex (IKK) contains two kinase subunits, IKKa and IKKb, necessary for IkB phosphorylation and NF-kB activation. Cell 1997;91:243–52.

[79] Hideshima T, Richardson P, Chauhan D, et al. The proteasome inhibitor PS-341 inhibits growth, induces apoptosis, and overcomes drug resistance in human multiple myeloma cells. Cancer Res 2001;61:3071–6.

[80] Mitsiades N, Mitsiades CS, Poulaki V, et al. Molecular sequelae of proteasome inhibition in human multiple myeloma cells. Proc Natl Acad Sci U S A 2002;99:14374–9.

[81] Mitsiades N, Mitsiades CS, Richardson PG, et al. The proteasome inhibitor PS-341 potentiates sensitivity of multiple myeloma cells to conventional chemotherapeutic agents: therapeutic applications. Blood 2003;101:2377–80.

[82] Hideshima T, Mitsiades C, Akiyama M, et al. Molecular mechanisms mediating antimyeloma activity of proteasome inhibitor PS-341. Blood 2003;101:1530–4.

[83] Lee AH, Iwakoshi NN, Anderson KC, et al. Proteasome inhibitors disrupt the unfolded protein response in myeloma cells. Proc Natl Acad Sci U S A 2003;100:9946–51.

[84] Hideshima T, Chauhan D, Hayashi T, et al. Proteasome inhibitor PS-341 abrogates IL-6 triggered signaling cascades via caspase-dependent downregulation of gp130 in multiple myeloma. Oncogene 2003;22:8386–93.

[85] Hideshima T, Chauhan D, Schlossman RL, et al. Role of TNF-a in the pathophysiology of human multiple myeloma: therapeutic applications. Oncogene 2001;20:4519–27.

[86] Hideshima T, Chauhan D, Richardson P, et al. NF-kB as a therapeutic target in multiple myeloma. J Biol Chem 2002;277:16639–47.

[87] Heider U, Kaiser M, Muller C, et al. Bortezomib increases osteoblast activity in myeloma patients irrespective of response to treatment. Eur J Haematol 2006;77:233–8.

[88] Giuliani N, Morandi F, Tagliaferri S, et al. The proteasome inhibitor bortezomib affects osteoblast differentiation in vitro and in vivo in multiple myeloma patients. Blood 2007;110:334–8.

[89] von Metzler I, Krebbel H, Hecht M, et al. Bortezomib inhibits human osteoclastogenesis. Leukemia 2007;21:2025–34.

[90] Chauhan D, Catley L, Li G, et al. A novel orally active proteasome inhibitor induces apoptosis in multiple myeloma cells with mechanisms distinct from Bortezomib. Cancer Cell 2005;8:407–19.

[91] Miller CP, Ban K, Dujka ME, et al. NPI-0052, a novel proteasome inhibitor, induces caspase-8 and ROS-dependent apoptosis alone and in combination with HDAC inhibitors in leukemia cells. Blood 2007;110:267–77.

[92] Demo SD, Kirk CJ, Aujay MA, et al. Antitumor activity of PR-171, a novel irreversible inhibitor of the proteasome. Cancer Res 2007;67:6383–91.

[93] O'Connor OA, Orlowski RZ, Alsina M, et al. Multicenter phase I studies to evaluate the safety, tolerability, and clinical response to intensive dosing with the proteasome Inhibitor PR-171 in patients with relapsed or refractory hematological malignancies. Blood 2006;108:687a.

[94] Hideshima T, Chauhan D, Shima Y, et al. Thalidomide and its analogues overcome drug resistance of human multiple myeloma cells to conventional therapy. Blood 2000;96:2943–50.

[95] LeBlanc R, Hideshima T, Catley LP, et al. Immunomodulatory drug costimulates T cells via the B7-CD28 pathway. Blood 2004;103:1787–90.

[96] Davies FE, Raje N, Hideshima T, et al. Thalidomide and immunomodulatory derivatives augment natural killer cell cytotoxicity in multiple myeloma. Blood 2001;98:210–6.

[97] Bolden JE, Peart MJ, Johnstone RW. Anticancer activities of histone deacetylase inhibitors. Nat Rev Drug Discov 2006;5:769–84.

[98] Finnin MS, Donigian JR, Cohen A, et al. Structures of a histone deacetylase homologue bound to the TSA and SAHA inhibitors. Nature 1999;401:188–93.

[99] Marks PA, Jiang X. Histone deacetylase inhibitors in programmed cell death and cancer therapy. Cell Cycle 2005;4:549–51.

[100] Marks PA, Dokmanovic M. Histone deacetylase inhibitors: discovery and development as anticancer agents. Expert Opin Investig Drugs 2005;14:1497–511.

[101] Lin RJ, Nagy L, Inoue S, et al. Role of the histone deacetylase complex in acute promyelocytic leukaemia. Nature 1998;391:811–4.

[102] Marks P, Rifkind RA, Richon VM, et al. Histone deacetylases and cancer: causes and therapies. Nat Rev Cancer 2001;1:194–202.

[103] Mitsiades N, Mitsiades CS, Richardson PG, et al. Molecular sequelae of histone deacetylase inhibition in human malignant B cells. Blood 2003;101:4055–62.

[104] Huang L, Sowa Y, Sakai T, et al. Activation of the p21WAF1/CIP1 promoter independent of p53 by the histone deacetylase inhibitor suberoylanilide hydroxamic acid (SAHA) through the Sp1 sites. Oncogene 2000;19:5712–9.

[105] Richon VM, Sandhoff TW, Rifkind RA, et al. Histone deacetylase inhibitor selectively induces p21WAF1 expression and gene-associated histone acetylation. Proc Natl Acad Sci U S A 2000;97:10014–9.

[106] Mitsiades CS, Mitsiades NS, McMullan CJ, et al. Transcriptional signature of histone deacetylase inhibition in multiple myeloma: biological and clinical implications. Proc Natl Acad Sci U S A 2004;101:540–5.

[107] Fandy TE, Shankar S, Ross DD, et al. Interactive effects of HDAC inhibitors and TRAIL on apoptosis are associated with changes in mitochondrial functions and expressions of cell cycle regulatory genes in multiple myeloma. Neoplasia 2005;7:646–57.

[108] Remiszewski SW, Sambucetti LC, Bair KW, et al. N-hydroxy-3-phenyl-2-propenamides as novel inhibitors of human histone deacetylase with in vivo antitumor activity: discovery of (2E)-N-hydroxy-3-[4-[[(2-hydroxyethyl)[2-(1H-indol-3-yl)ethyl]amino]methyl]phenyl]-2-propenamide (NVP-LAQ824). J Med Chem 2003;46:4609–24.

[109] Atadja P, Gao L, Kwon P, et al. Selective growth inhibition of tumor cells by a novel histone deacetylase inhibitor, NVP-LAQ824. Cancer Res 2004;64:689–95.

[110] Fiskus W, Pranpat M, Balasis M, et al. Histone deacetylase inhibitors deplete enhancer of zeste 2 and associated polycomb repressive complex 2 proteins in human acute leukemia cells. Mol Cancer Ther 2006;5:3096–104.

[111] Guo F, Sigua C, Tao J, et al. Cotreatment with histone deacetylase inhibitor LAQ824 enhances Apo-2L/tumor necrosis factor-related apoptosis inducing ligand-induced death inducing signaling complex activity and apoptosis of human acute leukemia cells. Cancer Res 2004;64:2580–9.

[112] Rosato RR, Maggio SC, Almenara JA, et al. The histone deacetylase inhibitor LAQ824 induces human leukemia cell death through a process involving XIAP down-regulation, oxidative injury, and the acid sphingomyelinase-dependent generation of ceramide. Mol Pharmacol 2006;69:216–25.

[113] Weisberg E, Catley L, Kujawa J, et al. Histone deacetylase inhibitor NVP-LAQ824 has significant activity against myeloid leukemia cells in vitro and in vivo. Leukemia 2004;18:1951–63.

[114] Qian DZ, Wang X, Kachhap SK, et al. The histone deacetylase inhibitor NVP-LAQ824 inhibits angiogenesis and has a greater antitumor effect in combination with the vascular endothelial growth factor receptor tyrosine kinase inhibitor PTK787/ZK222584. Cancer Res 2004;64:6626–34.

[115] Catley L, Weisberg E, Tai YT, et al. NVP-LAQ824 is a potent novel histone deacetylase inhibitor with significant activity against multiple myeloma. Blood 2003;102:2615–22.

[116] George P, Bali P, Annavarapu S, et al. Combination of the histone deacetylase inhibitor LBH589 and the hsp90 inhibitor 17-AAG is highly active against human CML-BC cells and AML cells with activating mutation of FLT-3. Blood 2005;105:1768–76.

[117] Fiskus W, Pranpat M, Bali P, et al. Combined effects of novel tyrosine kinase inhibitor AMN107 and histone deacetylase inhibitor LBH589 against Bcr-Abl-expressing human leukemia cells. Blood 2006;108:645–52.

[118] Geng L, Cuneo KC, Fu A, et al. Histone deacetylase (HDAC) inhibitor LBH589 increases duration of gamma-H2AX foci and confines HDAC4 to the cytoplasm in irradiated non-small cell lung cancer. Cancer Res 2006;66:11298–304.

[119] Yu C, Friday BB, Lai JP, et al. Abrogation of MAPK and Akt signaling by AEE788 synergistically potentiates histone deacetylase inhibitor-induced apoptosis through reactive oxygen species generation. Clin Cancer Res 2007;13:1140–8.

[120] Qian DZ, Kato Y, Shabbeer S, et al. Targeting tumor angiogenesis with histone deacetylase inhibitors: the hydroxamic acid derivative LBH589. Clin Cancer Res 2006;12:634–42.

[121] Maiso P, Carvajal-Vergara X, Ocio EM, et al. The histone deacetylase inhibitor LBH589 is a potent antimyeloma agent that overcomes drug resistance. Cancer Res 2006;66:5781–9.

[122] Catley L, Weisberg E, Kiziltepe T, et al. Aggresome induction by proteasome inhibitor bortezomib and alpha-tubulin hyperacetylation by tubulin deacetylase (TDAC) inhibitor LBH589 are synergistic in myeloma cells. Blood 2006;108:3441–9.

[123] Haggarty SJ, Koeller KM, Wong JC, et al. Domain-selective small-molecule inhibitor of histone deacetylase 6 (HDAC6)-mediated tubulin deacetylation. Proc Natl Acad Sci U S A 2003;100:4389–94.

[124] Garcia-Mata R, Gao YS, Sztul E. Hassles with taking out the garbage: aggravating aggresomes. Traffic 2002;3:388–96.

[125] Kawaguchi Y, Kovacs JJ, McLaurin A, et al. The deacetylase HDAC6 regulates aggresome formation and cell viability in response to misfolded protein stress. Cell 2003;115:727–38.

[126] Hideshima H, Bradner JE, Wong J, et al. Small molecule inhibition of proteasome and aggresome function induces synergistic anti-tumor activity in multiple myeloma. Proc Natl Acad Sci USA 2005;102:8567–72.

[127] Furumai R, Matsuyama A, Kobashi N, et al. FK228 (depsipeptide) as a natural prodrug that inhibits class I histone deacetylases. Cancer Res 2002;62:4916–21.

[128] Khan SB, Maududi T, Barton K, et al. Analysis of histone deacetylase inhibitor, depsipeptide (FR901228), effect on multiple myeloma. Br J Haematol 2004;125:156–61.

[129] Plumb JA, Finn PW, Williams RJ, et al. Pharmacodynamic response and inhibition of growth of human tumor xenografts by the novel histone deacetylase inhibitor PXD101. Mol Cancer Ther 2003;2:721–8.

[130] Feng R, Hager JH, Hassig CA, et al. A novel, mercaptoketone-based HDAC inhibitor, KD5170 exerts marked inhibition of osteoclast formation and anti-Myeloma activity in vitro. Blood 2006;108:991a.

[131] Chatterjee M, Jain S, Stuhmer T, et al. STAT3 and MAPK signaling maintain overexpression of heat shock proteins 90alpha and beta in multiple myeloma cells, which critically contribute to tumor-cell survival. Blood 2007;109:720–8.

[132] Mitsiades CS, Mitsiades NS, McMullan CJ, et al. Antimyeloma activity of heat shock protein-90 inhibition. Blood 2006;107:1092–100.

[133] Davenport EL, Moore HE, Dunlop AS, et al. Heat shock protein inhibition is associated with activation of the unfolded protein response (UPR) pathway in myeloma plasma cells. Blood 2007;110:2641–9.

[134] Sydor JR, Normant E, Pien CS, et al. Development of 17-allylamino-17-demethoxygeldanamycin hydroquinone hydrochloride (IPI-504), an anti-cancer agent directed against Hsp90. Proc Natl Acad Sci U S A 2006;103:17408–13.

[135] Tu Y, Gardner A, Lichtenstein A. The phosphatidylinositol 3-kinase/AKT kinase pathway in multiple myeloma plasma cells: roles in cytokine-dependent survival and proliferative responses. Cancer Res 2000;60:6763–70.

[136] Hideshima T, Catley L, Yasui H, et al. Perifosine, an oral bioactive novel alkylphospholipid, inhibits Akt and induces in vitro and in vivo cytotoxicity in human multiple myeloma cells. Blood 2006;107:4053–62.

[137] Gajate C, Mollinedo F. Edelfosine and perifosine induce selective apoptosis in multiple myeloma by recruitment of death receptors and downstream signaling molecules into lipid rafts. Blood 2007;109:711–9.

[138] Hideshima T, Catley L, Raje N, et al. Inhibition of Akt induces significant downregulation of survivin and cytotoxicity in human multiple myeloma cells. Br J Haematol 2007;138: 783–91.

[139] Shi Y, Hsu JH, Hu L, et al. Signal pathways involved in activation of p70S6K and phosphorylation of 4E-BP1 following exposure of multiple myeloma tumor cells to interleukin-6. J Biol Chem 2002;277:15712–20.

[140] Pene F, Claessens YE, Muller O, et al. Role of the phosphatidylinositol 3-kinase/Akt and mTOR/P70S6-kinase pathways in the proliferation and apoptosis in multiple myeloma. Oncogene 2002;21:6587–97.

[141] Stromberg T, Dimberg A, Hammarberg A, et al. Rapamycin sensitizes multiple myeloma cells to apoptosis induced by dexamethasone. Blood 2004;103:3138–47.

[142] Shi Y, Gera J, Hu L, et al. Enhanced sensitivity of multiple myeloma cells containing PTEN mutations to CCI-779. Cancer Res 2002;62:5027–34.

[143] Raje N, Kumar S, Hideshima T, et al. Combination of the mTOR inhibitor rapamycin and Revlimid™(CC-5013) has synergistic activity in multiple myeloma. Blood 2004;104: 4188–93.

[144] Frost P, Moatamed F, Hoang B, et al. In vivo antitumor effects of the mTOR inhibitor CCI-779 against human multiple myeloma cells in a xenograft model. Blood 2004;104:4181–7.

[145] Frost P, Shi Y, Hoang B, et al. AKT activity regulates the ability of mTOR inhibitors to prevent angiogenesis and VEGF expression in multiple myeloma cells. Oncogene 2007;26: 2255–62.

[146] van de Donk NW, de Weerdt O, Veth G, et al. G3139, a Bcl-2 antisense oligodeoxynucleotide, induces clinical responses in VAD refractory myeloma. Leukemia 2004;18: 1078–84.

[147] Badros AZ, Goloubeva O, Rapoport AP, et al. Phase II study of G3139, a Bcl-2 antisense oligonucleotide, in combination with dexamethasone and thalidomide in relapsed multiple myeloma patients. J Clin Oncol 2005;23:4089–99.

[148] Kline MP, Rajkumar SV, Timm MM, et al. ABT-737, an inhibitor of Bcl-2 family proteins, is a potent inducer of apoptosis in multiple myeloma cells. Leukemia 2007;21:1549–60.

[149] Chauhan D, Velankar M, Brahmandam M, et al. A novel Bcl-2/Bcl-X(L)/Bcl-w inhibitor ABT-737 as therapy in multiple myeloma. Oncogene 2007;26:2374–80.

[150] Trudel S, Stewart AK, Li Z, et al. The Bcl-2 family protein inhibitor, ABT-737, has substantial antimyeloma activity and shows synergistic effect with dexamethasone and melphalan. Clin Cancer Res 2007;13:621–9.

Hematol Oncol Clin N Am 21 (2007) 1093–1113

HEMATOLOGY/ONCOLOGY CLINICS
OF NORTH AMERICA

ELSEVIER
SAUNDERS

Monoclonal Gammopathy of Undetermined Significance and Smoldering Multiple Myeloma

Robert A. Kyle, MD[a,b],*, S. Vincent Rajkumar, MD[a,b]

[a]Division of Hematology, Mayo Clinic, 200 First Street SW, Rochester, MN 55905, USA
[b]College of Medicine, Mayo Clinic, 200 First Street SW, Rochester, MN 55905, USA

W aldenström introduced the term "essential hyperglobulinemia" to describe patients who had a small serum protein electrophoretic spike but no evidence of multiple myeloma (MM), Waldenström macroglobulinemia (WM), amyloidosis (AL), or related disorders [1]. He stressed the constancy of the size of the protein peak contrasting it with the increasing quantity of monoclonal protein in MM. Later many used the term "benign monoclonal gammopathy," but this is misleading because some patients develop symptomatic MM, WM, AL, or a related monoclonal plasma cell proliferative disorder with time. In 1978, the term "monoclonal gammopathy of undetermined significance" (MGUS) was introduced. MGUS is defined as a serum monoclonal (M) protein less than 3.0 g/dL; less than 10% plasma cells in the bone marrow, if done; little or no M protein in the urine; and absence of lytic bone lesions, anemia, hypercalcemia, or renal insufficiency [2].

RECOGNITION OF MONOCLONAL GAMMOPATHIES

Agarose gel electrophoresis is the preferred method of detection. Immunofixation must then be performed to confirm the presence of an M protein and to determine its heavy chain type and light chain class after a localized band or spike is recognized. In addition, immunofixation should always be performed when MM, WM, AL, or a related plasma cell disorder is suspected, even when a spike is not seen on serum protein electrophoresis. Measurement of the M spike is the preferred method of quantitation of the M protein. Quantitation of immunoglobulins may also be performed with a rate nephelometer. This instrument measures monoclonal and polyclonal immunoglobulins, but it is not affected by molecular size and accurately measures 7sIgM, polymers of IgA, and aggregates of IgG. The results of nephelometry may be 1 to 2 g/dL

Supported in part by grants CA62242 and CA107476 from the National Cancer Institute.

*Corresponding author. College of Medicine, Mayo Clinc, 200 First Street SW, Rochester, MN 55905. E-mail address: kyle.robert@mayo.edu (R.A. Kyle).

greater than expected from serum protein electrophoresis. Electrophoresis and immunofixation of a 24-hour urine specimen should also be performed in all patients who have MM, WM, AL, and heavy chain diseases or when these entities are expected. The 24-hour urine specimen is necessary because the amount of M protein provides an indirect measurement of the patient's tumor mass.

Measurement of the serum free light chain (FLC) is an automated nephelometric assay that measures the level of free κ and λ light chains in the serum. The normal ratio for FLC κ/λ is 0.26 to 1.65. The FLC ratio is useful for patients who have plasma cell disorders who do not have a measurable M spike in the serum or urine. In addition, the free light chain is of prognostic value in MGUS and solitary plasmacytoma of bone. It is also useful in monitoring patients who have nonsecretory MM.

Screening for the presence of an M protein may be done using only serum protein electrophoresis, immunofixation, and FLC quantitation. Only 2 of 428 patients who had a serum M protein and a monoclonal urinary protein at initial diagnosis were missed by performing the three serum studies [3] in which the serum FLC assay was used in place of urinary studies. If an M protein is found, total protein, electrophoresis, and immunofixation of a concentrated aliquot from a 24-hour urine specimen must be performed.

From 1960 through 2006, 36,392 cases of monoclonal plasma cell disorders were identified at Mayo Clinic: 21,256 (58.5%) of MGUS; 6408 (18%) of MM; 3389 (9%) of AL; 1157 (3%) of lymphoproliferative disorders; 1359 (4%) of smoldering multiple myeloma (SMM); 740 (2%) of solitary or extramedullary plasmacytoma; 824 (2%) of WM; and 1259 (3.5%) of other causes, including POEMS syndrome, idiopathic Bence Jones proteinuria, and light chain deposition disease (Fig. 1).

PREVALENCE OF MONOCLONAL GAMMOPATHY OF UNDETERMINED SIGNIFICANCE

M proteins without MM, WM, AL, or related plasma cell disorders have been reported in approximately 1% of people older than 50 years and in about 3% of those older than 70 years in Sweden [4], the United States [5], and in Western France [6]. The frequency of MGUS is higher among older patients and is higher among blacks than whites. In a study of 4 million African American and white men admitted to Veterans' Affairs Hospitals, the prevalence of MGUS was 0.98% in African Americans and 0.4% in whites. The age-adjusted prevalence of MGUS in the African Americans compared with whites was threefold greater [7].

The first population-based study using agarose gel electrophoresis and immunofixation to detect monoclonal proteins has been reported [8]. Serum samples were obtained from 21,463 (77%) of the 28,038 enumerated residents of Olmsted County, Minnesota, who were 50 years of age or older (Table 1). MGUS was found in 694 (3.2%) of these patients (3.7% of men and 2.9% of women, $P<.001$). The rate among men was similar to that among women

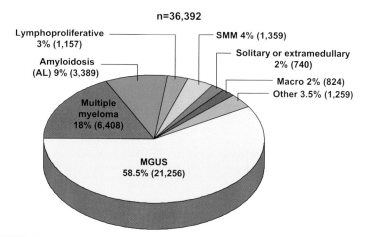

**Monoclonal Gammopathies
Mayo Clinic 1960-2006**

n=36,392

Lymphoproliferative 3% (1,157)
Amyloidosis (AL) 9% (3,389)
Multiple myeloma 18% (6,408)
SMM 4% (1,359)
Solitary or extramedullary 2% (740)
Macro 2% (824)
Other 3.5% (1,259)
MGUS 58.5% (21,256)

Fig. 1. Monoclonal gammopathies diagnosed at the Mayo Clinic during 2006. Macro, macroglobulinemia; MGUS, monoclonal gammopathy of undetermined significance; SMM, smoldering multiple myeloma.

a decade older. Caucasians accounted for 97.3%. In both sexes, the prevalence increased with advancing age and was almost four times as high among people 80 years of age or older as among those 50 to 59 years of age. In men older than 85 years, the prevalence of MGUS was 8.9%, whereas in women it was 7.0% (total 7.5%). There was no significant difference in the concentration of the M protein among the age groups.

IgG accounted for 68.9% of the 694 patients who had MGUS, IgM in 17.2%, IgA in 10.8%, and biclonal in 3%. κ was present in 62% and λ in 38%. The M protein concentration was small with 63% having an M spike less than 1.0 g/dL. The M spike was 1.0 to 1.49 g/dL in 16.6%, 1.5 to 1.99 g/dL in 15.4%, and 2.0 g/dL or greater in 4.5%. The M protein was too low to measure in 13.1%. The median size was 0.5 g/dL, but 0.7 g/dL if the unmeasurable proteins were excluded. The concentration of uninvolved (background, normal, or polyclonal) immunoglobulins was reduced in 124 (27.7%) of the 447 patients whose immunoglobulin concentration was measured. One of the two measured immunoglobulins was reduced in 21.9% and both were decreased in 5.8% of patients. A urinary M protein was found in 21.5% of the 79 patients who were tested. κ was present in 16.5% and λ in 5.0%.

LONG-TERM NATURAL HISTORY OF MONOCLONAL GAMMOPATHY OF UNDETERMINED SIGNIFICANCE

MGUS is a common finding in the medical practice of all physicians. It produces no symptoms and is found during laboratory testing of an apparently

Table 1
Prevalence of monoclonal gammopathy of undetermined significance according to age group and sex among residents of Olmsted County, Minnesota

Age (y)	Men no./total no. (%)[a]	Women no./total no. (%)[a]	Total no./total no. (%)[a]
50–59	82/4,038 (2.0)	59/4,335 (1.4)	141/8,373 (1.7)
60–69	105/2,864 (3.7)	73/3,155 (2.3)	178/6,019 (3.0)
70–79	104/1,858 (5.6)	101/2,650 (3.8)	205/4,508 (4.6)
≥80	59/709 (8.3)	110/1,854 (6.0)	170/2,563 (6.6)
Total	350/9,469 (3.7)[b]	343/11,994 (2.9)[b]	694/21,463 (3.2)[b,c]

[a]The percentage was calculated as the number of patients who had MGUS divided by the number who were tested.
[b]Prevalence was age-adjusted to the 2000 United States total population as follows: men, 4.0% (95% confidence interval [CI], 3.5–4.4); women, 2.7% (95% CI, 2.4–3.0); and total, 3.2% (95% CI, 3.0–3.5).
[c]Prevalence was age- and sex-adjusted to the 2000 United States total population.
From Kyle RA, Therneau TM, Rajkumar SV, et al. Prevalence of monoclonal gammopathy of undetermined significance. N Engl J Med. 2006;354(13):1366; with permission.

normal patient or during evaluation of an unrelated disorder. All practicing physicians see patients who have MGUS. It is important for the physician and the patient to determine whether the M protein will remain stable and benign or progress to MM or a related disorder.

Mayo Clinic Referral Patients

To determine the long-term outcome of patients who have MGUS, we reviewed the medical records of 241 patients who were examined at the Mayo Clinic in Rochester, Minnesota, between January 1, 1956, and December 31, 1970 [9]. After 3579 person-years (median 13.7 years; range 0–39 years), patients were classified a posteriori into one of four groups: Group 1: Patients still living without an increase in serum M protein; Group 2: Patients in whom the M protein had increased to 3.0 g/dL or higher or bone marrow plasma cells increased to 10% or more but who had not required therapy for their lymphoplasma cell disorder; Group 3: Patients who died of unrelated causes; and Group 4: Patients in whom MM, AL, WM, or a related lymphoplasma cell proliferative disorder had developed.

The cohort consisted of 140 men (58%) and 101 women (42%) with a median age of 64 years when MGUS was recognized. Only 4% were younger than 40 years of age, whereas one third were 70 years or older. IgG accounted for 73.5%, IgA 10.5%, and IgM 14%; 2% had a biclonal gammopathy. The light chain was κ in 63% and λ in 37%. Thirty-eight percent had reduction of uninvolved immunoglobulins, whereas only 7 patients had a urinary M protein at diagnosis. The number of living patients who had a stable M protein value (Group 1) consisted of 14 (6%) patients (Table 2). The median duration of follow-up in this subgroup was 33 years. Twenty-five patients (group 2) had a serum M protein value of 3.0 g/dL or higher but did not require chemotherapy for MM or WM. All 25 patients have died but no deaths were related to MM or WM. A total of 138 patients (57%) died without evidence of symptomatic MM, WM, AL, or other lymphoplasma cell proliferative disease (Group 3).

Table 2

Course of 241 patients who had monoclonal gammopathy of undetermined significance

Patient group	Description	No. (%) of patients at follow-up[a]
1	Living patients who had no substantial increase of monoclonal protein	14 (6)
2	Monoclonal protein value ≥3.0 g/dL but no myeloma or related disorder	25 (10)
3	Died of unrelated causes	138 (57)
4	Developed multiple myeloma, macroglobulinemia, amyloidosis, or related disorder	64 (27)
Total		241 (100)

[a]Person-years follow-up = 3579 (median 13.7 year per patient; range, 0–39 years).

From Kyle RA, Therneau TM, Rajkumar SV, et al. Long-term follow-up of 241 patients with monoclonal gammopathy of undetermined significance: the original Mayo Clinic series 25 years later. Mayo Clin Proc 2004;79(7):861; with permission.

Sixty-five patients survived more than 10 years after recognition of MGUS. Cardiac disease, cerebrovascular disease, and non–plasma cell malignancies accounted for most deaths.

MM, AL, WM, or a related malignant lymphoproliferative disorder developed in 64 patients (27%) (Group 4). The actuarial rate of progression was 17% at 10 years, 34% at 20 years, and 39% at 25 years, a rate of approximately 1.5% per year (Fig. 2). Of the 64 patients in this group, 44 (69%) developed MM. The interval from recognition of MGUS to progression was 10.4 years (range 1–32 years) (Table 3). The diagnosis of MM in 10 patients was made more than 20 years after the serum M protein was detected. Median survival after diagnosis of MM was 33 months. AL developed in 8 patients, and WM occurred in 7 patients; a lymphoproliferative disorder consisting of malignant lymphoma (3), chronic lymphocytic leukemia (1), and an atypical malignant lymphoproliferative disorder (1) was observed in 5 patients [9].

Follow-up of 1384 Patients from Southeastern Minnesota Who Had Monoclonal Gammopathy of Undetermined Significance

To confirm the findings of the 241 Mayo Clinic patients referred from the United States and other countries, which may be subject to referral bias, we studied 1384 patients who had MGUS from the 11 counties of southeastern Minnesota evaluated at Mayo Clinic from 1960 to 1994 [10]. The cohort included 753 men (54%) and 631 women (46%). The median age at the time of diagnosis was 72 years, but only 2% were younger than 40 years and 59% were 70 years or older. The M protein was IgG in 70%, IgA in 12%,

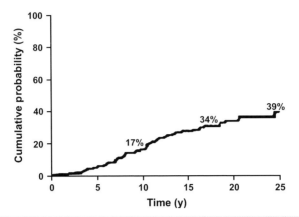

Fig. 2. Rate of development of MM or related disorders in 241 patients who had monoclonal gammopathy of undetermined significance.

IgM in 15%, and biclonal in 3%. κ light chain type was present in 61% and λ in 39%. The level of uninvolved (normal or background) immunoglobulins was reduced in 38% of 840 patients tested. Electrophoresis, immunoelectrophoresis, and immunofixation were performed on urine from 418 patients; 21% had a monoclonal κ light chain, whereas 10% had a λ light chain and 69% were negative for monoclonal light chain. The median percentage of bone marrow plasma cells was 3% (range 0 to 10%).

The 1384 patients were followed for 11,009 person-years (median 15 years; range 0–35 years), during which time 963 (70%) died. During follow-up, MM, lymphoma with an IgM protein, AL, WM, chronic lymphocytic leukemia (CLL), or plasmacytoma developed in 115 patients (8%) (Table 4). The cumulative probability of progression to one of those disorders was 10% at 10 years, 21% at 20 years, and 26% at 25 years. The overall risk for progression was approximately 1% per year. Patients were at risk for progression even after 25 years or more of stable MGUS (Fig. 3). In addition, 32 patients had an increase

Table 3

Development of multiple myeloma or related disorder in 64 patients who had monoclonal gammopathy of undetermined significance

	No. (%) of patients	Interval to disease, y	
		Median	Range
Multiple myeloma	44 (69)	10.6	1–32
Macroglobulinemia	7 (11)	10.3	4–16
Amyloidosis	8 (12)	9.0	6–19
Lymphoproliferative disease	5 (8)	8.0	4–19
Total	64 (100)	10.4	1–32

From Kyle RA, Therneau TM, Rajkumar SV, et al. Long-term follow-up of 241 patients with monoclonal gammopathy of undetermined significance: the original Mayo Clinic series 25 years later. Mayo Clin Proc 2004;79(7):862; with permission.

Table 4
Risk for progression among 1384 residents of southeastern Minnesota in whom monoclonal gammopathy of undetermined significance was diagnosed in 1960 through 1994

Type of progression	Observed no. of patients	Expected no. of patients[a]	Relative risk (95% CI)
Multiple myeloma	75	3.0	25.0 (20–32)
Lymphoma	19[b]	7.8	2.4 (2–4)
Primary amyloidosis	10	1.2	8.4 (4–16)
Macroglobulinemia	7	0.2	46.0 (19–95)
Chronic lymphocytic leukemia	3[c]	3.5	0.9 (0.2–3)
Plasmacytoma	1	0.1	8.5 (0.2–47)
Total	115	15.8	7.3 (6–9)

CI, confidence interval.

[a]Expected numbers of cases were derived from the age- and sex-matched white population of the Surveillance, Epidemiology, and End Results program in Iowa, except for primary amyloidosis for which data are from [69].

[b]All 19 patients had serum IgM monoclonal protein. If the 30 patients who had IgM, IgA, or IgG monoclonal protein and lymphoma were included, the relative risk would be 3.9 (95% CI, 2.6–5.5).

[c]All 3 patients had serum IgM monoclonal protein. If all 6 patients who had IgM, IgA, or IgG monoclonal protein and chronic lymphocytic leukemia were included, the relative risk would be 1.7 (95% CI, 0.6–3.7).

From Kyle RA, Therneau TM, Rajkumar SV, et al. A long-term study of prognosis in monoclonal gammopathy of undetermined significance. N Engl J Med. 2002;346(8):567; with permission.

of M protein to greater than 3 g/dL or percentage of plasma cells increased to more than 10% but symptomatic MM did not develop. At 20 years, the death rates for patients who had MGUS were 10% from plasma cell disorders and 72% from non–plasma cell disorders, such as cardiac disease, cerebrovascular events, or non–plasma cell malignancies (Fig. 4). The number of patients who had progression to a plasma cell neoplasm or related disorder (115 patients) was more than seven times that expected by incidence rates for those conditions in the general population (see Table 4). The risk for progression was 25-fold for MM, 46-fold for WM, and 8.4-fold for AL.

The MGUS disappeared without a known cause in 27 patients (2%). Only 6 of these 27 patients (0.4% of all patients) had a discrete, measurable spike on the densitometer tracing (median 1.2 g/dL).

The 75 patients in whom MM developed accounted for 65% of the 115 patients who had progressed. In 24 patients (32%), the diagnosis of MM was made more than 10 years after detection of the M protein and 5 (7%) were recognized after 20 years of follow-up. The characteristics of these 75 patients who had MM were comparable to those of the 1027 patients who had newly-diagnosed MM referred to the Mayo Clinic from 1985 to 1988, except that the southeastern Minnesota patients were older (median 72 versus 66 years) and less likely to be men (46% versus 60%) [11].

The findings in the Southeastern Minnesota cohort thus confirmed the results of the initial Mayo Clinic study of 241 referral patients.

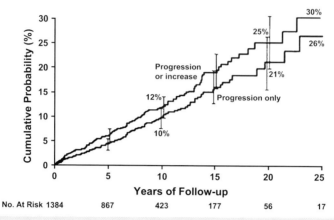

Fig. 3. Probability of progression among 1384 residents of southeastern Minnesota in whom MGUS was diagnosed from 1960 through 1994. The top curve shows the probability of progression to a plasma-cell cancer (115 patients) or of an increase in the monoclonal protein concentration to more than 3 g/dL or the proportion of plasma cells in bone marrow to more than 10% (32 patients). The bottom curve shows only the probability of progression of MGUS to multiple myeloma, IgM lymphoma, primary amyloidosis, macroglobulinemia, chronic lymphocytic leukemia, or plasmacytoma (115 patients). The bars show 95% confidence intervals. (*From* Kyle RA, Therneau TM, Rajkumar SV, et al. A long-term study of prognosis in monoclonal gammopathy of undetermined significance. N Engl J Med. 2002; 346(8):567; with permission.)

Other Series

Malignant disease developed in 13 of 128 patients who had MGUS who were followed up for a median of 56 months. The actuarial probability of the development of malignant disease was 8.5% at 5 years and 19.2% at 10 years [12]. Gregerson and colleagues [13] reported a cohort of 1324 patients who had MGUS in North Jutland, Denmark, in which malignant transformation was the cause of death in 97 patients compared with 4.9 deaths expected. In the Danish Cancer Registry, 64 new cases of malignancy (5 expected, relative risk 12.9) were found among 1229 patients who had MGUS [14]. The risk for development of MM was 34.3-fold, WM 63.8-fold, and non-Hodgkin lymphoma 5.9-fold. A related malignancy developed in 51 of 504 patients from Iceland who had MGUS [15]. In summary, most studies confirm that the risk for progression from MGUS to MM or related disorders is about 1% per year. They also agree that the risk does not disappear even after long-term follow-up.

PATHOPHYSIOLOGY OF PROGRESSION OF MONOCLONAL GAMMOPATHY OF UNDETERMINED SIGNIFICANCE

The events responsible for malignant transformation of MGUS to MM or a related plasma cell disorder are poorly understood. Genetic changes, various cytokines related to myeloma bone disease, bone marrow angiogenesis, and

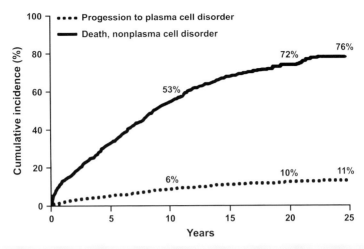

Fig. 4. Rate of death from non–plasma cell disorders compared with progression to plasma cell disorders in 1384 patients who had MGUS from southeastern Minnesota. (*From* Kyle RA, Rajkumar SV. Monoclonal gammopathies of undetermined significance. Immunol Rev 2003;194:125; with permission.)

infectious agents may all play a role in progression of MGUS. Unfortunately, the specific role of these alterations is not known [16].

Genetic Changes

Cytogenetic changes are common in MM and in MGUS. Approximately 60% of patients who have MM have IgH (14q32) translocations [17]. These same translocations are also present in MGUS. In one series, IgH translocations were found in 46% of patients who had MGUS [18]. IgH translocations consisting of t(11;14)(q13;q32) were found in 25%, t(4;14)(p16.3;q32) in 9%, and t(14;16)(q32;q23) in 5% among 59 patients who had MGUS studied with cytoplasmic Ig FISH. These translocations led to the dysregulation of oncogenes, such as cyclin D1 (11q13), c-maf (16q23), FGFR3/MMSET (fibroblastic growth factor receptor 3/MM SET domain) (4p16.3), and cyclin D3 (6p21), and may be involved with the initiation of the MGUS clone rather than progression of MGUS to MM. Most MGUS patients who lack IgH translocations have evidence of hyperdiploidy. In another report, 11 of 28 patients (40%) who had SMM or MGUS had hyperdiploidy, which is similar to the percentage of hyperdiploid MM reported in the literature [19].

Deletions of chromosome 13 have been found to have an adverse prognostic value in MM, but this abnormality is also present in MGUS [20]. It is not known, however, whether the rate of progression from MGUS to MM is increased because the frequency of deletion of chromosome 13 is similar in MGUS and MM.

K-RAS and N-RAS mutations were noted in 5% of MGUS, in contrast to 31% of MM, but this may or may not be a causal event in the progression of MGUS to MM [21].

Myeloma Bone Disease Associated Cytokines

Clinically, lytic bone lesions, osteopenia, hypercalcemia, and pathologic fractures differentiate MM from MGUS. We found a 2.7-fold increase in axial fractures but no increase in limb fractures in 488 Olmsted County residents who had MGUS [22].

Osteoclast activation and inhibition of osteoblast differentiation are responsible for bone lesions with progression of MGUS to MM. Osteoclast activation is caused by overexpression of various cytokines, such as receptor activator of nuclear factor κβ ligand (RANKL) and macrophage inflammatory protein 1-α (MIP-1α) [23]. RANKL is modulated by a decoy receptor, osteoprotegerin. Myeloma bone disease may occur from excess RANKL or reduced levels of osteoprotegerin [24].

Angiogenesis

Bone marrow angiogenesis is increased in MM [25]. The median microvessel density (vessels per high-power field) in 400 patients who had plasma cell disorders increased with disease stage in one study: 1.3 in the 42 normal controls, 1.7 in AL, 3 in MGUS, 4 in SMM, 11 in MM, and 20 in relapsed myeloma [26]. Loss of an endogenous angiogenesis inhibitor may be involved in the increased angiogenesis that occurs with disease progression. In one study, 63% of MGUS sera inhibited angiogenesis, whereas 43% of SMM and 4% of MM serum samples ($P<.001$) did so [27].

Helicobacter pylori

In one report, 68% of patients who had MGUS also had *Helicobacter pylori* infection, whereas eradication of the infection led to resolution of the monoclonal gammopathy in 11 of 39 patients [28]. On the other hand, 30% of 93 patients who had MGUS who were residents of Olmsted County, Minnesota, had positive serologic results for *H pylori*, as did 32% of 98 control patients from the same population. In addition, 33% of 154 patients from Mayo Clinic who had MGUS were positive for *H pylori*, as were 33% who did not have MGUS. The role of *H pylori* infection, if any, is controversial [29].

PREDICTORS OF PROGRESSION IN MONOCLONAL GAMMOPATHY OF UNDETERMINED SIGNIFICANCE

Prediction of patients who have MGUS who remain stable from those in whom progression develops is impossible at the time of diagnosis [30].

Size of Monoclonal Protein

The size of the M protein at recognition of MGUS was the most important predictor of progression in 1384 patients who had MGUS [10]. The risk for progression to MM or a related disorder 20 years after diagnosis of MGUS was 14% for patients who had an initial M protein level of 0.5 g/dL or less, 16%

for 1 g/dL, 25% for 1.5 g/dL, 41% for 2 g/dL, 49% for 2.5 g/dL, and 64% for 3.0 g/dL. The risk for progression with an M protein level of 1.5 g/dL was almost twice that in a patient who had an M protein level of 0.5 g/dL, whereas risk for progression with an M protein of 2.5 g/dL was 4.6 times that of a patient who had a 0.5 g/dL spike.

Type of Immunoglobulin
Patients who had IgM or IgA monoclonal protein had an increased risk for progression compared with those who had IgM protein ($P = .001$).

Number of Bone Marrow Plasma Cells
In a group of 1104 patients who had MGUS, more than 5% bone marrow plasma cells, presence of Bence Jones proteinuria, polyclonal immunoglobulin reduction, and elevated erythrocyte sedimentation rate were independent factors influencing MGUS transformation [31]. Malignant transformation occurred in 6.6% when the bone marrow plasma cell level was less than 10% and 37% in patients who had MGUS with a plasma cell level of 10% to 30% [32].

Abnormal Serum/FLC Ratio and Risk Stratification of Monoclonal Gammopathy of Undetermined Significance
Thirty-three percent of 1148 patients who had MGUS from southeastern Minnesota had an abnormal FLC ratio. The risk for progression was significantly higher than that in patients who had a normal FLC ratio (hazard ratio 3.5; $P<.001$) and was independent of the size and type of serum M protein [33]. A new risk stratification model using size and type of M protein and the FLC ratio was developed. In patients who had a serum M protein 1.5 g/dL or greater, presence of IgA or IgM monoclonal protein, and an abnormal serum FLC ratio, the risk for progression at 20 years was 58% compared with 5% when none of the risk factors were present (Table 5) [33].

LIFE EXPECTANCY AND CAUSE OF DEATH
Survival was shorter among 241 patients who had MGUS diagnosed between 1956 and 1971 compared with an age- and sex-adjusted 1980 United States population (13.7 versus 15.5 years) [9]. In the 1384-patient cohort who had MGUS, survival was 8.1 years compared with an expected 11.8 years ($P<.001$) for Minnesota residents of matched age and sex [10].

DIFFERENTIAL DIAGNOSIS
At the time of presentation, the differentiation of a patient who has MGUS from one who has MM may be difficult and is based on the clinical and laboratory findings. A radiographic bone survey is indicated to exclude myeloma in almost all patients. A bone marrow aspirate and biopsy should be done if myeloma is suspected and in all patients who have an M-protein value of 1.5 g/dL or more, an IgA or an IgM monoclonal protein, an abnormal FLC ratio, or unexplained anemia or elevation of creatinine or calcium

Table 5
Risk-stratification model to predict progression of monoclonal gammopathy of undetermined significance to myeloma or related disorders

Risk group	No. of patients	Relative risk	Absolute risk for progression at 20 y (%)	Absolute risk for progression at 20 y accounting for death as a competing risk (%)
Low risk (serum M protein <1.5 gm/dL, IgG subtype, normal FLC ratio [0.26–1.65])	449	1.0	5	2
Low-intermediate risk (any one factor abnormal)	420	5.4	21	10
High-intermediate risk (any two factors abnormal)	226	10.1	37	18
High risk (all three factors abnormal)	53	20.8	58	27

This table was originally published in Rajkumar SV, Kyle RA, Therneau TM, et al. Serum free light chain ratio is an independent risk factor for progression in monoclonal gammopathy of undetermined significance (MGUS). Blood 2005;106:812–7. © the American Society of Hematology.

values. The serum monoclonal protein level is of help because higher levels are associated with a greater likelihood of malignancy. Reduction of uninvolved immunoglobulins or the presence of an M protein in the urine (Bence Jones proteinuria) may be present in MGUS and are of little help in differentiation. Patients who have more than 10% bone marrow plasma cells or an M spike greater than 3 g/dL represent SMM. These patients have a higher risk for progression to malignancy than patients who have MGUS, but should be observed and not treated. The presence of osteolytic lesions suggests MM, but metastatic carcinoma may also produce lytic lesions, and if there is doubt a biopsy is required to make the distinction. An elevated plasma cell labeling index usually indicates symptomatic MM, but one third of patients who have symptomatic MM have a normal labeling index and the test is not widely available. Circulating plasma cells in the peripheral blood suggest symptomatic MM [34].

FISH studies are not helpful because abnormalities are found in MGUS and MM. Conventional cytogenetic studies are not useful because an abnormal karyotype is rare in MGUS because of the low proliferative rate and the small number of plasma cells.

In summary, the differentiation of active MM requiring therapy from MGUS or SMM depends primarily on the presence or absence of end-organ damage (CRAB: hypercalcemia, renal insufficiency, anemia, bone lesions) that is believed to be attributable to the underlying plasma cell proliferative disorder. MGUS and SMM are distinguished from each other based on the size of the serum M protein and the bone marrow plasma cell percentage.

MANAGEMENT

Serum protein electrophoresis should be repeated in 3 to 6 months to exclude MM; if results are stable and the patient has no clinical features of MM or AL and a serum M-protein value less than 1.5 g/dL, IgG type, and normal FLC ratio (low-risk MGUS), serum protein electrophoresis should be repeated at intervals of every 2 to 3 years. In this setting, bone marrow examination is rarely necessary.

If an asymptomatic patient has an M-protein value greater than 1.5 g/dL, IgA or IgM protein, or an abnormal FLC ratio, a bone marrow examination should be done. A bone marrow aspirate and biopsy should also be done in patients who have unexplained anemia, renal insufficiency, hypercalcemia, or bone lesions. If possible, cytogenetic studies (conventional and FISH), determination of the plasma cell labeling index, and a search for circulating plasma cells in the peripheral blood should be done. In the event of an IgM monoclonal protein, a bone marrow examination and a computed tomographic scan of the abdomen may be useful for recognizing retroperitoneal lymph nodes. Levels of β-2 microglobulin, lactate dehydrogenase, and C-reactive protein should be determined if there is evidence of MM or WM. If the results of these tests are satisfactory, serum protein electrophoresis should be repeated at 6-month intervals for a year and then at annual intervals. If there is any change in their clinical condition, patients must contact their physicians.

VARIANTS OF MONOCLONAL GAMMOPATHY OF UNDETERMINED SIGNIFICANCE

IgM Monoclonal Gammopathy of Undetermined Significance

IgM MGUS is defined as serum IgM monoclonal protein less than 3 gm/dL, bone marrow lymphoplasmacytic infiltration less than 10%, and no evidence of anemia, constitutional symptoms, hyperviscosity, lymphadenopathy, or hepatosplenomegaly [35]. Between 1956 and 1978, 430 patients who had an IgM monoclonal protein were seen at Mayo Clinic. MGUS was found in 56% [36]. Gobbi and colleagues [37] found an IgM MGUS in approximately 20% of patients who had MGUS and in 30% of patients who had an IgM paraprotein.

IgM MGUS was diagnosed in 213 Mayo Clinic patients who resided in the 11 counties of southeastern Minnesota [38]. Twenty-nine (14%) of these 213 patients developed non-Hodgkin lymphoma (N = 17), WM (N = 6), chronic lymphocytic leukemia (N = 3), or AL (N = 3), with relative risks of 15-, 262-, 6-, and 16-fold, respectively. The risk for progression was 1.5% per year. The level of the serum M protein and serum albumin values at diagnosis were independent predictors of progression. Morra and colleagues [39] reported progression in 14 (10%) of 138 patients who had IgM MGUS who had remained stable for 12 months. Overt WM or a related disorder developed in 8 of 83 patients who had an IgM-related disorder (type I cryoglobulinemia in 19, type II cryoglobulinemia in 56, peripheral neuropathy in 5, and idiopathic thrombocytopenia in 3) [40].

In another report of 217 patients who had IgM MGUS and 201 who had indolent WM, 15 of those who had IgM MGUS and 45 of those who had indolent WM progressed to symptomatic WM. The respective numbers were 2 and 6 for non-Hodgkin lymphoma and 0 and 3 for AL. The variables adversely related to progression were the initial M protein level, hemoglobin value, and gender in both groups [41].

IgD Monoclonal Gammopathy of Undetermined Significance

The presence of an IgD monoclonal protein almost always indicates MM, AL, or plasma cell leukemia. IgD MGUS has been reported in two patients who were followed up for 6 and 8 years, respectively, without evidence of progression.

Biclonal Gammopathy

Biclonal gammopathies have two different M proteins and occur in 3% to 6% of patients who have monoclonal gammopathies. They may result from the proliferation of two different clones of plasma cells or by production of two monoclonal proteins by a single clone of plasma cells. In a report of 57 patients who had biclonal gammopathy, 37 had biclonal gammopathy of undetermined significance. Two localized bands were found in only 18 patients with electrophoresis on cellulose acetate, whereas in the remainder the second M protein was not recognized until immunoelectrophoresis or immunofixation was performed. The clinical findings of biclonal gammopathies were similar to those of monoclonal gammopathies [42].

Triclonal Gammopathy

In a review of 24 patients who had triclonal gammopathy, 16 were associated with a malignant immunolymphoproliferative disorder, 5 occurred in nonhematologic disease, and 3 were of undetermined significance [43]. Three separate populations of M protein–producing cells were identified in a patient who had non-Hodgkin lymphoma [44].

Idiopathic Bence Jones Proteinuria

Seven patients have been described as having Bence Jones proteinuria (>1 g/24 h) but no M protein was found in the serum and there was no evidence of MM or a related disorder [45]. MM developed in two, SMM in one, AL in one, and two patients died of unrelated causes. One of these patients had excreted up to 1.8 g/24 h of κ light chain for 37 years without evidence of MM or AL at autopsy.

ASSOCIATION OF MONOCLONAL GAMMOPATHY WITH OTHER DISORDERS

The association of two diseases depends on the frequency with which each occurs independently. Valid epidemiologic and statistical methods must be used in evaluating these associations. It is essential that an appropriate control population be used. A recent review contains more detail concerning the association of M proteins with other diseases [16].

Lymphoproliferative Disorders

Malignant lymphoma has been associated with monoclonal gammopathies. Forty-four (7%) of 640 patients who had diffuse non-Hodgkin lymphoma or chronic lymphocytic leukemia had an M protein, whereas only 4 of 292 patients who had nodular lymphoma and 1 of 218 patients who had Hodgkin disease had an M protein [46].

In a cohort of 430 patients who had an IgM monoclonal protein seen at the Mayo Clinic, the following types were found: MGUS 56%, WM 17%, lymphoproliferative disease 14%, non-Hodgkin lymphoma 7%, chronic lymphocytic leukemia 5%, and AL 1% [36]. In a series of 382 patients who had a lymphoid neoplasm and an IgM monoclonal gammopathy, the following diagnoses were made: WM 59%, chronic lymphocytic leukemia 20%, marginal zone lymphoma 7%, follicular lymphoma 5%, mantle cell lymphoma 3%, diffuse large B cell lymphoma 2%, and miscellaneous 4% [47]. Seven (27%) of 26 patients who had extranodal marginal zone lymphoma had an M protein [48].

Leukemia

In a group of 100 patients who had chronic lymphocytic leukemia and an M protein in the serum or urine, IgM accounted for 38%, IgG 51%, IgA 1%, and light chain only 10% [49]. Monoclonal gammopathy has also been recognized in hairy cell leukemia, chronic myelocytic leukemia, chronic neutrophilic leukemia, acute leukemia, Sézary syndrome, and mycosis fungoides.

Other Hematologic Disorders

Monoclonal gammopathy has been reported in myelodysplastic syndrome, idiopathic myelofibrosis, polycythemia vera, paroxysmal nocturnal hemoglobinuria, and Gaucher disease. Acquired von Willebrand disease has been reported with MGUS [50]. On the other hand, thromboembolic events occurred in 19 (6.1%) of 310 patients who had MGUS [51]. Monoclonal gammopathies have also been reported with pernicious anemia and pure red cell aplasia.

Connective Tissue Disorders

M proteins have been reported with rheumatoid arthritis, lupus erythematosus, scleroderma, and polymyalgia rheumatica.

Neurologic Disorders

Sensorimotor peripheral neuropathy of unknown cause was found in 16 (6%) of 279 patients [52]. An association exists between MGUS and sensorimotor peripheral neuropathy. The incidence is variable and depends on patient selection bias, the vigor with which an M protein is sought, and whether the diagnosis of peripheral neuropathy is made on clinical or electrophysiologic grounds.

The most common M protein associated with peripheral neuropathy is IgM, followed by IgG and IgA. In approximately one half of patients who have an IgM monoclonal gammopathy and peripheral neuropathy, the M protein binds to myelin-associated glycoprotein (MAG). The role of antibodies and peripheral neuropathy has been reviewed [53]. In a series of 65 patients who had

MGUS and sensorimotor peripheral neuropathy, 31 had IgM, 24 had IgG, and 10 had IgA monoclonal proteins [54]. Neither the size of the monoclonal spike nor anti-MAG activity influenced the type and severity of neuropathy. MGUS neuropathies differ from that associated with AL in the following: (1) the lower extremities are more often involved in MGUS, but both upper and lower extremities are involved in AL; (2) the course of neuropathy in AL is always slowly progressive; and (3) autonomic features (hypotension, anhidrosis, bowel change, and so forth) and heart or kidney failure often occur.

Therapy of peripheral neuropathy and monoclonal gammopathy are challenging. Plasmapheresis has been of benefit in some patients, whereas chlorambucil has been helpful in some patients who have IgM monoclonal protein or melphalan and prednisone for IgG and IgA gammopathies. Fludarabine and rituximab have been reported as producing some benefit. Intravenous immunoglobulin infusions have been of little benefit. Treatment of neuropathies associated with monoclonal gammopathies has been recently reviewed [55]. Monoclonal gammopathy and motor neuron disease have been reported, but a casual effect has not been proven. Myasthenia gravis, ataxia-telangiectasia, and nemaline myopathy have all been reported with MGUS.

POEMS Syndrome (Osteosclerotic Myeloma)

POEMS syndrome is characterized by polyneuropathy, organomegaly, endocrinopathy, monoclonal protein, and skin changes. POEMS syndrome is defined by the presence of a monoclonal plasma cell disorder, peripheral neuropathy, and at least one of the following seven features: osteosclerotic myeloma, Castleman disease, organomegaly, endocrinopathy (excluding diabetes mellitus or hypothyroidism), edema, typical skin changes, and papilledema [35]. Not every patient meeting the above criteria has POEMS syndrome; the features should have a temporal relationship to each other and no other attributable cause. The presence of single or multiple osteosclerotic lesions are important features. The absence of either osteosclerotic myeloma or Castleman disease should make the diagnosis suspect. Hypertrichosis, hyperpigmentation, gynecomastia, and testicular atrophy may be present. Polycythemia or thrombocytosis may occur. Almost all have a monoclonal protein of the λ light chain type. The serum M protein is small and Bence Jones proteinuria, renal insufficiency, hypercalcemia, and skeletal fractures are rarely seen. The bone marrow usually contains fewer than 5% plasma cells. The median duration of survival was 13.8 years in a 99-patient cohort [56]. Elevated levels of interleukin-1β, tumor necrosis factor-alpha, interleukin-6, and vascular endothelial growth factor (VEGF) are frequently present.

Radiation therapy in tumoricidal doses is indicated if single or multiple sclerotic lesions are found in a limited area. If the lesions are widespread, systemic therapy similar to myeloma, such as autologous stem cell transplantation or alkylating therapy, is indicated.

Dermatologic Diseases

Lichen myxedematosus (scleromyxedema papular mucinosis) is a rare dermatologic condition usually associated with a cathodal IgG λ protein. Pyoderma gangrenosum and necrobiotic xanthogranuloma are frequently associated with an M protein. Schnitzler syndrome is characterized by the presence of chronic urticaria and an IgM monoclonal protein. Plain xanthomatosis or subcorneal pustular dermatosis has been associated with a monoclonal gammopathy. The association of monoclonal gammopathies and skin disorders has been reported [57].

Endocrine Disorders

The association of hyperparathyroidism and MGUS is controversial. Nine (1%) of 911 patients at Mayo Clinic had MGUS, which is similar to that in a normal population [58]. On the other hand, 20 of 101 patients with hyperparathyroidism had an M protein compared with only 2 of 127 controls [59].

Immunosuppression

Monoclonal proteins have been seen in patients who have acquired immunodeficiency syndrome. Monoclonal proteins are frequently seen after renal transplantation, liver transplantation [60], heart transplantation, or autologous bone marrow transplantation [61]. In a report of five patients who had MGUS undergoing transplantation, smoldering multiple myeloma developed in two and one other had an increase in the serum M protein [62].

Miscellaneous Conditions

Acquired C1 inhibitor deficiency [63] and capillary leak syndrome [64] have been reported with monoclonal gammopathy. Idiopathic segmental glomerulosclerosis may be associated with MGUS [65]. MGUS has been reported following silicone breast implants, but the frequency does not seem to be increased [66]. The monoclonal gammopathy may be bound to calcium, copper, transferrin, or serum phosphorus. Monoclonal proteins may be associated with antibody activity [67].

SMOLDERING (ASYMPTOMATIC) MULTIPLE MYELOMA

SMM is defined as a serum IgG or IgA M protein of 3 g/dL or higher or 10% or more plasma cells in the bone marrow but no evidence of end-organ damage (hypercalcemia, renal insufficiency, anemia, or skeletal lesions) [35]. It accounts for approximately 15% of all cases of newly diagnosed MM [68]. Almost all patients who have SMM seem to have evidence of genomic instability manifested as IgH translocations or hyperdiploidy on molecular genetic testing. SMM is differentiated from MM in the same manner as MGUS, based on the presence or absence of end-organ damage. Differentiation between MGUS and SMM was discussed previously.

Natural History of Smoldering Multiple Myeloma

SMM, similar to MGUS, is an asymptomatic condition. The risk for progression to myeloma or related malignancy is much higher in SMM compared with

MGUS: 1% per year versus 10% to 20% per year, respectively. In a recent study, we found that the risk for progression was 10% per year for the first 5 years, 3% per year for the next 5 years, and then 1% to 2% per year for the following 10 years.

The type of monoclonal protein, the amount of Bence Jones proteinuria, and the presence of circulating plasma cells in the peripheral blood are all risks for progression.

Therapy

The current standard care is close follow-up every 3 to 6 months. There is no evidence that early treatment of SMM or stage I MM improves overall survival. The recommendation to observe closely without treatment until progression is also based on the toxic effects of therapy and that the disease may not progress for years.

References

[1] Waldenström J. Abnormal proteins in myeloma. Adv Intern Med 1952;5:398–440.

[2] Kyle RA. Monoclonal gammopathy of undetermined significance. Natural history in 241 cases. Am J Med 1978;64(5):814–26.

[3] Katzmann JA, Dispenzieri A, Kyle RA, et al. Elimination of the need for urine studies in the screening algorithm for monoclonal gammopathies by using serum immunofixation and free light chain assays. Mayo Clin Proc 2006;81(12):1575–8.

[4] Axelsson U, Bachmann R, Hallen J. Frequency of pathological proteins (M-components) in 6,995 sera from an adult population. Acta Med Scand 1966;179(2):235–47.

[5] Kyle RA, Finkelstein S, Elveback LR, et al. Incidence of monoclonal proteins in a Minnesota community with a cluster of multiple myeloma. Blood 1972;40(5):719–24.

[6] Saleun JP, Vicariot M, Deroff P, et al. Monoclonal gammopathies in the adult population of Finistere, France. J Clin Pathol 1982;35(1):63–8.

[7] Landgren O, Gridley G, Turesson I, et al. Risk of monoclonal gammopathy of undetermined significance (MGUS) and subsequent multiple myeloma among African American and white veterans in the United States. Blood 2006;107(3):904–6.

[8] Kyle RA, Therneau TM, Rajkumar SV, et al. Prevalence of monoclonal gammopathy of undetermined significance. N Engl J Med 2006;354(13):1362–9.

[9] Kyle RA, Therneau TM, Rajkumar SV, et al. Long-term follow-up of 241 patients with monoclonal gammopathy of undetermined significance: the original Mayo Clinic series 25 years later. Mayo Clin Proc 2004;79(7):859–66.

[10] Kyle RA, Therneau TM, Rajkumar SV, et al. A long-term study of prognosis in monoclonal gammopathy of undetermined significance. N Engl J Med 2002;346(8):564–9.

[11] Kyle RA, Gertz MA, Witzig TE, et al. Review of 1027 patients with newly diagnosed multiple myeloma. Mayo Clin Proc 2003;78(1):21–33.

[12] Blade J, Lopez-Guillermo A, Rozman C, et al. Malignant transformation and life expectancy in monoclonal gammopathy of undetermined significance. Br J Haematol 1992;81(3):391–4.

[13] Gregersen H, Ibsen J, Mellemkjoer L, et al. Mortality and causes of death in patients with monoclonal gammopathy of undetermined significance. Br J Haematol 2001;112(2):353–7.

[14] Gregersen H, Mellemkjaer L, Salling Ibsen J, et al. Cancer risk in patients with monoclonal gammopathy of undetermined significance. Am J Hematol 2000;63(1):1–6.

[15] Ogmundsdottir HM, Haraldsdottir V. Monoclonal gammopathy in Iceland: a population-based registry and follow-up. Br J Haematol 2002;118(1):166–73.

[16] Kyle RA, Rajkumar SV. Monoclonal gammopathy of undetermined significance. Br J Haematol 2006;134(6):573–89.

[17] Avet-Loiseau H, Li JY, Facon T, et al. High incidence of translocations t(11;14)(q13;q32) and t(4;14)(p16;q32) in patients with plasma cell malignancies. Cancer Res 1998;58(24): 5640–5.

[18] Avet-Loiseau H, Facon T, Daviet A, et al. 14q32 translocations and monosomy 13 observed in monoclonal gammopathy of undetermined significance delineate a multistep process for the oncogenesis of multiple myeloma. Intergroupe Francophone du Myelome. Cancer Res 1999;59(18):4546–50.

[19] Chng WJ, Van Wier SA, Ahmann GJ, et al. A validated FISH trisomy index demonstrates the hyperdiploid and nonhyperdiploid dichotomy in MGUS. Blood 2005;106(6):2156–61.

[20] Avet-Loiseau H, Li JY, Morineau N, et al. Monosomy 13 is associated with the transition of monoclonal gammopathy of undetermined significance to multiple myeloma. Intergroupe Francophone du Myelome. Blood 1999;94(8):2583–9.

[21] Rasmussen T, Kuehl M, Lodahl M, et al. Possible roles for activating RAS mutations in the MGUS to MM transition and in the intramedullary to extramedullary transition in some plasma cell tumors. Blood 2005;105(1):317–23.

[22] Melton LJ 3rd, Rajkumar SV, Khosla S, et al. Fracture risk in monoclonal gammopathy of undetermined significance. J Bone Miner Res 2004;19(1):25–30.

[23] Roodman III GD. Biology of myeloma bone disease. In: Broudy VC, Abkowitz JL, Vose JM, editors. Hematology 2002: American Society of Hematology Education Program Book. Washington, DC:Blood; 2002. p. 227–32.

[24] Croucher PI, Shipman CM, Lippitt J, et al. Osteoprotegerin inhibits the development of osteolytic bone disease in multiple myeloma. Blood 2001;98(13):3534–40.

[25] Vacca A, Ribatti D, Roncali L, et al. Bone marrow angiogenesis and progression in multiple myeloma. Br J Haematol 1994;87(3):503–8.

[26] Rajkumar SV, Mesa RA, Fonseca R, et al. Bone marrow angiogenesis in 400 patients with monoclonal gammopathy of undetermined significance, multiple myeloma, and primary amyloidosis. Clin Cancer Res 2002;8(7):2210–6.

[27] Kumar S, Witzig TE, Timm M, et al. Bone marrow angiogenic ability and expression of angiogenic cytokines in myeloma: evidence favoring loss of marrow angiogenesis inhibitory activity with disease progression. Blood 2004;104(4):1159–65.

[28] Malik AA, Ganti AK, Potti A, et al. Role of *Helicobacter pylori* infection in the incidence and clinical course of monoclonal gammopathy of undetermined significance. Am J Gastroenterol 2002;97(6):1371–4.

[29] Rajkumar SV, Kyle RA, Plevak MF, et al. Helicobacter pylori infection and monoclonal gammopathy of undetermined significance. Br J Haematol 2002;119(3):706–8.

[30] Kyle RA. "Benign" monoclonal gammopathy—after 20 to 35 years of follow-up. Mayo Clin Proc 1993;68(1):26–36.

[31] Cesana C, Klersy C, Barbarano L, et al. Prognostic factors for malignant transformation in monoclonal gammopathy of undetermined significance and smoldering multiple myeloma. J Clin Oncol 2002;20(6):1625–34.

[32] Baldini L, Guffanti A, Cesana BM, et al. Role of different hematologic variables in defining the risk of malignant transformation in monoclonal gammopathy. Blood 1996;87(3): 912–8.

[33] Rajkumar SV, Kyle RA, Therneau TM, et al. Serum free light chain ratio is an independent risk factor for progression in monoclonal gammopathy of undetermined significance. Blood 2005;106(3):812–7.

[34] Kumar S, Rajkumar SV, Kyle RA, et al. Prognostic value of circulating plasma cells in monoclonal gammopathy of undetermined significance. J Clin Oncol 2005;23(24):5668–74.

[35] Rajkumar SV, Dispenzieri A, Kyle RA. Monoclonal gammopathy of undetermined significance, Waldenström macroglobulinemia, AL amyloidosis, and related plasma cell disorders: diagnosis and treatment. Mayo Clin Proc 2006;81(5):693–703.

[36] Kyle RA, Garton JP. The spectrum of IgM monoclonal gammopathy in 430 cases. Mayo Clin Proc 1987;62(8):719–31.

[37] Gobbi PG, Baldini L, Broglia C, et al. Prognostic validation of the international classification of immunoglobulin M gammopathies: a survival advantage for patients with immunoglobulin M monoclonal gammopathy of undetermined significance? Clin Cancer Res 2005;11(5): 1786–90.

[38] Kyle RA, Therneau TM, Rajkumar SV, et al. Long-term follow-up of IgM monoclonal gammopathy of undetermined significance. Blood 2003;102(10):3759–64.

[39] Morra E, Cesana C, Klersy C, et al. Prognostic factors for transformation in asymptomatic immunoglobulin M monoclonal gammopathies. Clin Lymphoma 2005;5(4):265–9.

[40] Cesana C, Barbarano L, Miqueleiz S, et al. Clinical characteristics and outcome of immunoglobulin M-related disorders. Clin Lymphoma 2005;5(4):261–4.

[41] Baldini L, Goldaniga M, Guffanti A, et al. Immunoglobulin M monoclonal gammopathies of undetermined significance and indolent Waldenström's macroglobulinemia recognize the same determinants of evolution into symptomatic lymphoid disorders: proposal for a common prognostic scoring system. J Clin Oncol 2005;23(21):4662–8.

[42] Kyle RA, Robinson RA, Katzmann JA. The clinical aspects of biclonal gammopathies. Review of 57 cases. Am J Med 1981;71(6):999–1008.

[43] Grosbois B, Jego P, de Rosa H, et al. [Triclonal gammopathy and malignant immunoproliferative syndrome] [review]. Revue de Medecine Interne 1997;18(6):470–3 [in French].

[44] Tirelli A, Guastafierro S, Cava B, et al. Triclonal gammopathy in an extranodal non-Hodgkin lymphoma patient. Am J Hematol 2003;73(4):273–5.

[45] Kyle RA, Greipp PR. "Idiopathic" Bence Jones proteinuria: long-term follow-up in seven patients. N Engl J Med 1982;306(10):564–7.

[46] Alexanian R. Monoclonal gammopathy in lymphoma. Arch Intern Med 1975;135(1): 62–6.

[47] Lin P, Hao S, Handy BC, et al. Lymphoid neoplasms associated with IgM paraprotein: a study of 382 patients. Am J Clin Pathol 2005;123(2):200–5.

[48] Asatiani E, Cohen P, Ozdemirli M, et al. Monoclonal gammopathy in extranodal marginal zone lymphoma (ENMZL) correlates with advanced disease and bone marrow involvement. Am J Hematol 2004;77(2):144–6.

[49] Noel P, Kyle RA. Monoclonal proteins in chronic lymphocytic leukemia. Am J Clin Pathol 1987;87(3):385–8.

[50] Lamboley V, Zabranieki L, Sie P, et al. Myeloma and monoclonal gammopathy of uncertain significance associated with acquired von Willebrand's syndrome. Seven new cases with a literature review. Joint Bone Spine 2002;69(1):62–7.

[51] Sallah S, Husain A, Wan J, et al. The risk of venous thromboembolic disease in patients with monoclonal gammopathy of undetermined significance. Ann Oncol 2004;15(10): 1490–4.

[52] Kelly JJ Jr, Kyle RA, O'Brien PC, et al. Prevalence of monoclonal protein in peripheral neuropathy. Neurology 1981;31(11):1480–3.

[53] Quarles RH, Weiss MD. Autoantibodies associated with peripheral neuropathy [review]. Muscle Nerve 1999;22(7):800–22.

[54] Gosselin S, Kyle RA, Dyck PJ. Neuropathy associated with monoclonal gammopathies of undetermined significance. Ann Neurol 1991;30(1):54–61.

[55] Nobile-Orazio E. Treatment of dys-immune neuropathies. J Neurol 2005;252(4):385–95.

[56] Dispenzieri A, Kyle RA, Lacy MQ, et al. POEMS syndrome: definitions and long-term outcome. Blood 2003;101(7):2496–506.

[57] Daoud MS, Lust JA, Kyle RA, et al. Monoclonal gammopathies and associated skin disorders [review]. J Am Acad Dermatol 1999;40(4):507–35.

[58] Mundis RJ, Kyle RA. Primary hyperparathyroidism and monoclonal gammopathy of undetermined significance. Am J Clin Pathol 1982;77(5):619–21.

[59] Arnulf B, Bengoufa D, Sarfati E, et al. Prevalence of monoclonal gammopathy in patients with primary hyperparathyroidism: a prospective study. Arch Intern Med 2002;162(4): 464–7.

[60] Badley AD, Portela DF, Patel R, et al. Development of monoclonal gammopathy precedes the development of Epstein-Barr virus-induced posttransplant lymphoproliferative disorder. Liver Transpl Surg 1996;2(5):375–82.

[61] Zent CS, Wilson CS, Tricot G, et al. Oligoclonal protein bands and Ig isotype switching in multiple myeloma treated with high-dose therapy and hematopoietic cell transplantation. Blood 1998;91(9):3518–23.

[62] Rostaing L, Modesto A, Abbal M, et al. Long-term follow-up of monoclonal gammopathy of undetermined significance in transplant patients. Am J Nephrol 1994;14(3):187–91.

[63] Pascual M, Widmann JJ, Schifferli JA. Recurrent febrile panniculitis and hepatitis in two patients with acquired complement deficiency and paraproteinemia. Am J Med 1987;83(5):959–62.

[64] Droder RM, Kyle RA, Greipp PR. Control of systemic capillary leak syndrome with aminophylline and terbutaline. Am J Med 1992;92(5):523–6.

[65] Dingli D, Larson DR, Plevak MF, et al. Focal and segmental glomerulosclerosis and plasma cell proliferative disorders. Am J Kidney Dis 2005;46(2):278–82.

[66] Karlson EW, Tanasijevic M, Hankinson SE, et al. Monoclonal gammopathy of undetermined significance and exposure to breast implants. Arch Intern Med 2001;161(6):864–7.

[67] Merlini G, Farhangi M, Osserman EF. Monoclonal immunoglobulins with antibody activity in myeloma, macroglobulinemia and related plasma cell dyscrasias [review]. Semin Oncol 1986;13(3):350–65.

[68] Dimopoulos MA, Moulopoulos LA, Maniatis A, et al. Solitary plasmacytoma of bone and asymptomatic multiple myeloma. Blood 2000;96(6):2037–44.

[69] Kyle RA, Linos A, Beard CM, et al. Incidence and natural history of primary systemic amyloidosis in Olmsted County, Minnesota, 1950 through 1989. Blood 1992;79(7):1817–22.

Hematol Oncol Clin N Am 21 (2007) 1115–1140

Prognostic Factors and Staging in Multiple Myeloma

Rafael Fonseca, MD[a,b,*], Jesus San Miguel, MD, PhD[a,b]

[a]Mayo Clinic Arizona, 13208 East Shea Boulevard, Collaborative Research Building, 3-006,
Scottsdale, AZ 85259-5494, USA
[b]Hematology Department, University Hospital of Salamanca, Center for Cancer Research,
Salamanca, Spain

Multiple myeloma (MM) is a clonal B-cell disorder in which malignant plasma cells (PCs) expand and accumulate in the bone marrow (BM) leading to cytopenias, bone resorption, and the production (in most cases) of the characteristic monoclonal protein [1]. MM is a heterogeneous disease; some patients die within a few weeks of diagnosis, whereas others live for longer than 10 years. The reason for this heterogeneity is compound and involves interaction between host factors and features intrinsic to disease biology. Throughout this article we review current knowledge regarding the effect those factors have in determining the likelihood of a better or worse outcome for patients who have newly diagnosed disease. It should be immediately noted that the validity of most prognostic factors has been tested predominantly in the new diagnosis setting and little validation exists for the same factors in the case of relapsed and refractory disease. It is quite possible that some of the biologic factors that can predict outcome at diagnosis have much lessened effect when tested in patients receiving third-line chemotherapy. For instance, although it is generally accepted that patients entered into clinical trials for relapsed/refractory disease carry the worst outcome, this is generally not true if one estimates survival since time of diagnosis. Patients who have the most dire host factors or the most aggressive biologic variants of MM do not live long enough to be enrolled in these clinical trials. A patient entering a clinical trial for third-line therapy is likely to have had an overall more favorable outcome, even if at the time of study entry the prospective survival is limited.

There are many reasons an accurate prognostic determination is paramount for high-quality clinical practice and research. It allows the physician to engage in a more direct discussion with the patient regarding disease threat and likelihood of survival (eg, at 5 or 10 years). This risk stratification also allows for

*Corresponding author. Mayo Clinic Arizona, 13208 East Shea Boulevard, Collaborative Research Building, 3-006, Scottsdale, AZ 85259-5494. E-mail address: fonseca.rafael@mayo.edu (R. Fonseca).

0889-8588/07/$ – see front matter
doi:10.1016/j.hoc.2007.08.010

a more rational selection of therapy approaches. The genetic framework now allows us to predict patients likely to have short remission after treatment with high-dose chemotherapy followed by stem cell support (HDT) [2–5]. Although this information does not yet preclude the application of HDT as upfront treatment, it suggests that reserving it as back-up strategy is reasonable [6] and allows for other therapies to be explored. This prognostic classification is essential to better understand the composition of patients entered into clinical trials, and also allows, albeit with the usual statistical limitations, cross-comparison of different clinical trial populations. Indirectly this prognostic classification can also provide relevance to new biologic factors proposed as significant in disease pathogenesis, but biologic factors considered crucial in the pathogenesis do not need to necessarily have prognostic associations.

In this article, we discuss two predominant categories of prognostic factors: those related to the host and those intrinsic to disease biology. Although undoubtedly a large fraction of disease heterogeneity can be determined by the genetic subtypes of MM [2,7], an important component in determining outcome is related to host features. For instance, it is clear that during the first 6 to 12 months after the diagnosis host factors predominate in distinguishing outcome (Fig. 1), whereas the relevance of genetic factors becomes more evident later on [2,7]. Also, as the patients become more distanced from the original diagnosis, secondary genetic (progression) events are likely to emerge along with discriminators of outcome. Host factors also influence the likelihood of survival at all times. For example, it has been recently shown that young patients who have MM have a better outcome than older individuals (see later discussion). This finding would seem paradoxical, because in general younger patients are enriched for the higher-risk genetic features, such as t(4;14)(p16;q32), whereas older individuals tend to be more associated with the indolent (eg, hyperdiploid) variant [8]. Most likely this is because of a better overall health and ability to withstand therapy by younger patients.

PROGNOSTIC AND STAGING SYSTEMS
Since the introduction of HDT and new drugs, such as thalidomide, bortezomib, and lenalidomide among others, clinicians have a wide array of therapeutic tools for patients who have MM. It would be desirable, as in other disorders, such as acute lymphoblastic leukemia and non-Hodgkin lymphoma, to have an international classification system for patients who have MM based on risk group categories, defined according to new independent prognostic factors. This system would assist us to individualize treatment according to patients' characteristics and to help in clinical decision-making. In addition, prognostic factors could represent a valuable tool for the evaluation of results of new treatment strategies. In this context, experimental therapies should be assayed on homogeneous cohorts of patients identified according to prognostic factors. Moreover, on evaluating randomized trials for the balance of the two arms, it would be important to take into account not only the individual prognostic

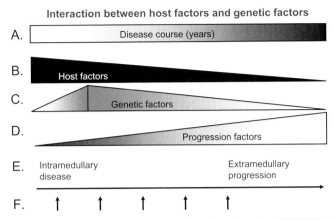

Fig. 1. Interaction between host factors and genetic factors. Effect on prognosis of the various determining factors according to time of disease evolution (A). Shortly after diagnosis the major influence on outcome relates to host features (B). Patients who are advanced in age or have poor renal function are less likely to receive adequate therapy. In addition debilitated patients or those who have more comorbid conditions are likely to be at greater risk for complications, such as pneumonia, other infections, or venous thrombosis. After that initial period of time the disease biology and the primary genetic events play a predominant role in determining prognosis (C). The negative effect on prognosis for the high-risk translocations becomes apparent and results in disease resistance, rapid relapse, and early death for many patients harboring these abnormalities. At this point some of the progression genetic events already are evident (D). For instance, whereas only a minority of cases display p53 loss/mutation at diagnosis (<10%), these small subset of patients have a dire prognosis. With further passing of time the effect of primary genetic events becomes less clear (C). Some patients in the more benign genetic categories will acquire additional genetic mutations resulting in aggressive disease (eg, hyperdiploid with cancer testis antigens signature, aggressive t(11;14) cases). Other patients who have high-risk genetic features have had such biology that allowed them to live through the initial phases of treatment and thus have lowered the risk imposed by their baseline genetic category (eg, t(4;14) with low β_2-microglobulin). With time the effect of secondary genetic events becomes more evident on prognosis (eg, chromosome 1 amplification). For example, patients who have p53 abnormalities progress to rapidly progressive extramedullary disease (E). Other genetic progression events are likely to have the same influence. Throughout the course of the patient's disease host factors remain important, and rise to the forefront because of therapy complications. Although all patients are grouped clinically as "new diagnosis MM" this stage can represent a broad spectrum of genetic evolution; in some cases the disease is barely progressing from monoclonal gammopathy of undetermined significance or smoldering multiple myeloma, and in others a full-blown clonally aggressive disease is evident (eg, plasma cell leukemia cases). The bottom arrows (F) show that those categorized as new-diagnosis disease patients can present at various stages of clonal evolution.

factors but also the possible additive effect of two or three prognostic factors within a particular therapeutic arm.

According to these statements, a new International Staging System (ISS) has recently been proposed [9]. It derives from a multicenter study collecting a total of 11,171 patients compiled from American, Asian, and European cooperative groups and large individual institutions. The ISS is based on the levels of β_2-microglobulin and albumin (Table 1), and it allows discriminating three risk groups regardless of age, geographic region, or standard or HDT. Further efforts are underway to improve this staging system with the inclusion of other parameters, such as cytogenetics and molecular markers. Although this latter classification will not be widely applicable because these parameters are only available at selected centers, it may be of great value in evaluating new treatment strategies at large cooperative groups and referral institutions. This classification, although extensively validated, has the shortfall that is not primarily based on biology and thus may accurately predict outcome but not ultimately influence management strategies. For instance (and ironically), patients who have stage 3 disease (elevated β_2-microglobulin) because of renal failure are at higher risk for death shortly after diagnosis; however, they may require dose reduction rather than therapy intensification, and may have indolent disease from the MM perspective and only developed renal failure because of the nephrotoxic nature of the monoclonal protein.

CLASSIFICATION SCHEMES BASED ON MULTIPLE MYELOMA BIOLOGY
Classification Schemes for Multiple Myeloma
Because prognosis is inextricably linked to disease subtype, it is worth discussing in detail the multiple classification schemes and prognostic allocation groups in MM. It is now clear that MM is not one disease but rather many, with each one of the subtypes largely defined by the specific genetic an cytogenetic aberrations (see Fig. 1) [2,7]. The genetic classification systems are relevant not only to further our understanding of disease biology but also because of their practical applicability as prognostic tools. Classifications can be proposed at three levels.

Biologic classification
This classification scheme is mostly driven by biology-based considerations. Usually it has clinical prognostic implications, but does not necessarily have to. Classic examples of this include the hyperdiploid versus non-hyperdiploid classification, specific chromosome translocations, and so forth [10–12]. Markers predictive of response to specific therapies are likely to be primarily derived from direct application of biology factors.

Table 1
International staging system for multiple myeloma

Stage	Parameters	Median survival
1	β_2M<3.5 mg/L and albumin>3.5 g/dL	62 months
2	β_2M<3.5 mg/L and albumin<3.5 g/dL, or β_2M 3.5–5.5	44 months
3	β_2M>5.5 mg/L	29 months

Prognostic classification

This scheme incorporates major biologic classifiers and additional markers in an effort to discriminate the ultimate outcome of patients [2,4,13]. The markers capable of discerning prognosis usually serve, albeit with dissimilar penetrance, in prognosticating patients treated with multiple treatment modalities. For instance, the t(4;14)(p16;q32) has always been associated with more aggressive disease, and in the series in which it has been tested it always shortens survival of patients (Table 2) [2–5,13–17].

Biology Classification ("Enduring")

As in most other hematologic neoplasms, the genetic and genomic aberrations of tumor cells are believed to the primary prognostic factors for MM. We believe that a comprehensive cytogenetic evaluation should be performed in all

Table 2
Prognostic implications for t(4;14)(p16;q32)

Author	Prevalence	Treatment	OS	Assay	HR
Avet-Loiseau et al [13]	100/714 (14%)	HDT	41 versus 79	iFISH	2.79
Gutierrez et al [37]	29/260 (11%)	HDT	24 versus 48	clg-FISH	2.6
Gertz et al [5]	26/153 (17%)	HDT	19 versus 44	clg-FISH	2.1
Fonseca et al [4]	42/332 (13%)	Conventional	26 versus 45	clg-FISH	1.78
Moreau et al [3]	22/168 (13%)	HDT	23 versus 66	iFISH	NA
Keats et al [14]	31/208 (14.9%)	Conventional and HDT	21 versus 42	RT-PCR IgH/ MMSET	2.0
Chang et al [61]	15/120 (12.5%)	HDT	18 versus 48	clg-FISH	NA
Dewald et al [32]	10/154 (6.5%)	Conventional and HDT	13 versus 45	IgH FGFR3	NA
Jaksic et al [15]	19/124 (15%)	HDT	24 months	clg-FISH	NA
Chieccio et al [38]	28/535 (5%)	Conventional and HDT	9 versus 41	CC	NA
	85/729 (12%)		19 versus NR	iFISH	NA
	59/490 (12%)		19 versus 44	Combined	NA
Chang et al [16]	6/41 (15%)	Velcade	9 versus 15	clg-FISH	NA
Chang et al [17]	16/85 (19%)	HDT	19 versus 46	clg-FISH IHC FGFR3	NA

Abbreviations: CC, conventional chemotherapy; FGFR3, fibroblast growth factor receptor 3; HR, hazard ratio; IHC, immunohistochemistry; MMSET, multiple myeloma SET domain gene; NA, not available; OS, overall survival; RT-PCR, reverse transcriptase PCR.

cases at the time of diagnosis, and should include at a minimum interphase fluorescent in situ hybridization (FISH) in purified PCs or in combination with immunofluorescent detection of light-chain restricted PCs (cIg-FISH) [18]. We have recently published a consensus guideline whereby using cIg-FISH alone allows for the prognostic classification of patients (Fig. 2) [19].

Primary genetic events

A biologic classification of MM is unlikely to change dramatically given the current knowledge of disease pathogenesis [20]. For more details regarding the genetics of MM please refer to other articles in this issue. For example, we know that 15% of all MM are t(11;14)(q13;q32) and that the baseline features associated with this subtype are always the same [21]. So even if curative therapy for MM were designed, this prevalence would remain the same. A key requirement for biology classifying factors is that they result from intrinsic genetic defects and correlate with some clinicopathologic features at presentation. Again, as an example, MM with t(11;14) is associated with CD20 expression, lymphoplasmacytic morphology, hyposecretory disease, and lambda light chain usage [22,23]. Although these features are not unique to t(11;14)(q13;q32) MM, the entity seems unique; nonetheless, it is neutral with regard to prognosis [13,21].

Overall MM is divided into two major categories: hyperdiploid MM (with a low prevalence of IgH translocations) and non-hyperdiploid MM (encompassing hypodiploid, pseudodiploid, and near-tetraploid MM, and highly enriched for IgH translocations) [10,11,24]. Several groups have demonstrated that t(4;14)(p16;q32) and t(14;16)(q32;q23) are associated with poor survival, irrespective of the treatment modality [4,13]. In contrast, the t(11;14)(q13;q32) seems to be associated overall with a slightly more favorable outcome, although the net effect is small and usually statistically insignificant [4,13]. This finding

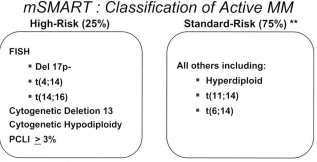

mSMART : Classification of Active MM

High-Risk (25%)

FISH
- Del 17p-
- t(4;14)
- t(14;16)

Cytogenetic Deletion 13
Cytogenetic Hypodiploidy
PCLI $\geq$ 3%

Standard-Risk (75%) **

All others including:
- Hyperdiploid
- t(11;14)
- t(6;14)

**Low risk with β-2 microglobulin > 5.5 (in absence of renal failure)or LDH >upper limit of normal may be at higher risk.

Mayo Clin Proc 2007;82:323-341

Fig. 2. mSmart classification. (*Data from* Dispenzieri A, Rajkumar SV, Gertz MA, et al. Treatment of newly diagnosed multiple myeloma based on Mayo stratification of myeloma and risk-adapted therapy (mSMART): consensus statement. Mayo Clin Proc 2007;82:323–41.)

has lead most to consider t(11;14)(q13;q32) cases as prognostically neutral. Hyperdiploidy in general is associated with a better outcome, with some series showing neutrality in this effect [25–27].

We have recently re-examined the role of chromosome 13 as a biologic factor versus a surrogate marker of aggressive disease. The field of MM genetics was invigorated by the observation first that cases with abnormal metaphase cytogenetics were associated with a shortened survival, and later by the observation that chromosome 13 deletions were also associated with a shorter survival [4,28–32]. In the case of chromosome 13 abnormalities, they are detected in 50% of patients [33–36]. Of all cases with chromosome 13 abnormalities, 85% constitute monosomy and the remaining 15% are interstitial deletions [33–36]. There is no known difference in effect for prognosis for deletions versus monosomy. The prognostic significance for chromosome 13 likely emanates from its close association with high-risk genetic features (eg, t(4;14)(p16;q32)) [4,13,37,38]. Chromosome 13 deletion is not significant in discriminating prognosis for non-hyperdiploid patients [38] and is not capable of distinguishing prognosis for hyperdiploid patients [27]. Its prognostic significance is thus now believed to be a surrogate of its association with non-hyperdiploid MM. Does that mean that chromosome 13 has no biologic importance [38]? More and more data suggest a crucial role for chromosome 13 as prerequisite for clonal expansion for tumors: nearly 90% of cases with t(4;14)(p16;q32) harbor chromosome 13 deletion [33–36]. We have recently found that chromosome 13 loss is associated with diminished regulatory function of *Rb*, and we believe this is a key factor promoting clonal expansion and malignant phenotype (Rafael Fonseca, MD, unpublished data, 2007).

Secondary genetic events

Tumor clone development is believed to be a consequence of a multistep process that accumulates sequential genetic changes [20]. The specific steps associated with disease progression and their association with the different cytogenetic subtypes has not been well defined. Some of the genetic abnormalities that seem to reflect progression include deletions at 17p13, chromosome 1 abnormalities (1p deletion and 1q amplification), and C-*myc* translocations. It is also likely that some of the best prognostic markers come from the complete understanding of secondary (progression) events.

Deletions of 17p13. The most important molecular cytogenetic factor for prognostication is deletion of 17p13 (the locus for the tumor suppressor gene *p53*) [4,13,39]. In all series tested, 17p13 deletions confer a negative effect on survival. We and others have shown that patients who have 17p13 deletions have an overall shorter survival, more aggressive disease, higher prevalence of extramedullary disease (such as plasmacytomas), and hypercalcemia [4,13,39]. Deletions of 17p13 predict for a short duration of response after HDT and involvement of the central nervous system [40,41]. We have recently shown that extramedullary disease is likely a consequence of defective *p53*, because most cases of plasma cell leukemia (primary and secondary) have abnormalities in the *p53* pathway (Rafael Fonseca, MD, unpublished data, 2007). In support of this we know that most, if not all, human MM cell lines have *p53* deficiency (M Kuehl, personal communication, 2007). Our hypothesis is that plasma cells are indeed capable of surviving at extramedullary locations, but that they usually undergo apoptosis in the presence of an intact p53 response.

Ras mutation and p16 *methylation.* Other studies have shown an adverse outcome for patients who have K-*ras* mutations but not those who have N-*ras* mutations [37,42–44] (Rafael Fonseca, MD, unpublished data, 2007). This observation is interesting because *ras* mutations cluster more among patients who have t(11;14)(q13;q32) and are likely important factors for disease progression for this subtype [44] (Rafael Fonseca, MD, unpublished data, 2007). The issue is less clear for *p16* methylation. Although some original studies had suggested negative associations with prognosis [45–50], recent data on large datasets suggest that *p16* methylation is prognostically neutral [51]. It has been recently found that a low transcription of the *p16* gene measured by reverse transcriptase-PCR is associated with short survival, however, which suggests a possible impact of this gene in the MM pathogenesis [52].

The fundamental observation that MM is characterized by up-regulation of any one of the three cyclin D genes [53] resulted in the observation that some patients lacking the aforementioned primary translocations are characterized, at the gene expression level, by augmented expression of CCND2 (with or without concurrent CCND1 expression). It is possible one unifying genetic mechanism explains CCND2 elevation, but also that multiple abnormalities ultimately lead to increased CCND2 expression. Another subgroup identified by this classification is the "none" group. This group is characterized by minimal expression of *RB1* (50%) complimenting a model consistent with hyperactivity of cyclin D or down-regulation of checkpoints (*RB1*) mediating G1/S transition (Rafael Fonseca, MD, unpublished data, 2007).

Chromosome 1 abnormalities. Chromosome 1 abnormalities have been long known to be highly prevalent in MM. Most of these abnormalities involve rearrangements located in the pericentromeric regions and frequently in the form of jumping translocations. Chromosome 1 abnormalities have been recently proposed as major prognostic factors for MM [54]. Regarding chromosome 1, it should be noted that 1q gain and 1p loss are so closely related that it is hard to provide differentiation [10,12,55]. We had previously reported that abnormalities of the short and long arm of chromosome 1 were associated with shorter survival [10]. In one study by Shaughnessy and colleagues [54] a gene expression signature for high-risk disease was found and validated. This signature is enriched disproportionately for genes located in chromosome 1. This finding also builds on previous studies showing that chromosome 1 abnormalities are associated with an adverse outcome. Although an initial search suggested that CKS1B might be the responsible gene for this association, other studies have failed to validate this notion [56]. Two recent series have failed to confirm the overriding negative prognostic association with chromosome 1 amplification detected by FISH [13,56]. It is thus still unclear how chromosome 1 participates biologically in generating more aggressive clones.

Non-canonical nuclear factor-κB activation. Our group has recently shown, using multiple primary genetic mechanisms, that there is constitutive activation of the non-canonical nuclear factor-κB (NF-κB) pathway in at least 50% of MM cases [57]. This activation is a consequence of inactivation of suppressors by either biallelic deletion of deletion/mutation combinations or hyperactivity as a consequence of amplification or chromosome translocations. The summary of these effects (epistatic mutations) is readily detectable by gene expression profiling. All of these aberrations ultimately result in increased processing of p100 to p52 and consequent NF-κB nuclear hyperactivity. These genetic events have not been fully positioned in the process of disease progression, but likely are secondary genetic events as they transcend the primary genetic categories.

Predictive factors

Predictive factors are biomarkers capable of detecting meaningful likelihood of clinical benefit with specific interventions. Although they can be quite similar (and sometimes the same as plain prognostic markers), predictive markers have the added ability of being therapy-specific and usually linked closely to biology. Traditionally, most predictive factors have focused on likelihood of response and, to a lesser extent, on outcome prediction (overall and event-free survival). With the increasing armamentarium against MM, the need for these markers will become pressing as sequence of treatments could be of critical importance. Little is known now with regard to specific prognostic markers, and more clinical correlative studies are needed. One study by Mulligan and colleagues [58] evaluated the ability of gene expression profiling in predicting clinical outcome for patients treated with bortezomib. Although the authors were able to identify subsets of patients who had dissimilar outcomes, additional validation is needed [58].

In another study, Mateos and colleagues [59] have looked at the outcome of patients treated with bortezomib in combination with melphalan and prednisone. They have data showing abrogation of the negative prognostic effects of IgH translocations and Rb deletion when bortezomib is included as primary therapy. The reason we consider this predictive is that there unequivocal evidence of the negative influence on prognosis of t(4;14)(p16;q32) for patients treated with melphalan-based chemotherapy. Longer follow-up is needed to fully understand the abrogation of this effect, however. The prevailing interpretation of these data is that for patients who have high-risk disease one should consider early introduction of bortezomib (as opposed to the usual route of induction followed by HDT). The main clinical problem for patients who have t(4;14)(p16;q32) is not primary refractory disease but rather rapid and refractory relapse [60]. The clinical benefit of early bortezomib introduction thus ultimately depends on the sustainability of the responses. Based on these considerations and despite data shortcomings, our group has incorporated bortezomib early on in the treatment course of patients who have high-risk disease because of the shorter benefit of HDT (recommendations available at mSMART.org).

One example of prediction is our aforementioned recent observation of non-canonical NF-κB activation in a subset of patients. We have found that the likelihood of responsiveness to bortezomib, and sustainability of responses, seem higher among patients who have intrinsic activation of this pathway [57]. In our study, those who had a low level of TRAF3 gene expression had a much higher likelihood of response to bortezomib (90%) as opposed to all others (30%).

Prognostic Classifications

Although it is now clear that much of the major prognostic variation of MM is dictated by primary genetic categories, secondary changes can also have a profound influence in outcome by providing clonal survival/proliferation advantages. Some of the basic genetic categories have not resulted (yet) in specific clinical outcome difference, yet define unique subtypes (eg, t(11;14)(q13;q32)) [4,13]. The clinical consequences of secondary genetic changes tend not to be related to therapy administered. One possible way to define prognostic markers is that they associate with baseline features of aggressiveness (pathobiology) and should exert their influence if patients are not treated (natural history) (Table 3). It is possible that these markers also identify patients more likely to progress from the premalignant stages of the disease. In general, the effect on overall outcome for validated prognostic markers is evident irrespective of treatment modality, even when the hazard ratios for their influence may vary. For example, we cite the negative implications for outcome for the t(4;14)(p16;q32) as it identifies patients who have shorter clinical benefit from standard and HDT(see Table 2). Although it seems that some of the prognostic ability can be challenged with novel agents, it is still too early to negate prognostication ability for

Table 3
Prognostic and predictive factors

Classification	Definitive categories	Need additional data or series
Biologic	t(11;14)(q13;q32)	CCND2
	t(4;14)(p16;q32)	Chromosome 1
	t(14;16)(q32;q23)	Non-canonical NF-κB ↑
	Hyperdiploidy	C-myc
	Deletions of 13	
	17p13 deletions	
Prognostic	t(4;14)(p16;q32)	Hyperdiploidy
	t(14;16)(q32;q23)	UAMS gene signature
	−17p13	Proliferation signature
	Deletions 13 by metaphase	CTA
	Hypodiploidy by metaphase	Centrosome signature

t(4;14)(p16;q32) for patients receiving such agents as bortezomib [59]. The same negative effect for prognosis is evident for the t(14;16)(q32;q23); two series using conventional therapy (Eastern Cooperative Oncology Group [ECOG]) and HDT (University of Arkansas for the Medical Sciences [UAMS]) have shown the deleterious effect on survival [2,4]. Minimal data are available regarding the other MAF variants.

Other prognostic markers exert effects across the major biologic subtypes of MM. Some are well established, including the aforementioned effect of 17p13 in prognosis [4,13,39]. Using high-throughput genomic tools is likely to unravel novel means of predicting patient outcome. A major effort at the University of Arkansas has identified a set of 70 genes (signature) capable of predicting high-risk MM [54]. The team further shows that a simplified list of 17 genes is capable of providing the same prognostic discrimination [54]. This last model discriminates high-risk disease with unprecedented ability. This high-risk profile was indeed enriched for genes located in chromosome 1. It is possible that RT-PCR or immunohistochemistry-based strategies can be used to derive clinically applicable prognostication models for the disease. Other markers could include proliferation index by gene expression profiling (GEP), centrosome index by GEP, and cancer testis antigens (CTA) [27,53,61].

OTHER PROGNOSTIC FACTORS INTRINSIC TO THE CELL

DNA Ploidy Studies and Proliferative Activity of Plasma Cells

As mentioned above, hyperdiploidy is usually associated with a more favorable outcome [2,53], whereas hypodiploidy is associated with a poor response to treatment and short survival [10,62,63], consistent with the high incidence of hypodiploid cases reported in plasma cell leukemia [62,64]. In our experience, DNA hyperdiploidy can be readily detectable by flow cytometry analysis, and these patients who have MM show a significantly better outcome as compared with the non-hyperdiploid cases [65,66]. In contrast, the chromosome count of MM with hypodiploidy is not very different from diploid cases, and therefore detection of hypodiploidy using flow cytometry is difficult [67]. Using standard karyotype analysis and comparative genomic hybridization, we have shown that several monosomies, not only that of chromosome 13, have important negative prognostic implications, consistent with the clinical observation of the poor outcome of hypodiploid MM [10,68]. Because hypodiploidy is also associated tightly with chromosome 13 monosomy, this further elucidates the challenge of dissecting the specific contribution of each genetic factor [27].

Tumor growth rate is a composite of proliferation and attrition, because of cell death resulting in an increase in tumor burden and subsequent disease complications. This notion leads to the early introduction of proliferations assays as prognostic tools for MM. The growth rate has been classically measured using the PC labeling index (PCLI), a slide-based assay capable of estimating cells undergoing DNA replication (ie, cells in S-phase of the cell cycle) [69]. Joshua and colleagues [70] have shown that the proliferative activity is almost entirely attributable to an increase of the proliferation of immature PCs.

Initial proliferation studies were based on in vitro radioactive labeling, and they were therefore difficult to apply in routine laboratories. Because of these limitations, nonradioactive approaches, such as the use of bromodeoxyuridine, another thymidine analog, have been developed showing a similar prognostic impact [69]. The use of propidium iodide (PI) staining for PCs and its subsequent analysis at flow cytometry permits the discrimination of PC distribution along the different cell cycle phases using appropriate mathematical models. This discrimination requires the simultaneous identification of the neoplastic PCs (CD38$^+$ and CD138$^+$) present in the sample so that their cell cycle distribution can be analyzed separately from that of the normal hematopoietic residual cells [71]. With this method, we have found a clear correlation between a high percentage of S-phase PCs (>3%) and poor outcome [66,72].

Recently, the availability of GEP has allowed the use of a new concept for PCLI, because the proliferative activity of PCs can be estimated using the normalized value of 11 genes associated with proliferation (*TOP2A, BIRC5, CCNB2, NEK2, ANAPC7, STK6, BUB1, CDC2, C10orf3, ASPM,* and *CDCA1*) [2,53]. This system has been validated by comparing PCs from healthy donors, patients who have MM, and MM cell lines, but it has not yet been tested for survival analysis.

Morphology

In contrast to other hematologic malignancies in which the morphologic features of the malignant cells are quite significant for classification and prognosis, little attention is yet paid to the morphology of tumor PCs. Nevertheless, an immature or plasmablastic morphology is associated with a poor outcome and has independent prognostic significance [73–75].

Immunophenotype

Discrepant results have been reported regarding the prognostic implications of the antigenic profile of PCs [76–82], which may be because of inappropriate study design, small series of patients not uniformly treated, and technical pitfalls (use of single versus multiparametric labeling, differences in the clones of monoclonal antibodies and fluorochromes, criteria for definition of positivity, and strategy of analysis). Some studies suggest that markers associated with an early PC phenotype (CD20$^+$, CD45$^+$, sIg) correlate with a poor outcome [76,77,83]. Down-regulation of CD56 and a greater expression of CD44 have been associated with an extramedullary spreading of malignant PCs [78,79]. The expression of CD28 has been related to disease activity, probably confined to highly proliferative accelerated phases of the disease [78–80,84]. An additional observation is that certain cancer testis antigens are frequently expressed in MM PCs as tumor-specific antigens, providing the basis for immunotherapeutic approaches [85–89]. Moreover, expression of some of these cancer testis antigens, such as SSX1, SSX4, SSX5, and especially SSX2, is associated with reduced survival [90].

In recent years, CD45 expression has been extensively studied by the French group, and lack of CD45 expression was associated with adverse prognosis

[83,91]. The proliferating MM compartment was restricted to the CD45[bright] minor subset in the BM [92]. This finding could be explained because this compartment depends directly on interleukin-6 (IL-6), and CD45 is as a phosphatase required for IL-6–mediated growth [93–95]. Our group has obtained similar results in relationship between a high percentage of CD45[+] cells and indolent forms of the disease or better prognosis in symptomatic MM [96].

In a large series of more than 600 uniformly treated (HDT) patients, we have not detected any prognostic influence for CD45 antigen expression (Mateo and colleagues, unpublished data). In fact, the only antigens that correlated with disease outcome were: CD19, CD28, and CD117, the expression of the first two associated with adverse prognosis and acquisition of CD117 associated with a favorable outcome. In addition, lack or down-regulation of CD56 showed a trend toward adverse prognosis. The most important prognostic information came from the combination of CD28 and CD 117 antigens, which allows the discrimination of three risk categories: favorable (CD28[-] CD 117[+]), intermediate (either both + or −), and adverse (CD28[+] CD117[-]) with median overall survival not reached, 68 and 42 months, respectively. Moreover, this antigenic profile remained an independent prognostic factor on multivariate analysis. Immunophenotyping can also assist in the differential diagnosis between monoclonal gammopathy of undetermined significance (MGUS) and MM [97–99], to monitor changes in the PC compartment after treatment (minimal residual disease) [100,101], and to predict the risk for transformation from MGUS or smoldering MM into symptomatic MM.

HOST FACTORS AND THEIR INTERACTIONS
Prognostic Factors Depending on the Host
Among host factors, the favorable influence of a good performance status and young age are well established. Very advanced age is a poor prognostic factor; thus, we have observed that patients older than 80 years of age have a much worse prognosis than patients between 65 and 80 years of age, independently of other prognostic factors [72]. An age younger than 60 to 70 years is associated with prolonged survival [8,102–106]. Moreover, it has been reported that patients younger than 40 years old who have normal renal function and low β_2-microglobulin have a median survival of more than 8 years [107]. These findings are highly reflective of why host factors are important, because overall a higher-risk MM is more common among younger individuals. Nevertheless, several groups support that age is not an independent prognostic factor [108] and in fact recommend HDT to patients older than 70 years who have MM [109]. A poor performance status (ECOG scale of 2 to 4) clearly confers a poor prognosis [102], but this parameter is rather subjective and is usually excluded from prognostic factor analysis.

As far as ethnicity and race are concerned, the initial information from a Southwest Oncology Group (SWOG) study showed that African Americans and whites have similar survival [110], but another more recent United States study suggests a better response and longer survival for African American patients [111]. The possibility to evaluate thousands of polymorphisms through single nucleotide polymorphism technology opens a new area for analyses of genomic polymorphisms and MM outcome. Accordingly, the influence of constitutional genomics will be reinvestigated, because the study of genetic polymorphisms has recognized several conditions that can be correlated not only with a predisposition to develop MM [112–117] but also with the tolerance to the therapy and the probability to develop complications [118,119].

The prognostic influence of immune surveillance is highly relevant in tumor development; patients who have MM might develop T-cell clones that can recognize autologous idiotypic Ig structures as tumor-specific antigens. In fact, the occurrence of expanded T-cell cytotoxic clones within the $CD8^+CD57^+CD28^-$ compartment is associated with an improved prognosis [120,121]. The number of peripheral blood $CD4^+$ cells is significantly reduced in patients who have MM, particularly in those who have advanced clinical stages. The reduction mainly affects memory and not naive $CD4^+$ cells. Moreover, patients who have low $CD4^+$ levels ($<700 \times 10^6$ cells/L) display a short survival, although this is not an independent prognostic factor [71]. Similar results have been reproduced by the ECOG [122,123].

Tumor Burden and Disease Complications

Tumor burden and disease activity

The proportion of PCs in BM and the pattern of BM infiltration and the presence of circulating PCs partially reflect the tumor burden. A high number of PCs in BM and a diffuse pattern of infiltration are generally associated with a poor prognosis [72]. They are not consistent prognostic factors, however, probably because of the heterogeneous distribution of PCs in BM. The detection of circulating PCs, identified either by morphology or immunophenotyping, is associated with advanced disease, and it has been reported that the presence of high levels of circulating PCs (>4% PCs) is an independent adverse prognostic factor [124].

The Durie and Salmon [125] classification was the first comprehensive attempt to measure the tumor burden. The system was obtained with mathematic models that established a relevant relationship between the tumor mass and the M component size. The amount of M component is not usually recognized as a prognostic factor. Regarding the isotype of the monoclonal immunoglobulin, the British group has reviewed 2592 patients and observed that light chain only (LCO) patients had the worst median survival (1.9 years) compared with 2.3 and 2.5 year in patients who had IgA and IgG paraproteins [126], respectively. IgA and IgG patients who had levels of LC excretion similar to those of LCO patients also had poor survival times because of renal failure, resulting in worse survival during induction therapy and at relapse. Patients included in this series were treated a long time ago, reflecting the short survival that these patients exhibit [126].

There is a wide array of biochemical markers associated with tumor burden and or disease activity. β_2-microglobulin levels increase as a result of tumor burden growth and renal function deterioration. β_2-microglobulin is a very sensitive indicator of renal function that is affected by renal function, MM, age, infections, or other kidney problems, which is why β_2-microglobulin abrogates the independent prognostic value of other renal indicators (creatinine, urea, and so forth) in multivariate analyses. Several threshold values for β_2-microglobulin (3 to 6 mg/dL) have been used to discriminate prognostic subgroups [66,69,127–130], but β_2-microglobulin can also be used as a continuous variable because the higher the β_2-microglobulin value, the shorter the survival. In contrast, β_2-microglobulin is not helpful for monitoring the course of the disease, because there are patients who relapse without a previous increase in β_2-microglobulin level (false negative), whereas others show increased values without any evidence of disease progression [127,131]. This finding makes mandatory the assessment of serum β_2-microglobulin levels at diagnosis in MM, along with the albumin, because they are the two parameters that define the three stages of the new ISS [9].

Interleukin-6 (IL6) is a major PC growth factor, and elevated serum levels have been described to be associated with short survival [132,133]. Similarly, high levels of its soluble receptor (sIL-6R) correlate with poor prognosis [134–136]. Nevertheless, discrepant results have also been reported, so these two markers are not extensively used in clinical practice to asses the prognosis in patients who have MM [137]. Moreover, IL-6 influences the hepatic synthesis of several acute-phase reactant proteins, such as C-reactive protein (CRP) and α1-antitrypsin (α_1-AT), that could be used in its place. Serum CRP levels actually represent a surrogate marker for IL-6 concentration [138], and the same could be applied for α1AT [139]. The use of CRP together with β_2-microglobulin constitutes a useful combination to predict survival in patients who have MM, allowing stratification of these patients into three groups according to CRP and β_2-microglobulin serum levels [138]. Finally, the Nordic MM Study Group reported that patients who had high serum soluble syndecan-1 or CD138 ($\geq$1170 units/mL) display a short survival (20 months versus 44 months) [140], data that have been recently confirmed by the group from Birmingham in an extensive series of 324 cases [141]. Other markers of disease activity, such as thymidine-kinase, neopterin, and lactate dehydrogenase, do not usually remain as independent prognostic factors in multivariate analyses [142].

Disease complications
Skeletal lesions have usually been evaluated by radiograph and their prognostic impact remains debatable. More recently, MRI has shown usefulness as a prognostic factor. The Greek group has evaluated 142 symptomatic patients who had MM with MRI [143]. Focal BM lesions were identified in 50% of patients, diffuse BM replacement in 28%, a variegated pattern in 14%, and normal pattern in 8%. These patterns were of prognostic value, because median survival was only 24 months for patients who had the diffuse pattern, whereas it was longer than 50 months for those with the remaining patterns ($P = .001$) [143]. In addition, this information added prognostic information to the ISS

stages. Other groups have found a close relationship between the MRI and duration of response, because those patients who have signs of BM infiltration quickly relapse [144]. Similar results have also been reported by using whole-body positron emission tomography (PET) with (18)F-FDG [145,146]. Bone resorption markers, such as urinary levels of pyridinoline and deoxypyridinoline, are augmented in patients who have advanced clinical stages and progressive disease, and they are correlated with CRP, creatinine, and albumin levels, but the relationship with survival is not very close [147–149]. In addition, cytokines influence bone lesions and can be related with the prognosis. As previously mentioned, high levels of IL-6 or metalloproteinase-9 are associated with advanced bone disease [150,151]. Elevated serum levels of stromal-derived factor-1alpha have been described to be associated with increased osteoclast activity and osteolytic bone disease in multiple patients who have MM [152]. In addition, soluble receptor activator of nuclear κB (sRANKL) is elevated in patients who have advanced bone disease, and the ratio between sRANKL and osteoprotegerin is a very good predictor for survival [153]. In the same line, proinflammatory enzymes, such as cyclooxygenase-2 [154], can be produced by MM cells to support local inflammation, and high expression is associated with poor outcome [154]. Disease complications, such as anemia, thrombocytopenia, and renal insufficiency, have a relevant influence on disease outcome [102]. Moderate anemia is present at diagnosis in 50% of patients who have MM, and 20% present with severe anemia (hemoglobin <8 g/dL). By contrast, thrombocytopenia is observed in only 10% to 15% of patients at diagnosis. Around 20% of patients who have MM have creatinine values greater than 2 mg/dL at diagnosis, and the proportion of patients who have renal impairment doubles during disease evolution.

RESPONSE TO INITIAL TREATMENT

In most hematologic malignancies, response to front-line therapy is one, if not the most, important prognostic factor. Traditionally this has not been the case in MM, although the concept is currently being challenged. Until the introduction of HDT, complete remission (CR) was rare and the only available comparison was between responding patients (achieving partial or minor responses) and nonresponding patients, the former category having a better outcome [155]. The meta-analysis for melphalan-based clinical trails showed prolongation in event-free survival but failed to show superiority in overall survival for those patients achieving a partial or minor response as compared with nonresponding patients. The introduction of HDT and novel agents, such as immunomodulatory drugs and bortezomib [156,157], have resulted in an increase in response rate, including CR [59]. Using the European Bone Marrow Transplant Registry/International Bone Marrow Transplant Registry criteria, several groups have shown that CR is a surrogate marker for survival [156–163]. Notable examples now also include the recent results of the Intergroup Francophone du Myelome 99-06 and Italian study in which the improvement in response of MPT versus MP resulted in survival prolongation [156].

Using a landmark analysis, ECOG has shown that even among cases treated with conventional chemotherapy, achieving a CR results in improvements in survival [163]. Another study by the Spanish PETHEMA/GEM group has made a similar observation for patients treated with HDT [162]. A third study at the M.D. Anderson Cancer Center also confirms these observations [160]. In contrast, the SWOG has reported that time to first progression is a more important outcome predictor that response to front-line therapy [164]. In addition, the Arkansas Group using HDT and thalidomide have shown that higher CR rates are associated with prolonged event-free but not overall survival [165]. An important difficulty in addressing the impact of response is related to our inability to measure amplitude in the quality of response in patients achieving CR; therefore, more sensitive techniques are needed.

A new sensitive test is now part of the standard disease-monitoring tools used in the clinic, the serum free light chain (FLC) assay [166]. It is expected that this test will complement and expand our ability to qualify CR states, although in our opinion it is unlikely to provide greater amplitude of measurement. It is now clear that discordant cases of CR exist when FLC is introduced; some patients can attain immunofixation (IF)–negative CR but still have detectable FLC, but just as many seem to normalize the FLC and still remain IF-positive. The International Working Group has introduced the term stringent complete remission, defined as CR-negative immunofixation in the serum and urine, disappearance of any soft tissue plasmacytomas, 5% or fewer PCs in BM, plus normal FLC ratio and absence of clonal cells in BM by immunohistochemistry or immunofluorescence as a new response category [167].

Two alternative techniques can be used to measure minimal residual disease. These include: (1) multiparametric flow cytometry evaluation of residual phenotypically aberrant plasma cells ($CD56^+CD19^-CD45^-$ or $CD28^+$ or $CD117^+$), and (2) the use of PCR, clone-specific assays, such as the ASO-PCR or RQ-allele specific oligonucleotide-PCR. These latter techniques are highly specific in that they are derived from the clone-specific sequence but have limited applicability in that successful application is only possible in a subset of patients. By contrast, immunophenotyping can be applied to the vast majority of patients. In addition, we should also measure residual disease outside the BM, and for this purpose imaging techniques, such as MRI or PET, could be most valuable. In any case, we believe that in MM, similarly to other hematologic malignancies, achievement of CR should be a priority, but clearly improved criteria for definition of CR (both in and outside of the BM milieu) are urgently required. Those patients who return to a "MGUS-like status" following intensive treatment can enjoy a prolonged survival despite having a residual M component, and therefore the definition of the underlying biologic and genetic characteristics of these patients needs to be elucidated in future investigations. The availability of highly efficient rescue treatments, based on novel agents, makes it more and more difficult to analyze the role of response to initial therapy in the final overall survival.

SUMMARY

The field of MM prognostication is replete with studies that have shown the value of independent predictors in determining clinical outcome. It is clear that host factors and factors intrinsic to the cells are the ultimate determinants of prognosis. In the immediate period after diagnosis, those factors related to the host are likely to be more relevant (eg, renal failure), whereas with passing time factors intrinsic to the cells predominate. At a minimum, we recommend that a comprehensive molecular cytogenetic assessment (FISH $\pm$ karyotype) should be performed at diagnosis, together with conventional evaluation, including β_2-microglobulin and albumin (ISS). In addition, information on proliferative activity of PCs may be of value. The introduction of novel methods of prognostication (eg, gene expression profiling) should be strongly considered in all clinical trials, but will need translation into practical diagnostic tools.

References

[1] Kyle RA, Rajkumar SV. Multiple myeloma. [see comment][erratum appears in N Engl J Med. 2005 Mar 17;352(11):1163]. N Engl J Med 2004;351:1860–73.

[2] Zhan F, Huang Y, Colla S, et al. The molecular classification of multiple myeloma. Blood 2006;108:2020–8.

[3] Moreau P, Facon T, Leleu X, et al. Recurrent 14q32 translocations determine the prognosis of multiple myeloma, especially in patients receiving intensive chemotherapy. Blood 2002;100:1579–83.

[4] Fonseca R, Blood E, Rue M, et al. Clinical and biologic implications of recurrent genomic aberrations in myeloma. Blood 2003;101:4569–75.

[5] Gertz MA, Lacy MQ, Dispenzieri A, et al. Clinical implications of t(11;14)(q13;q32), t(4;14)(p16.3;q32), and -17p13 in myeloma patients treated with high-dose therapy. Blood 2005;106:2837–40.

[6] Fermand JP, Ravaud P, Chevret S, et al. High-dose therapy and autologous peripheral blood stem cell transplantation in multiple myeloma: up-front or rescue treatment? Results of a multicenter sequential randomized clinical trial. Blood 1998;92:3131–6.

[7] Fonseca R. Many and multiple myeloma(s). Leukemia 2003;17:1943–4.

[8] Ross FM, Ibrahim AH, Vilain-Holmes A, et al. Age has a profound effect on the incidence and significance of chromosome abnormalities in myeloma. Leukemia 2005;19: 1634–42.

[9] Greipp PR, San Miguel J, Durie BG, et al. International staging system for multiple myeloma. J Clin Oncol 2005;23:3412–20.

[10] Debes-Marun C, Dewald G, Bryant S, et al. Chromosome abnormalities clustering and its implications for pathogenesis and prognosis in myeloma. Leukemia 2003;17:427–36.

[11] Smadja NV, Fruchart C, Isnard F, et al. Chromosomal analysis in multiple myeloma: cytogenetic evidence of two different diseases. Leukemia 1998;12:960–9.

[12] Carrasco DR, Tonon G, Huang Y, et al. High-resolution genomic profiles define distinct clinico-pathogenetic subgroups of multiple myeloma patients. Cancer Cell 2006;9: 313–25.

[13] Avet-Loiseau H, Attal M, Moreau P, et al. Genetic abnormalities and survival in multiple myeloma: the experience of the Intergroupe Francophone du Myelome. Blood 2007.

[14] Keats JJ, Reiman T, Maxwell CA, et al. In multiple myeloma, t(4;14)(p16;q32) is an adverse prognostic factor irrespective of FGFR3 expression. Blood 2003;101:1520–9.

[15] Jaksic W, Trudel S, Chang H, et al. Clinical outcomes in t(4;14) multiple myeloma: a chemotherapy-sensitive disease characterized by rapid relapse and alkylating agent resistance. J Clin Oncol 2005.

[16] Chang H, Trieu Y, Qi X, et al. Bortezomib therapy response is independent of cytogenic abnormalities in relapsed/refractory multiple myeloma. Leuk Res 2007;31:779–82.

[17] Chang H, Qi XY, Samiee S, et al. Genetic risk identifies multiple myeloma patients who do not benefit from autologous stem cell transplantation. Bone Marrow Transplant 2005.

[18] Ahmann GJ, Jalal SM, Juneau AL, et al. A novel three-color, clone-specific fluorescence in situ hybridization procedure for monoclonal gammopathies. Cancer Genet Cytogenet 1998;101:7–11.

[19] Dispenzieri A, Rajkumar SV, Gertz MA, et al. Treatment of newly diagnosed multiple myeloma based on Mayo stratification of myeloma and risk-adapted therapy (mSMART): consensus statement. Mayo Clin Proc 2007;82:323–41.

[20] Kuehl WM, Bergsagel PL. Multiple myeloma: evolving genetic events and host interactions. Nat Rev Cancer 2002;2:175–87.

[21] Fonseca R, Harrington D, Oken M, et al. Myeloma and the t(11;14)(q13;q32) represents a uniquely defined biological subset of patients. Blood 2002;99:3735–41.

[22] Hoyer JD, Hanson CA, Fonseca R, et al. The (11;14)(q13;q32) translocation in multiple myeloma. A morphologic and immunohistochemical study. Am J Clin Pathol 2000;113:831–7.

[23] Garand R, Avet-Loiseau H, Accard F, et al. t(11;14) and t(4;14) translocations correlated with mature lymphoplasmocytoid and immature morphology, respectively, in multiple myeloma. Leukemia 2003; [this issue].

[24] Fonseca R, Debes-Marun CS, Picken EB, et al. The recurrent IgH translocations are highly associated with nonhyperdiploid variant multiple myeloma. Blood 2003;102: 2562–7.

[25] Smadja NV, Bastard C, Brigaudeau C, et al. Hypodiploidy is a major prognostic factor in multiple myeloma. Blood 2001;98:2229–38.

[26] Fassas AB, Spencer T, Sawyer J, et al. Both hypodiploidy and deletion of chromosome 13 independently confer poor prognosis in multiple myeloma. Br J Haematol 2002;118:1041–7.

[27] Chng WJ, Santana-Davila R, Van Wier SA, et al. Prognostic factors for hyperdiploid-myeloma: effects of chromosome 13 deletions and IgH translocations. Leukemia 2006;20: 807–13.

[28] Tricot G, Barlogie B, Jagannath S, et al. Poor prognosis in multiple myeloma is associated only with partial or complete deletions of chromosome 13 or abnormalities involving 11q and not with other karyotype abnormalities. Blood 1995;86:4250–6.

[29] Tricot G, Sawyer JR, Jagannath S, et al. Unique role of cytogenetics in the prognosis of patients with myeloma receiving high-dose therapy and autotransplants. J Clin Oncol 1997;15:2659–66.

[30] Perez-Simon JA, Garcia-Sanz R, Tabernero MD, et al. Prognostic value of numerical chromosome aberrations in multiple myeloma: a FISH analysis of 15 different chromosomes. Blood 1998;91:3366–71.

[31] Zojer N, Konigsberg R, Ackermann J, et al. Deletion of 13q14 remains an independent adverse prognostic variable in multiple myeloma despite its frequent detection by interphase fluorescence in situ hybridization. Blood 2000;95:1925–30.

[32] Dewald GW, Therneau T, Larson D, et al. Relationship of patient survival and chromosome anomalies detected in metaphase and/or interphase cells at diagnosis of myeloma. Blood 2005;106:3553–8.

[33] Fonseca R, Oken MM, Harrington D, et al. Deletions of chromosome 13 in multiple myeloma identified by interphase FISH usually denote large deletions of the q arm or monosomy. Leukemia 2001;15:981–6.

[34] Fonseca R, Harrington D, Oken M, et al. Biologic and prognostic significance of interphase FISH detection of chromosome 13 abnormalities (D13) in multiple myeloma: an Eastern Cooperative Oncology Group (ECOG) Study. Cancer Res 2002;62:715–20.

[35] Avet-Loiseau H, Li JY, Morineau N, et al. Monosomy 13 is associated with the transition of monoclonal gammopathy of undetermined significance to multiple myeloma. Intergroupe Francophone du Myelome. Blood 1999;94:2583–9.

[36] Avet-Loiseau H, Daviet A, Saunier S, et al. Chromosome 13 abnormalities in multiple myeloma are mostly monosomy 13. Br J Haematol 2000;111:1116–7.

[37] Gutierrez NC, Castellanos MV, Martin ML, et al. Prognostic and biological implications of genetic abnormalities in multiple myeloma undergoing autologous stem cell transplantation: t(4;14) is the most relevant adverse prognostic factor, whereas RB deletion as a unique abnormality is not associated with adverse prognosis. Leukemia 2007;21:143–50.

[38] Chiecchio L, Protheroe RK, Ibrahim AH, et al. Deletion of chromosome 13 detected by conventional cytogenetics is a critical prognostic factor in myeloma. Leukemia 2006;20: 1610–7.

[39] Drach J, Ackermann J, Fritz E, et al. Presence of a p53 gene deletion in patients with multiple myeloma predicts for short survival after conventional-dose chemotherapy. Blood 1998;92:802–9.

[40] Chang H, Qi C, Yi QL, et al. p53 gene deletion detected by fluorescence in situ hybridization is an adverse prognostic factor for patients with multiple myeloma following autologous stem cell transplantation. Blood 2005;105:358–60.

[41] Chang H, Sloan S, Li D, et al. Multiple myeloma involving central nervous system: high frequency of chromosome 17p13.1 (p53) deletions. Br J Haematol 2004;127:280–4.

[42] Liu P, Leong T, Quam L, et al. Activating mutations of N- and K-ras in multiple myeloma show different clinical associations: analysis of the Eastern Cooperative Oncology Group Phase III Trial. Blood 1996;88:2699–706.

[43] Bezieau S, Devilder MC, Avet-Loiseau H, et al. High incidence of N and K-Ras activating mutations in multiple myeloma and primary plasma cell leukemia at diagnosis. Hum Mutat 2001;18:212–24.

[44] Rasmussen T, Kuehl M, Lodahl M, et al. Possible roles for activating RAS mutations in the MGUS to MM transition and in the intramedullary to extramedullary transition some plasma cell tumors. Blood 2005;105:317–23.

[45] Urashima M, Teoh G, Ogata A, et al. Characterization of p16(INK4A) expression in multiple myeloma and plasma cell leukemia. Clin Cancer Res 1997;3:2173–9.

[46] Tasaka T, Asou H, Munker R, et al. Methylation of the p16INK4A gene in multiple myeloma. Br J Haematol 1998;101:558–64.

[47] Mateos MV, Garcia-Sanz R, Lopez-Perez R, et al. Methylation is an inactivating mechanism of the p16 gene in multiple myeloma associated with high plasma cell proliferation and short survival. Br J Haematol 2002;118:1034–40.

[48] Chen W, Wu Y, Zhu J, et al. Methylation of p16 and p15 genes in multiple myeloma. Chin Med Sci J 2002;17:101–5.

[49] Guillerm G, Depil S, Wolowiec D, et al. Different prognostic values of p15(INK4b) and p16(INK4a) gene methylations in multiple myeloma. Haematologica 2003;88: 476–8.

[50] Uchida T, Kinoshita T, Ohno T, et al. Hypermethylation of p16 INK4A gene promoter during the progression of plasma cell dyscrasia. Leukemia 2001;15:157–65.

[51] Gonzalez-Paz N, Chng WJ, McClure RF, et al. Tumor suppressor p16 methylation in multiple myeloma: biological and clinical implications. Blood 2006.

[52] Sarasquete ME, Garcia-Sanz R, Armellini A, et al. The association of increased p14ARF/ p16INK4a and p15INK4a gene expression with proliferative activity and the clinical course of multiple myeloma. Haematologica 2006;91:1551–4.

[53] Bergsagel PL, Kuehl WM, Zhan F, et al. Cyclin D dysregulation: an early and unifying pathogenic event in multiple myeloma. Blood 2005;106:296–303.

[54] Shaughnessy JD Jr, Zhan F, Burington BE, et al. A validated gene expression model of high-risk multiple myeloma is defined by deregulated expression of genes mapping to chromosome 1. Blood 2007;109:2276–84.

[55] Sawyer JR, Tricot G, Mattox S, et al. Jumping translocations of chromosome 1q in multiple myeloma: evidence for a mechanism involving decondensation of pericentromeric heterochromatin. Blood 1998;91:1732–41.

[56] Fonseca R, Van Wier SA, Chng WJ, et al. Prognostic value of chromosome 1q21 gain by fluorescent in situ hybridization and increase CKS1B expression in myeloma. Leukemia 2006;20:2034–40.

[57] Keats JJ, Fonseca R, Chesi M, et al. Promiscuous mutations activate the noncanonical NF-κB pathway in multiple myeloma. Cancer Cell 2007;12:131–44.

[58] Mulligan G, Mitsiades C, Bryant B, et al. Gene expression profiling and correlation with outcome in clinical trials of the proteasome inhibitor bortezomib. Blood 2007;109:3177–88.

[59] Mateos MV, Hernandez JM, Hernandez MT, et al. Bortezomib plus melphalan and prednisone in elderly untreated patients with multiple myeloma: results of a multicenter phase I/II study. Blood 2006.

[60] Chang H, Sloan S, Li D, et al. The t(4;14) is associated with poor prognosis in myeloma patients undergoing autologous stem cell transplant. Br J Haematol 2004;125:64–8.

[61] Chng WJ, Ahmann GJ, Henderson K, et al. Clinical implication of centrosome amplification in plasma cell neoplasm. Blood 2006;107:3669–75.

[62] Garcia-Sanz R, Orfao A, Gonzalez M, et al. Primary plasma cell leukemia: clinical, immunophenotypic, DNA ploidy, and cytogenetic characteristics. Blood 1999;93:1032–7.

[63] Morgan RJ Jr, Gonchoroff NJ, Katzmann JA, et al. Detection of hypodiploidy using multiparameter flow cytometric analysis: a prognostic indicator in multiple myeloma. Am J Hematol 1989;30:195–200.

[64] Shimazaki C, Gotoh H, Ashihara E, et al. Immunophenotype and DNA content of myeloma cells in primary plasma cell leukemia. Am J Hematol 1992;39:159–62.

[65] Garcia-Sanz R, Orfao A, Gonzalez M, et al. Prognostic implications of DNA aneuploidy in 156 untreated multiple myeloma patients. Castelano-Leones (Spain) Cooperative Group for the Study of Monoclonal Gammopathies. Br J Haematol 1995;90:106–12.

[66] San Miguel JF, Garcia-Sanz R, Gonzalez M, et al. A new staging system for multiple myeloma based on the number of S-phase plasma cells. Blood 1995;85:448–55.

[67] Greipp PR, Trendle MC, Leong T, et al. Is flow cytometric DNA content hypodiploidy prognostic in multiple myeloma? Leuk Lymphoma 1999;35:83–9.

[68] Gutierrez NC, Garcia JL, Hernandez JM, et al. Prognostic and biologic significance of chromosomal imbalances assessed by comparative genomic hybridization in multiple myeloma. Blood 2004;104:2661–6.

[69] Greipp PR, Lust JA, O'Fallon WM, et al. Plasma cell labeling index and beta 2-microglobulin predict survival independent of thymidine kinase and C-reactive protein in multiple myeloma [see comments]. Blood 1993;81:3382–7.

[70] Joshua D, Petersen A, Brown R, et al. The labelling index of primitive plasma cells determines the clinical behaviour of patients with myelomatosis. Br J Haematol 1996;94:76–81.

[71] San Miguel JF, Garcia-Sanz R, Gonzalez M, et al. Immunophenotype and DNA cell content in multiple myeloma. Baillieres Clin Haematol 1995;8:735–59.

[72] Garcia-Sanz R, Gonzalez-Fraile MI, Mateo G, et al. Proliferative activity of plasma cells is the most relevant prognostic factor in elderly multiple myeloma patients. Int J Cancer 2004;112:884–9.

[73] Bartl R, Frisch B, Fateh MA, et al. Histologic classification and staging of multiple myeloma. A retrospective and prospective study of 674 cases. Am J Clin Pathol 1987;87:342–55.

[74] Rajkumar SV, Fonseca R, Lacy MQ, et al. Plasmablastic morphology is an independent predictor of poor survival after autologous stem-cell transplantation for multiple myeloma. J Clin Oncol 1999;17:1551–7.

[75] Greipp PR, Leong T, Bennett JM, et al. Plasmablastic morphology—an independent prognostic factor with clinical and laboratory correlates: Eastern Cooperative Oncology Group (ECOG) myeloma trial E9486 report by the ECOG Myeloma Laboratory Group. Blood 1998;91:2501–7.

[76] Omede P, Boccadoro M, Fusaro A, et al. Multiple myeloma: 'early' plasma cell phenotype identifies patients with aggressive biological and clinical characteristics. Br J Haematol 1993;85:504–13.

[77] San Miguel JF, Gonzalez M, Gascon A, et al. Immunophenotypic heterogeneity of multiple myeloma: influence on the biology and clinical course of the disease. Castellano-Leones (Spain) Cooperative Group for the Study of Monoclonal Gammopathies. Br J Haematol 1991;77:185–90.

[78] Pellat-Deceunynck C, Bataille R, Robillard N, et al. Expression of CD28 and CD40 in human myeloma cells: a comparative study with normal plasma cells. Blood 1994;84: 2597–603.

[79] Pellat-Deceunynck C, Barille S, Puthier D, et al. Adhesion molecules on human myeloma cells: significant changes in expression related to malignancy, tumor spreading, and immortalization. Cancer Res 1995;55:3647–53.

[80] Robillard N, Jego G, Pellat-Deceunynck C, et al. CD28, a marker associated with tumoral expansion in multiple myeloma. Clin Cancer Res 1998;4:1521–6.

[81] Mateo G, Corral M, Almeida J, et al. Immunophenotypic analysis of peripheral blood stem cell harvests from patients with multiple myeloma. 2003;88:1013–21.

[82] Sahara N, Takeshita A. Prognostic significance of surface markers expressed in multiple myeloma: CD56 and other antigens. Leuk Lymphoma 2004;45:61–5.

[83] Moreau P, Robillard N, Avet-Loiseau H, et al. Patients with CD45 negative multiple myeloma receiving high-dose therapy have a shorter survival than those with CD45 positive multiple myeloma. Haematologica 2004;89:547–51.

[84] Shapiro VS, Mollenauer MN, Weiss A. Endogenous CD28 expressed on myeloma cells up-regulates interleukin-8 production: implications for multiple myeloma progression. Blood 2001;98:187–93.

[85] Wang Z, Zhang Y, Mandal A, et al. The spermatozoa protein, SLLP1, is a novel cancer-testis antigen in hematologic malignancies. Clin Cancer Res 2004;10:6544–50.

[86] Lim SH, Wang Z, Chiriva-Internati M, et al. Sperm protein 17 is a novel cancer-testis antigen in multiple myeloma. Blood 2001;97:1508–10.

[87] Dhodapkar MV, Osman K, Teruya-Feldstein J, et al. Expression of cancer/testis (CT) antigens MAGE-A1, MAGE-A3, MAGE-A4, CT-7, and NY-ESO-1 in malignant gammopathies is heterogeneous and correlates with site, stage and risk status of disease. Cancer Immun 2003;3:9.

[88] Pellat-Deceunynck C, Mellerin MP, Labarriere N, et al. The cancer germ-line genes MAGE-1, MAGE-3 and PRAME are commonly expressed by human myeloma cells. Eur J Immunol 2000;30:803–9.

[89] van Baren N, Brasseur F, Godelaine D, et al. Genes encoding tumor-specific antigens are expressed in human myeloma cells. Blood 1999;94:1156–64.

[90] Taylor BJ, Reiman T, Pittman JA, et al. SSX cancer testis antigens are expressed in most multiple myeloma patients: co-expression of SSX1, 2, 4, and 5 correlates with adverse prognosis and high frequencies of SSX-positive PCs. J Immunother (1997) 2005;28:564–75.

[91] Bataille R, Jego G, Robillard N, et al. The phenotype of normal, reactive and malignant plasma cells. Identification of "many and multiple myelomas" and of new targets for myeloma therapy. Haematologica 2006;91:1234–40.

[92] Robillard N, Pellat-Deceunynck C, Bataille R. Phenotypic characterization of the human myeloma cell growth fraction. Blood 2005;105:4845–8.

[93] Mahmoud MS, Ishikawa H, Fujii R, et al. Induction of CD45 expression and proliferation in U-266 myeloma cell line by interleukin-6. Blood 1998;92:3887–97.

[94] Liu S, Ishikawa H, Tsuyama N, et al. Increased susceptibility to apoptosis in CD45(+) myeloma cells accompanied by the increased expression of VDAC1. Oncogene 2006;25: 419–29.

[95] kulas DT, Freund GG, Mooney RA. The transmembrane protein-tyrosine-phosphatase CD45 is associated with decreased insulin-receptor signaling. J Biol Chem 1996;271: 755–60.

[96] Kumar S, Rajkumar SV, Kimlinger T, et al. CD45 expression by bone marrow plasma cells in multiple myeloma: clinical and biological correlations. Leukemia 2005;19:1466–70.

[97] Ocqueteau M, Orfao A, Almeida J, et al. Immunophenotypic characterization of plasma cells from monoclonal gammopathy of undetermined significance patients. Implications for the differential diagnosis between MGUS and multiple myeloma. Am J Pathol 1998;152:1655–65.

[98] Harada H, Kawano MM, Huang N, et al. Phenotypic difference of normal plasma cells from mature myeloma cells. Blood 1993;81:2658–63.

[99] Kumar S, Rajkumar SV, Kyle RA, et al. Prognostic value of circulating plasma cells in monoclonal gammopathy of undetermined significance. J Clin Oncol 2005;23:5668–74.

[100] Rawstron AC, Davies FE, DasGupta R, et al. Flow cytometric disease monitoring in multiple myeloma: the relationship between normal and neoplastic plasma cells predicts outcome after transplantation. Blood 2002;100:3095–100.

[101] San Miguel JF, Almeida J, Mateo G, et al. Immunophenotypic evaluation of the plasma cell compartment in multiple myeloma: a tool for comparing the efficacy of different treatment strategies and predicting outcome. Blood 2002;99:1853–6.

[102] San Miguel JF, Garcia-Sanz R. Prognostic features of multiple myeloma. Best Pract Res Clin Haematol 2005;18:569–83.

[103] Mileshkin L, Prince HM. The adverse prognostic impact of advanced age in multiple myeloma. Leuk Lymphoma 2005;46:951–66.

[104] Mileshkin L, Biagi JJ, Mitchell P, et al. Multicenter phase 2 trial of thalidomide in relapsed/refractory multiple myeloma: adverse prognostic impact of advanced age. Blood 2003;102:69–77.

[105] Lenhoff S, Hjorth M, Holmberg E, et al. Impact on survival of high-dose therapy with autologous stem cell support in patients younger than 60 years with newly diagnosed multiple myeloma: a population-based study. Nordic Myeloma Study Group. Blood 2000;95:7–11.

[106] Janssen-Heijnen ML, Houterman S, Lemmens VE, et al. Prognostic impact of increasing age and co-morbidity in cancer patients: a population-based approach. Crit Rev Oncol Hematol 2005;55:231–40.

[107] Blade J, Kyle RA, Greipp PR. Presenting features and prognosis in 72 patients with multiple myeloma who were younger than 40 years. Br J Haematol 1996;93:345–51.

[108] Siegel DS, Desikan KR, Mehta J, et al. Age is not a prognostic variable with autotransplants for multiple myeloma. Blood 1999;93:51–4.

[109] Badros A, Barlogie B, Siegel E, et al. Autologous stem cell transplantation in elderly multiple myeloma patients over the age of 70 years. Br J Haematol 2001;114:600–7.

[110] Modiano MR, Villarwerstler P, Crowley J, et al. Evaluation of race as a prognostic factor in multiple-myeloma—An ancillary of Southwest-Oncology-Group Study 8229. J Clin Oncol 1996;14:974–7.

[111] Saraf S, Chen YH, Dobogai LC, et al. Prolonged responses after autologous stem cell transplantation in African-American patients with multiple myeloma. Bone Marrow Transplant 2006;37:1099–102.

[112] Davies FE, Rollinson SJ, Rawstron AC, et al. High-producer haplotypes of tumor necrosis factor alpha and lymphotoxin alpha are associated with an increased risk of myeloma and have an improved progression-free survival after treatment. J Clin Oncol 2000;18:2843–51.

[113] Parker KM, Ma MH, Manyak S, et al. Identification of polymorphisms of the IkappaBalpha gene associated with an increased risk of multiple myeloma. Cancer Genet Cytogenet 2002;137:43–8.

[114] Roddam PL, Rollinson S, O'Driscoll M, et al. Genetic variants of NHEJ DNA ligase IV can affect the risk of developing multiple myeloma, a tumour characterised by aberrant class switch recombination. J Med Genet 2002;39:900–5.

[115] Morgan GJ, Adamson PJ, Mensah FK, et al. Haplotypes in the tumour necrosis factor region and myeloma. Br J Haematol 2005;129:358–65.

[116] Spink CF, Gray LC, Davies FE, et al. Haplotypic structure across the I kappa B alpha gene (NFKBIA) and association with multiple myeloma. Cancer Lett 2007;246:92–9.

[117] Lincz LF, Scorgie FE, Robertson R, et al. Genetic variations in benzene metabolism and susceptibility to multiple myeloma. Leuk Res 2006.

[118] Neben K, Mytilineos J, Moehler TM, et al. Polymorphisms of the tumor necrosis factor-alpha gene promoter predict for outcome after thalidomide therapy in relapsed and refractory multiple myeloma. Blood 2002;100:2263–5.

[119] Dasgupta RK, Adamson PJ, Davies FE, et al. Polymorphic variation in GSTP1 modulates outcome following therapy for multiple myeloma. Blood 2003;102:2345–50.

[120] Sze DM, Giesajtis G, Brown RD, et al. Clonal cytotoxic T cells are expanded in myeloma and reside in the CD8(+)CD57(+)CD28(−) compartment. Blood 2001;98:2817–27.

[121] Brown RD, Yuen E, Nelson M, et al. The prognostic significance of T cell receptor beta gene rearrangements and idiotype-reactive T cells in multiple myeloma. Leukemia 1997;11:1312–7.

[122] Kay NE, Leong T, Kyle RA, et al. Circulating blood B cells in multiple myeloma: analysis and relationship to circulating clonal cells and clinical parameters in a cohort of patients entered on the Eastern Cooperative Oncology Group phase III E9486 clinical trial. Blood 1997;90:340–5.

[123] Kay NE, Leong TL, Bone N, et al. Blood levels of immune cells predict survival in myeloma patients: results of an Eastern Cooperative Oncology Group phase 3 trial for newly diagnosed multiple myeloma patients. Blood 2001;98:23–8.

[124] Witzig TE, Gertz MA, Lust JA, et al. Peripheral blood monoclonal plasma cells as a predictor of survival in patients with multiple myeloma. Blood 1996;88:1780–7.

[125] Durie BG, Salmon SE. A clinical staging system for multiple myeloma. Correlation of measured myeloma cell mass with presenting clinical features, response to treatment, and survival. Cancer 1975;36:842–54.

[126] Drayson M, Begum G, Basu S, et al. Effects of paraprotein heavy and light chain types and free light chain load on survival in myeloma: an analysis of patients receiving conventional-dose chemotherapy in Medical Research Council UK multiple myeloma trials. Blood 2006;108:2013–9.

[127] Boccadoro M, Omede P, Frieri R, et al. Multiple myeloma: beta-2-microglobulin is not a useful follow-up parameter. Acta Haematol 1989;82:122–5.

[128] Garewal H, Durie BG, Kyle RA, et al. Serum beta 2-microglobulin in the initial staging and subsequent monitoring of monoclonal plasma cell disorders. J Clin Oncol 1984;2:51–7.

[129] Bataille R, Grenier J, Sany J. Unexpected normal serum beta-microglobulin (B2M) levels in multiple myeloma. Anticancer Res 1987;7:513–5.

[130] Cuzick J, De SBL, Cooper EH, et al. Long-term prognostic value of serum beta 2 microglobulin in myelomatosis. Br J Haematol 1990;75:506–10.

[131] Greipp PR. Monoclonal gammopathies: new approaches to clinical problems in diagnosis and prognosis. Blood Rev 1989;3:222–36.

[132] Papadaki H, Kyriakou D, Foudoulakis A, et al. Serum levels of soluble IL-6 receptor in multiple myeloma as indicator of disease activity. Acta Haematol 1997;97:191–5.

[133] Klein B, Zhang XG, Jourdan M, et al. Paracrine rather than autocrine regulation of myeloma-cell growth and differentiation by interleukin-6. Blood 1989;73:517–26.

[134] Greipp PR, Gaillard JP, Kalish LA, et al. Independent prognostic value for serum soluble interleukin-6 receptor (sIL-6R) in Eastern Cooperative Oncology Group (ECOG) myeloma trial E9487 [meeting abstract]. Proceedings of the Annual Meeting of the American Society of Clinical Oncology 1993;12.

[135] Greipp PR, Gaillard JP, Klein B, et al. Independent prognostic value for plasma cell labeling index (PCLI), immunofluorescence microscopy plasma cell percent (IMPCP), beta 2-microglobulin (B2M), soluble interleukin-6 receptor (sIL-6R), and c-reactive protein (CRP) in myeloma trial E9487 [meeting abstract]. Blood 1994;84.

[136] Pulkki K, Pelliniemi TT, Rajamaki A, et al. Soluble interleukin-6 receptor as a prognostic factor in multiple myeloma. Finnish Leukaemia Group. Br J Haematol 1996;92:370–4.

[137] Ohtani K, Ninomiya H, Hasegawa Y, et al. Clinical significance of elevated soluble interleukin-6 receptor levels in the sera of patients with plasma cell dyscrasias [see comments]. Br J Haematol 1995;91:116–20.

[138] Bataille R, Boccadoro M, Klein B, et al. C-reactive protein and beta-2 microglobulin produce a simple and powerful myeloma staging system. Blood 1992;80:733–7.

[139] Merlini G, Perfetti V, Gobbi PG, et al. Acute phase proteins and prognosis in multiple myeloma. Br J Haematol 1993;83:595–601.

[140] Seidel C, Sundan A, Hjorth M, et al. Serum syndecan-1: a new independent prognostic marker in multiple myeloma. Blood 2000;95:388–92.

[141] Lovell R, Dunn JA, Begum G, et al. Soluble syndecan-1 level at diagnosis is an independent prognostic factor in multiple myeloma and the extent of fall from diagnosis to plateau predicts for overall survival. Br J Haematol 2005;130:542–8.

[142] San Miguel JF, Sanchez J, Gonzalez M. Prognostic factors and classification in multiple myeloma. Br J Cancer 1989;59:113–8.

[143] Moulopoulos LA, Gika D, Anagnostopoulos A, et al. Prognostic significance of magnetic resonance imaging of bone marrow in previously untreated patients with multiple myeloma. Ann Oncol 2005;16:1824–8.

[144] Baur-Melnyk A, Buhmann S, Durr HR, et al. Role of MRI for the diagnosis and prognosis of multiple myeloma. Eur J Radiol 2005;55:56–63.

[145] Durie BG, Waxman AD, D'Agnolo A, et al. Whole-body (18)F-FDG PET identifies high-risk myeloma. J Nucl Med 2002;43:1457–63.

[146] Orchard K, Barrington S, Buscombe J, et al. Fluoro-deoxyglucose positron emission tomography imaging for the detection of occult disease in multiple myeloma. Br J Haematol 2002;117:133–5.

[147] Fonseca R, Trendle MC, Leong T, et al. Prognostic value of serum markers of bone metabolism in untreated multiple myeloma patients. Br J Haematol 2000;109:24–9.

[148] Hernandez JM, Suquia B, Queizan JA, et al. Bone remodelation markers are useful in the management of monoclonal gammopathies. Hematol J 2004;5:480–8.

[149] Pecherstorfer M, Seibel MJ, Woitge HW, et al. Bone resorption in multiple myeloma and in monoclonal gammopathy of undetermined significance: quantification by urinary pyridinium cross-links of collagen. Blood 1997;90:3743–50.

[150] Demacq C, Montenegro MF. Systemic matrix metalloproteinase-9 (MMP-9) levels as prognostic indexes of bone disease in patients with multiple myeloma. Clin Chem Lab Med 2006;44:232 [author reply: 233].

[151] Sfiridaki A, Miyakis S, Tsirakis G, et al. Systemic levels of interleukin-6 and matrix metalloproteinase-9 in patients with multiple myeloma may be useful as prognostic indexes of bone disease. Clin Chem Lab Med 2005;43:934–8.

[152] Zannettino AC, Farrugia AN, Kortesidis A, et al. Elevated serum levels of stromal-derived factor-1alpha are associated with increased osteoclast activity and osteolytic bone disease in multiple myeloma patients. Cancer Res 2005;65:1700–9.

[153] Terpos E, Szydlo R, Apperley JF, et al. Soluble receptor activator of nuclear factor kappaB ligand-osteoprotegerin ratio predicts survival in multiple myeloma: proposal for a novel prognostic index. Blood 2003;102:1064–9.

[154] Ladetto M, Vallet S, Trojan A, et al. Cyclooxygenase-2 (COX-2) is frequently expressed in multiple myeloma and is an independent predictor of poor outcome. Blood 2005;105:4784–91.

[155] Blade J, Lopez-Guillermo A, Bosch F, et al. Impact of response to treatment on survival in multiple myeloma: results in a series of 243 patients. Br J Haematol 1994;88:117–21.

[156] Facon T, Mary J, Harousseau J, et al. Superiority of melphalan-prednisone (MP) + thalidomide (THAL) over MP and autologous stem cell transplantation in the treatment of newly

diagnosed elderly patients with multiple myeloma [abstract: 1]. ASCO Annual Meeting Proceedings Part I 2006;24.

[157] Palumbo A, Bringhen S, Caravita T, et al. Oral melphalan and prednisone chemotherapy plus thalidomide compared with melphalan and prednisone alone in elderly patients with multiple myeloma: randomised controlled trial. Lancet 2006;367:825–31.

[158] Child JA, Morgan GJ, Davies FE, et al. High-dose chemotherapy with hematopoietic stem-cell rescue for multiple myeloma. N Engl J Med 2003;348:1875–83.

[159] Attal M, Harousseau JL, Stoppa AM, et al. A prospective, randomized trial of autologous bone marrow transplantation and chemotherapy in multiple myeloma. Intergroupe Francais du Myelome. N Engl J Med 1996;335:91–7.

[160] Alexanian R, Weber D, Giralt S, et al. Impact of complete remission with intensive therapy in patients with responsive multiple myeloma. Bone Marrow Transplant 2001;27:1037–43.

[161] Barlogie B, Jagannath S, Desikan KR, et al. Total therapy with tandem transplants for newly diagnosed multiple myeloma. Blood 1999;93:55–65.

[162] Lahuerta JJ, Martinez-Lopez J, Serna JD, et al. Remission status defined by immunofixation vs. electrophoresis after autologous transplantation has a major impact on the outcome of multiple myeloma patients. Br J Haematol 2000;109:438–46.

[163] Kyle RA, Leong T, Li S, et al. Complete response in multiple myeloma: clinical trial E9486, an Eastern Cooperative Oncology Group study not involving stem cell transplantation. Cancer 2006;106:1958–66.

[164] Durie BG, Jacobson J, Barlogie B, et al. Magnitude of response with myeloma frontline therapy does not predict outcome: importance of time to progression in southwest oncology group chemotherapy trials. J Clin Oncol 2004;22:1857–63.

[165] Barlogie B, Tricot G, Anaissie E, et al. Thalidomide and hematopoietic-cell transplantation for multiple myeloma. N Engl J Med 2006;354:1021–30.

[166] Bradwell AR, Carr-Smith HD, Mead GP, et al. Serum test for assessment of patients with Bence Jones myeloma. Lancet 2003;361:489–91.

[167] Durie BG, Harousseau JL, Miguel JS, et al. International uniform response criteria for multiple myeloma. Leukemia 2006;20:1467–73.

HEMAT●L■GY/●N■■L■GY ■INICS
OF NORTH AMERICA

ELSEVIER
SAUNDERS

Management of Newly Diagnosed Myeloma

S. Vincent Rajkumar, MD[a,b,*], Antonio Palumbo, MD[c]

[a]Division of Hematology, Department of Internal Medicine, Mayo Clinic and Foundation, 200 First Street SW, Rochester, MN 55905, USA
[b]College of Medicine, Mayo Clinic, 200 First Street SW, Rochester, MN 55905, USA
[c]Division of Hematology, University of Turin, Azienda Ospedaliera S. Giovanni Battista, Ospedale Molinette, Turin, Italy

Multiple myeloma (MM) accounts for approximately 10% of hematologic malignancies [1,2]. Many patients evolve from an asymptomatic premalignant stage termed monoclonal gammopathy of unknown significance (MGUS). MGUS is present in approximately 3% of the population older than 50 years, and progresses to myeloma or related malignancy at a rate of 1% per year [3,4]. In some patients, an intermediate asymptomatic but more advanced premalignant stage referred to as smoldering multiple myeloma can be recognized. At diagnosis, most patients are older than 65 years; about 35% of myeloma patients are younger than 65 years, 28% are 65 to 74 years, and 37% are older than 75 [5]. The current changes of the demographic curves will probably increase the incidence of elderly patients in the near future. In newly diagnosed myeloma patients younger than 65 years, high-dose melphalan followed by autologous stem cell transplantation (ASCT) is considered the standard of care. In elderly patients, usually older than 65 years, oral melphalan and prednisone (MP) has been considered the standard until recently.

The discovery of new drugs, such as thalidomide, lenalidomide, and the proteasome inhibitor bortezomib, targeting the myeloma cells and the bone marrow microenvironment have significantly increased the clinical efficacy of the old chemotherapy regimens. The challenge is now to define the optimal sequence and combination of these drugs to significantly impact the natural history of the disease.

SVR has received research support to cover the cost of clinical trials at Mayo Clinic from Celgene Corporation. AP has received scientific advisory board and lecture fees from Pharmion, Celgene, and Janssen-Cilag. Also supported by grants CA 62242, CA107476, CA 100080, and CA 93842 from the National Cancer Institute, Bethesda, Maryland, USA to SVR. Supported in part by the Università degli Studi di Torino; Fondazione Neoplasie Sangue Onlus, Associazione Italiana Leucemie, Compagnia di S Paolo, Fondazione Cassa di Risparmio di Torino, Ministero dell'Università e della Ricerca (MIUR), and Consiglio Nazionale delle Ricerche (CNR); Italy.

*Corresponding author. Division of Hematology, Mayo Clinic, 200 First Street SW, Rochester, MN 55905. E-mail address: rajks@mayo.edu (S.V. Rajkumar).

0889-8588/07/$ – see front matter
doi:10.1016/j.hoc.2007.08.008

DIAGNOSIS

A monoclonal (M) protein can be detected by serum protein electrophoresis alone in 82% of patients and by serum immunofixation in 93%; a combination of serum and urine protein immunofixation studies improve the sensitivity to 97% [6]. In the work-up of a patient who has suspected myeloma, screening urine electrophoresis and immunofixation can be eliminated by using the serum free light chain assay instead. Less than 3% of patients have no evidence of monoclonal paraproteins (nonsecretory myeloma). The diagnosis of myeloma requires 10% or more plasma cells on bone marrow examination (or biopsy-proven plasmacytoma), M protein in the serum or urine (except in patients who have true nonsecretory myeloma), and evidence of organ damage (hypercalcemia, renal insufficiency, anemia, or bone lesions) believed secondary to the underlying plasma cell disorder.

RISK STRATIFICATION

The specific prognostic factors used to stratify patients at the Mayo Clinic into high-risk and standard-risk myeloma to guide therapeutic strategy are deletion 13 or hypodiploidy on metaphase cytogenetic studies, deletion 17p- or immunoglobulin heavy chain (IgH) translocations t(4;14) or t(14;16), or plasma cell labeling index of 3% or higher. Presence of any one or more of the above high-risk factors classifies a patient as having high-risk MM. The median survival of high-risk MM is less than 2 to 3 years even with tandem stem cell transplantation, compared with more than 6 to 7 years in patients who have average-risk MM [2].

TREATMENT

There is no evidence that early treatment of patients who have asymptomatic (smoldering) multiple myeloma prolongs survival compared with therapy at the time of symptoms. Clinical trials are ongoing to determine if newer agents can delay progression, however. An approach to treatment of symptomatic newly diagnosed multiple myeloma at Mayo Clinic is outlined in Fig. 1. It is not clear if high-risk patients need to be treated differently from standard-risk patients as outlined in this approach, however, and this requires further study. New regimens for myeloma are given in Table 1.

Treatment of Myeloma in Patients Eligible for Transplantation

Initial therapy for patients who have standard-risk disease depends on eligibility for ASCT. Eligibility is determined by age, performance status, and coexisting comorbidities. Protracted melphalan-based therapy should be avoided in patients who have newly diagnosed myeloma who are considered eligible for ASCT, because it can interfere with adequate stem cell mobilization. Typically patients are treated with approximately two to four cycles of induction therapy before stem cell harvest. This treatment includes patients who are transplant candidates but who wish to reserve ASCT as a delayed option for relapsed refractory disease. Such patients can resume induction therapy following stem cell collection until a plateau phase is reached, reserving ASCT for relapse.

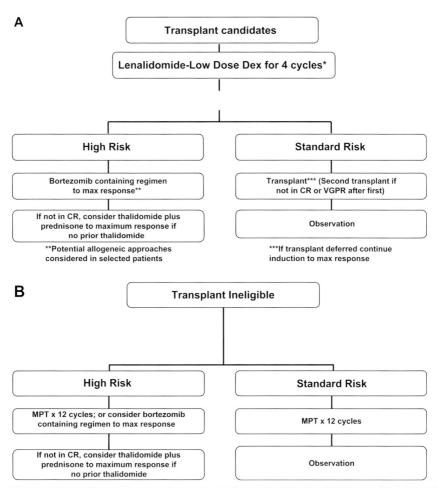

Fig. 1. Treatment of newly diagnosed myeloma. Mayo Stratification for Myeloma and Risk-Adapted Therapy (mSMART) approach to the treatment of newly diagnosed multiple myeloma in patients who are eligible for stem cell transplantation (A) and not eligible for transplantation (B). Clinical trials are preferred at every stage; the algorithm is for off-study therapy when a suitable clinical trial is not available. CR, complete response; Dex, dexamethasone; max, maximum; MPT, melphalan-prednisone-thalidomide; VGPR, very good partial response. (From Dispenzieri A, Rajkumar SV, Gertz MA, et al. Treatment of newly diagnosed multiple myeloma based on Mayo Stratification of Myeloma and Risk-Adapted Therapy (mSMART): Consensus statement. Mayo Clin Proc 2007;82:325; with permission.)

Vincristine, doxorubicin, dexamethasone (VAD) was used for many years as pretransplant induction therapy for patients considered candidates for ASCT. VAD has drawbacks, however, such as needing an intravenous indwelling catheter, and neurotoxicity from vincristine, which can limit the future use of thalidomide and bortezomib. Recently, Cavo and colleagues [7] in a matched

Table 1
New regimens for the treatment of newly diagnosed multiple myeloma

Regimen	Schedule[a]
Thalidomide-dexamethasone (Thal/Dex) [13]	Thalidomide 200 mg oral d 1–28
	Dexamethasone 40 mg oral d 1–4
	Repeated every 4 wk × 4 cycles as pretransplant induction therapy; or continued until plateau or progression if used as primary therapy
Lenalidomide-dexamethasone (Rev/low-dose dexamethasone) [21]	Lenalidomide 25 mg oral d 1–21 every 28 d
	Dexamethasone 40 mg oral d 1, 8, 15, 22 every 28 d
	Repeated every 4 wk × 4 cycles as pretransplant induction therapy; or continued until plateau or progression if used as primary therapy
Bortezomib-dex (Vel/Dex) [24]	Bortezomib 1.3 mg/m^2 intravenous d 1, 4, 8, 11
	Dexamethasone 40 mg oral d 1–4
	Repeated every 3 wk × 4 cycles as pretransplant induction therapy
Melphalan-prednisone-thalidomide (MPT) [27]	Melphalan 0.25 mg/kg oral d 1–4
	Prednisone 2 mg/kg oral d 1–4
	Thalidomide 100–200 mg oral d 1–28
	Repeated every 6 wk × 12 cycles
Melphalan-prednisone-bortezomib (MPV) [28]	Melphalan 9 mg/m^2 oral d 1–4
	Prednisone 60 mg/m^2 oral d 1 to 4
	Bortezomib 1.3 mg/m^2 intravenous d 1, 4, 8, 11, 22, 25, 29, 32
	Repeated every 42 d × 4 cycles followed by maintenance therapy as given below:
	Melphalan 9 mg/m^2 oral d 1–4
	Prednisone 60 mg/m^2 oral d 1 to 4
	Bortezomib 1.3 mg/m^2 intravenous d 1, 8, 15, 22
	Repeated every 35 d × 5 cycles
Melphalan-prednisone-lenalidomide (MPR) [39]	Melphalan 0.18 mg/kg oral d 1–4
	Prednisone 2 mg/kg oral d 1–4
	Lenalidomide 10 mg oral d 1–21
	Repeated every 4–6 wk × 9 cycles
Bortezomib-thalidomide-dexamethasone (VTD) [32]	Bortezomib 1.3 mg/m^2 intravenous d 1, 4, 8, 11
	Thalidomide 100–200 mg oral d 1–21
	Dexamethasone 20 mg/m^2 oral d 1–4
	Repeated every 4 wk × 4 cycles as pretransplant induction therapy

[a]Starting and subsequent doses need to be adjusted for performance status, renal function, blood counts, and other toxicities. Recommended dose of dexamethasone has been reduced from the published series to no more than four doses per month based on recent results of a trial comparing lenalidomide plus high-dose dexamethasone versus lenalidomide plus low-dose dexamethasone.

case-control study of 200 patients demonstrated that response rates with VAD were significantly lower compared with Thal/Dex; 76% versus 52%, respectively. Preliminary results from randomized trials confirm these findings [8,9]. As a result, VAD is no longer recommended as initial therapy. Thalidomide-dexamethasone (Thal/Dex) has increasingly been used in place of VAD. When thalidomide was incorporated into the high-dose therapy followed by autologous transplantation, a higher CR rate (62% versus 43%) and improved 5-year event-free survival (56% versus 44%) was observed compared with high-dose therapy without thalidomide [10]. Unfortunately, the 5-year overall survival was similar in both groups ($P = .9$). In the thalidomide group, a higher rate of thromboembolism (30% versus 17%) and peripheral neuropathy (27% versus 17%) were reported.

Dexamethasone alone has also been used as induction therapy. Objective response rates are approximately 45% [11], significantly lower compared with newer induction regimens. In randomized trials the early mortality rate associated with dexamethasone is more than 10% in the first 4 months of therapy, reflecting the toxicity and ineffectiveness of this regimen. Consequently, single-agent dexamethasone is no longer recommended as initial therapy.

The main choices for initial therapy are thalidomide-dexamethasone (Thal/Dex), bortezomib-based regimens, and lenalidomide-dexamethasone (Rev/Dex) (Table 2). All of these regimens act rapidly, and are associated with high response rates; Thal/Dex and Rev/Dex have the added advantage of being orally administered. Thal/Dex and Rev/Dex are associated with an increased risk for deep vein thrombosis (DVT), necessitating routine thromboprophylaxis.

Thalidomide-dexamethasone
The first clinical trial with thalidomide demonstrated a response rate of 25% in heavily pretreated patients who had relapsed refractory disease [12]. Response rates in relapsed disease are about 25% to 35% with single-agent thalidomide, 50% with thalidomide plus corticosteroids, and more than 65% with a three-drug combination of thalidomide, corticosteroids, and alkylators.

The use of Thal/Dex in newly diagnosed myeloma was initially based on three phase II clinical trials [13–15]. The Eastern Cooperative Oncology Group (ECOG) recently compared Thal/Dex to dexamethasone in 207 patients [11]. The best response within four cycles of therapy was significantly higher with Thal/Dex compared with dexamethasone alone: 63% versus 41%, respectively, $P = .0017$. Stem cell harvest was successful in 90% of patients in each arm. DVT was more frequent with Thal/Dex (17% versus 3%). Overall, grade 3 or higher nonhematologic toxicities were seen in 67% of patients within four cycles with Thal/Dex and 43% with dexamethasone alone ($P < .001$). Early mortality (first 4 months) was 7% with Thal/Dex and 11% with dexamethasone alone. Based on this trial, the US Food and Drug Administration (FDA) granted accelerated approval for Thal/Dex for the treatment of newly diagnosed myeloma.

Table 2
New induction regimens tested in patients younger than 65 years of age who had myeloma

Therapy	No. of patients	Median age (range)	≥PR (%)	CR (%)	Progression-free survival	Overall survival	Peripheral neuropathy, grade 3–4 (%)	DVT/embolism, grade 3–4 (%)	Infection, grade 3–4 (%)	References
TD	103	65 (38–83)	63	4	50% at 22 mo	72% at 2 y	7	17	6	[11]
TD	100	54 (49–59)	76	10	ND	ND	4	15	4	[7]
ASCT-T	323	ND	ND	62	56% at 5 y[a]	65% at 5 y	27[b]	30[b]	ND	[10]
RD	34	64 (32–78)	91	18	74% at 2 y	91% at 2 y	ND	3	6	[21]
VD	79	55 (ND)	82	9	ND	ND	3	3	4	[28]

Abbreviations: ASCT-T, autologous stem cell transplant + thalidomide; CR, complete response; DVT, deep vein thrombosis; ND, not determined; PR, partial response; RD, lenalidomide + dexamethasone; TD, thalidomide + dexamethasone; VD, bortezomib + dexamethasone.
[a]Event-free survival.
[b]Greater than grade 2.

Preliminary results are available from a separate randomized, double-blind, placebo-controlled study comparing Thal/Dex versus dexamethasone alone as primary therapy in 470 patients who had newly diagnosed myeloma (MM) [16]. Among 470 patients enrolled, time to progression (TTP) was significantly superior with Thal/Dex, $P < .001$. As in the ECOG trial, DVT and other grade 3 to 4 events were more frequent with Thal/Dex.

Patients receiving thalidomide in combination with high-dose steroids or chemotherapy need routine thromboprophylaxis with Coumadin (target INR 2–3) or low–molecular weight heparin (equivalent of enoxaparin 40 mg once daily). Aspirin can be used instead in patients receiving only low doses of dexamethasone (40 mg, 4 days a month or lower) or prednisone in combination with thalidomide, provided no concomitant erythropoietic agents are used.

Lenalidomide-dexamethasone
Richardson and colleagues [17] tested lenalidomide in a multicenter randomized phase II trial of 102 patients who had relapsed/refractory myeloma. Overall response rate with single-agent lenalidomide was 17%. Two large phase III trials have since shown significantly superior time to progression with Rev/Dex compared with placebo plus dexamethasone in relapsed myeloma [18,19]. Rev/Dex is currently approved by the FDA for the treatment of myeloma in patients who have received one prior therapy.

In newly diagnosed myeloma, a phase II trial conducted at the Mayo Clinic demonstrated remarkably high activity with the Rev/Dex regimen. Thirty-one of 34 patients (91%) achieved an objective response, including 2 (6%) achieving complete response (CR), and 11 (32%) meeting criteria for very good partial response (VGPR) [20]. With longer follow-up, 56% of patients achieved VGPR or better. In the subset of 21 patients receiving Rev/Dex as primary therapy without ASCT, 67% achieved VGPR or better [21]. Approximately 50% of patients experienced grade 3 or higher nonhematologic toxicity.

ECOG tested Rev/Dex as administered in the Mayo Phase II trial (and in the regulatory relapsed refractory myeloma studies) versus Rev/low-dose dexamethasone (40 mg dexamethasone once weekly) [22]. Results so far show that toxicity rates are significantly higher with Rev/high-dose dexamethasone compared with Rev/low-dose dexamethasone. Early (first 4 months) mortality rates were low in both arms, 5% and 0.5%, respectively. The early mortality rate in the Rev/low-dose dexamethasone arm is probably the lowest reported in any large phase III newly diagnosed trial in which enrollment was not restricted by age or eligibility for stem cell transplantation; DVT rates are also low, making this one of the safest pretransplant induction regimens for myeloma. Based on this Rev/low-dose dexamethasone is currently the regimen of choice at Mayo Clinic outside the setting of a clinical trial. This ECOG study was recently closed by the data monitoring committee because of significantly superior overall survival in patients receiving Rev/low-dose dexamethasone compared with Rev/high-dose dexamethasone. As a result, doses of dexamethasone in excess of 40 mg for 4 days each month should be avoided in patients who have newly diagnosed myeloma, either as a single agent or in combination with other agents.

The incidence of DVT is low with single-agent lenalidomide or lenalidomide plus low-dose dexamethasone, but increases markedly when the agent is combined with high-dose dexamethasone. Recommendations for thromboprophylaxis are similar to those discussed previously with Thal/Dex; aspirin alone is probably sufficient for patients receiving lenalidomide plus low-dose dexamethasone.

Bortezomib-based regimens

Bortezomib is a novel proteasome inhibitor approved for the treatment of patients who have relapsed and refractory multiple myeloma. In relapsed/refractory MM, approximately one third of patients respond to bortezomib therapy with an average response duration of 1 year [23]. Progression-free survival (PFS) is superior with bortezomib compared with dexamethasone alone in patients who have relapsed, refractory MM [24]. Bortezomib is currently approved by the FDA for the treatment of myeloma in patients who have failed one prior therapy.

In newly diagnosed myeloma, bortezomib has shown response rates of approximately 40% as a single agent [25]. Significantly higher response rates (approximately 70%–90%) have been observed with bortezomib plus dexamethasone (Vel/Dex) [26,27], bortezomib, thalidomide, dexamethasone (VTD), and other bortezomib-based combinations. The CR plus VGPR rate is approximately 25% to 30% with Vel/Dex in one study. No adverse effect on stem cell mobilization has been noted. The most common grade 2 or higher adverse events in one study were sensory neuropathy (31%), constipation (28%), myalgia (28%), and fatigue (25%) [26]. Harousseau and colleagues [28] recently reported preliminary results of a randomized trial comparing VAD versus Vel/Dex as pretransplant induction therapy. With more than 400 patients enrolled, preliminary results show superior response rates and long-term outcome with Vel/Dex compared with VAD. DVT risk is low with bortezomib (<5%).

The main drawback of bortezomib-based regimens is the need for intravenous therapy. Bortezomib-based regimens may be of value in patients who have renal failure, however, and in patients who have high-risk myeloma (see later discussion).

Other induction regimens

The role of other pretransplant induction regimens, such as those containing doxorubicin or liposomal doxorubicin, need to be weighed in terms of the added side effects that can affect quality of life and should be considered investigational until future studies show that the addition of these agents improves long-term outcome compared with the regimens discussed previously.

Transplantation in Newly Diagnosed Myeloma

The role of transplantation (autologous and allogeneic) in myeloma is discussed elsewhere in this issue. An increasing number of patients are opting for delayed transplantation. There is also new interest in allografting. In a recent trial, patients who had newly diagnosed multiple myeloma received an ASCT followed by an allograft from an HLA-identical sibling or a tandem ASCT. Patients who had an HLA-identical sibling then received nonmyeloablative total-body irradiation and stem cells from the sibling. Patients who did not have an HLA-identical sibling received two consecutive myeloablative doses of melphalan, each of which was followed by autologous stem cell rescue. The median overall survival and event-free survival were longer in patients who had HLA-identical siblings than in those who did not have HLA-identical siblings (80 months versus 54 months, $P = .01$; and 35 months versus 29 months, $P = .02$, respectively). These data suggest that survival in recipients of a hematopoietic stem cell autograft followed by a stem cell allograft from an HLA-identical sibling may be superior to that in recipients of tandem stem cell autografts [29]. Further studies are needed to confirm these findings in the context of improved initial therapeutic approaches discussed later in this article.

New Maintenance Approaches

The role of maintenance therapy remains controversial in myeloma. After conventional or high-dose therapy, maintenance with interferon alpha provided marginal benefits. In patients who responded to conventional chemotherapy, maintenance therapy with 50 mg alternate-day prednisone significantly improved progression-free and overall survival compared with 10 mg alternate-day prednisone [30].

In a large randomized study conducted by the IFM group, patients younger than 65 years were randomly assigned to receive no maintenance, pamidronate, or pamidronate plus thalidomide [31]. The 3-year post-randomization probability of event-free survival ($P < .009$) and the 4-year overall survival ($P < .04$) were significantly prolonged in patients who received thalidomide. The proportion of patients who had skeletal events was not influenced by the administration of pamidronate. Grade 3 to 4 neuropathy (7%), fatigue (6%), and constipation (1%) were more prominent in the thalidomide group. The incidence of thromboembolic events was not significantly different in the three arms. More recently, a randomized trial compared thalidomide-prednisone versus prednisone alone as maintenance therapy after autologous stem cell transplantation: the 1-year progression-free survival was 91% versus 69%, and the 2-year overall survival was 90% versus 81%, respectively. Neurologic side effects were more common with thalidomide, but no differences were observed in the incidence of thromboembolic events [32]. Additional studies are needed to determine the role of routine maintenance in myeloma, especially the use of lenalidomide, which has a better safety profile than thalidomide for long-term maintenance.

Treatment of Myeloma in Patients Not Eligible for Autologous Stem Cell Transplantation

Patients who are not transplant candidates are treated with standard alkylating agent therapy. For decades this has meant therapy with melphalan plus prednisone (MP) [1]. Over the years, despite better response rates, no survival benefit has been reported with any of the more aggressive combination chemotherapy regimens compared with MP. In a recent randomized trial, four treatment regimens have been evaluated: MP, melphalan and dexamethasone, high-dose dexamethasone, and high-dose dexamethasone plus interferon alpha [33]. Response rate was significantly higher among patients receiving melphalan-dexamethasone. Median progression-free survival was 21 and 23 months after MP or melphalan and dexamethasone, but only 12 and 15 months after high-dose dexamethasone or high-dose dexamethasone plus interferon alpha, respectively. No difference in overall survival was reported among the four different groups, however. Melphalan should be incorporated in the induction regimen for elderly patients who are not candidates for autologous transplant.

In patients older than 65 years, melphalan 200 mg/m^2 followed by autologous transplant is too toxic, whereas intermediate-dose melphalan (100–140 mg/m^2) seems more suitable. In one study, patients were aged 65 to 70 years and melphalan 100 mg/m^2 was superior to MP [34]. In another study, patients were aged 65 to 75 years and melphalan 100 mg/m^2 was superior to MP in response rate but not in progression-free and overall survival [35]. In the first study, 22% of patients did not complete the assigned treatment; in the second trial, 37% of patients did not complete it. According to these data, the age of 70 years may be suggested as the age limit for intermediate-dose melphalan.

Recently three new combinations have emerged: melphalan, prednisone, thalidomide; melphalan, prednisone, lenalidomide; and melphalan, prednisone, bortezomib (Table 3).

Melphalan, prednisone, thalidomide
Two randomized studies show that melphalan, prednisone, thalidomide (MPT) improves response and event-free survival compared with MP [35,36]; an overall survival advantage has been reported in one of the two trials [35]. Although results with melphalan, prednisone, lenalidomide (MPR) and melphalan, prednisone, bortezomib (MPV) are promising, randomized trials are needed to determine if MPR or MPV is superior to MPT.

In the Italian randomized trial, oral MPT was compared with MP in patients aged 60 to 85 years [36]. The partial response (PR) rates were 76% in patients treated with MPT and 47.6% in those treated with MP; near-CR or CR rates were 27.9% and 7.2%, respectively. The 2-year event-free survival rates were 54% for MPT and 27% for MP ($P = .0006$). The 3-year survival rates were 80% and 64%, respectively ($P = .19$). Compared with the MP regimen MPT was associated with a higher risk for grade 3 to 4 neurologic adverse events (10% versus 1%), infections (10% versus 2%, $P = .001$), cardiac toxicity (7% versus 4%), and thromboembolism (12% versus 2%). Introduction of enoxaparin prophylaxis significantly reduced the rate of thromboembolism from 20% to 3% ($P = .005$).

In the French phase III trial, MPT was compared with MP and with intermediate-dose melphalan (100 mg/m^2) followed by ASCT. A higher PR rate

Table 3
New induction regimens tested in patients older than 65 years of age who had myeloma

Therapy	No. of patients	Median age (range)	>65 years (%)	≥PR (%)	CR (%)	Progression-free survival	Overall survival	Peripheral neuropathy, grade 3–4 (%)	DVT/embolism, grade 3–4 (%)	Infection, grade 3–4 (%)	References
MPT	124	ND (65–75)	100	81	16	50% at 28 mo	78% at 2 y	6	12	13	[35]
MPT	129	72 (60–85)	97	76	16	54% at 2 y[a]	80% at 3 y	8	12	10	[36]
MPR	54	71 (57–77)	96	85	24	91% at 2 y	92% at 2 y	0	6	8	[39]
VMP	60	75 (65–85)	100	89	32	91% at 16 mo	90% at 16 mo	17	ND	16	[38]

Abbreviations: CR, complete response; DVT, deep vein thrombosis; MPR, melphalan + prednisone + lenalidomide; MPT, melphalan + prednisone + thalidomide; ND, not determined; PR, partial response; VMP, bortezomib + melphalan + prednisone.
[a]Event-free survival.

was seen in the MPT and in the melphalan 100 mg/m^2 arms, compared with MP (81% versus 73% versus 40%, respectively) [35]. Similarly, the CR rates were significantly higher with MPT and intermediate-dose melphalan compared with MP. Progression-free survival was superior in the patients treated with MPT compared with MP ($P < .001$) and autologous transplantation ($P = .001$). Furthermore, overall survival was significantly improved in the MPT group in comparison with MP ($P = .001$) and autologous transplantation ($P = .004$). MPT was associated with a higher risk for grade 3 to 4 neutropenia, infections, thrombocytopenia, thromboembolic complications, peripheral neuropathy, constipation, and cardiac events. These data, along with the Italian study, strongly support the use of MPT as standard of care in elderly patients who have newly diagnosed myeloma.

Antithrombotic prophylaxis is recommended when using MPT. At present there is no evidence of the best prophylaxis: low–molecular weight heparin, therapeutic doses of warfarin, or daily aspirin are the preferred options [37].

Melphalan, prednisone, bortezomib
The Spanish cooperative group conducted a large phase I/II trial of MPV [38]. The association showed encouraging results: PR rate was 89%, including 32% immunofixation-negative CR, and half achieved immunophenotypic remission (no detectable plasma cells at 10^{-4} to 10^{-5} sensitivity). Progression-free survival at 16 months of patients treated with bortezomib, melphalan, and prednisone (VMP) was significantly prolonged in comparison with historical controls treated with MP only (91% versus 66%); similarly, overall survival at 16 months was improved (90% versus 62%). Interestingly, response rate, progression-free survival, and overall survival were similar among patients who did or did not have chromosome 13 deletion or IgH translocations. Grade 3 to 4 adverse events were thrombocytopenia, neutropenia, peripheral neuropathy, infections, and diarrhea. The treatment seemed more toxic in patients older than 75 years and during early cycles. Bortezomib may induce transient thrombocytopenia and peripheral neuropathy. Pre-existing neuropathy or previous neurotoxic therapy increases the risk for peripheral neuropathy, which can be reduced or resolved by timely dose adjustment of the drug. Bortezomib may enhance the incidence of infections, in particular herpes zoster reactivation, and prophylactic antiviral medications are highly recommended.

Melphalan, prednisone, lenalidomide
In a phase I/II trial dosing, safety, and efficacy of MPR were studied in newly diagnosed elderly patients who had myeloma [39]. Aspirin was administered as antithrombotic prophylaxis. At the maximum tolerated dose (lenalidomide 10 mg plus melphalan 0.18 mg/kg), 85% of patients achieved at least a PR and 23.8% immunofixation-negative CR. The 1-year event-free and overall survivals were 92% and 100%, respectively. The corresponding 1-year event-free and overall survivals were 78% and 87.4%, respectively, in historical MPT-treated control patients. Grade 3 to 4 adverse events were mainly related to hematologic toxicities (neutropenia 66%). Severe nonhematologic side effects

were less frequent and included febrile neutropenia (8%), cutaneous rash (10%), and thromboembolism (6%). Preliminary results showed that the event-free survival of patients who had deletion of chromosome 13 or chromosomal translocation (4;14) was not significantly different from those who did not have such abnormalities. By contrast, patients who had high levels of serum β2-microglobulin experienced a shorter event-free survival compared with those who showed low levels of β2-microglobulin.

Neutropenia and DVT are the major complications with lenalidomide; the addition of aspirin markedly reduced the risk for thromboembolic events in newly diagnosed patients treated with lenalidomide in association with dexamethasone or chemotherapy. Although the optimal prophylaxis strategy has not been established, aspirin seems to be the preferred choice.

Treatment of High-Risk Myeloma

Patients who have high-risk myeloma tend to do poorly with median overall survival of approximately 2 years even with tandem ASCT. One option for these patients is novel therapeutic strategies [2]. For example, bortezomib-containing regimens can be considered early in the disease course as primary therapy, with stem cell transplantation reserved for relapse. In at least three separate studies, bortezomib seems to overcome the adverse effect of deletion 13 [40,41].

Allogeneic approaches may be an option in selected patients (eg, ASCT followed by nonmyeloablative allogeneic transplantation). The recent IFM 99 trial in patients who had deletion 13 and high β2-microglobulin levels has not shown significant benefit with this strategy compared with tandem ASCT [42]. In case patients are treated similar to standard-risk patients, routine maintenance therapy should be considered (eg, thalidomide plus prednisone), given the high risk for relapse. Clearly clinical trials and new agents specifically designed for high-risk myeloma are needed.

SUMMARY

High-dose melphalan followed by ASCT in younger patients and oral MPT in the elderly are the standard of care for the initial therapy of myeloma. Survival after transplant seems to be related to the achievement of CR or VGPR. Improved response rate after induction treatment, before transplant, could translate into better results after high-dose therapy and into a prolonged survival. In younger patients, combinations incorporating thalidomide or lenalidomide or bortezomib significantly increase the pretransplant CR rate before high-dose melphalan and autologous transplantation. These combinations may further improve the CR rate achieved after transplant.

Cytogenetic abnormalities, such as deletion of chromosome 13 or chromosomal translocation (4;14), are considered negative prognostic factors. Unfortunately, most of the studies reported to date have not prospectively stratified patients based on cytogenetic abnormalities, making a firm conclusion difficult. In patients treated with MPV, and in a smaller cohort of patients treated with MPR, the event-free survival of patients who had deletion of chromosome

13 or chromosomal translocation (4;14) was not significantly different from those who did not show such abnormalities. If these data are confirmed, it seems likely that a cytogenetically adapted strategy will represent the most rational, molecularly targeted approach to myeloma therapy.

References

[1] Kyle RA, Rajkumar SV. Multiple myeloma. N Engl J Med 2004;351:1860–73.

[2] Rajkumar SV, Kyle RA. Multiple myeloma: diagnosis and treatment. Mayo Clin Proc 2005;80:1371–82.

[3] Kyle RA, Therneau TM, Rajkumar SV, et al. A long-term study of prognosis of monoclonal gammopathy of undetermined significance. N Engl J Med 2002;346:564–9.

[4] Kyle RA, Therneau TM, Rajkumar SV, et al. Prevalence of monoclonal gammopathy of undetermined significance. N Engl J Med 2006;354:1362–9.

[5] Ries LAG, Eisner MP, Kosary CL, et al, editors. SEER cancer statistics review, 1975–2000. Bethesda (MD): National Cancer Institute. Available at: http://seer.cancer.gov//csr/1975_2001. Accessed September 7, 2004.

[6] Kyle RA, Gertz MA, Witzig TE, et al. Review of 1,027 patients with newly diagnosed multiple myeloma. Mayo Clin Proc 2003;78:21–33.

[7] Cavo M, Zamagni E, Tosi P, et al. Superiority of thalidomide and dexamethasone over vincristine-doxorubicin-dexamethasone (VAD) as primary therapy in preparation for autologous transplantation for multiple myeloma. Blood 2005;106:35–9.

[8] Fermand J-P, Jaccard A, Macro M, et al. A randomized comparison of dexamethasone + thalidomide (Dex/Thal) vs Dex + Placebo (Dex/P) in patients (pts) with relapsing multiple myeloma (MM). Blood 2006;108:3563.

[9] Macro M, Divine M, Uzunhan Y, et al. Dexamethasone + thalidomide (Dex/Thal) compared to VAD as a pre-transplant treatment in newly diagnosed multiple myeloma (MM): a randomized trial. Blood 2006;108:57.

[10] Barlogie B, Tricot G, Anaissie E, et al. Thalidomide and hematopoietic-cell transplantation for multiple myeloma. N Engl J Med 2006;354:1021–30.

[11] Rajkumar SV, Blood E, Vesole DH, et al. Phase III clinical trial of thalidomide plus dexamethasone compared with dexamethasone alone in newly diagnosed multiple myeloma: a clinical trial coordinated by the Eastern Cooperative Oncology Group. J Clin Oncol 2006;24:431–6.

[12] Singhal S, Mehta J, Desikan R, et al. Antitumor activity of thalidomide in refractory multiple myeloma [see comments]. N Engl J Med 1999;341:1565–71.

[13] Rajkumar SV, Hayman S, Gertz MA, et al. Combination therapy with thalidomide plus dexamethasone for newly diagnosed myeloma. J Clin Oncol 2002;20:4319–23.

[14] Weber DM, Gavino M, Delasalle K, et al. Thalidomide alone or with dexamethasone for multiple myeloma. Blood 1999;94(Suppl 1):604a, (A 2686).

[15] Cavo M, Zamagni E, Tosi P, et al. First-line therapy with thalidomide and dexamethasone in preparation for autologous stem cell transplantation for multiple myeloma. Haematologica 2004;89:826–31.

[16] Rajkumar SV, Hussein M, Catalano J, et al. A randomized, double-blind, placebo-controlled trial of thalidomide plus dexamethasone versus dexamethasone alone as primary therapy for newly diagnosed multiple myeloma. Blood 2006;108:795.

[17] Richardson PG, Blood E, Mitsiades CS, et al. A randomized phase 2 study of lenalidomide therapy for patients with relapsed or relapsed and refractory multiple myeloma 10.1182/blood-2006-04-015909. Blood 2006;108:3458–64.

[18] Dimopoulos MA, Spencer A, Attal M, et al. Study of lenalidomide plus dexamethasone versus dexamethasone alone in relapsed or refractory multiple myeloma (MM): results of a phase 3 study (MM-010). Blood 2005;106:6.

[19] Weber DM, Chen C, Niesvizky R, et al. Lenalidomide plus high-dose dexamethasone provides improved overall survival compared to high-dose dexamethasone alone for relapsed

or refractory multiple myeloma (MM): results of a North American phase III study (MM-009). Proceedings of the American Society of Clinical Oncology 2006;24:A7521.

[20] Rajkumar SV, Hayman SR, Lacy MQ, et al. Combination therapy with lenalidomide plus dexamethasone (Rev/Dex) for newly diagnosed myeloma. Blood 2005;106: 4050–3.

[21] Lacy M, Gertz M, Dispenzieri A, et al. Lenalidomide plus dexamethasone (Rev/Dex) in newly diagnosed myeloma: response to therapy, time to progression, and survival. Blood 2006;108:798.

[22] Rajkumar SV, Jacobus S, Callander N, et al. A randomized phase III trial of lenalidomide plus high-dose dexamethasone versus lenalidomide plus low-dose dexamethasone in newly diagnosed multiple myeloma (E4A03): a trial coordinated by the Eastern Cooperative Oncology Group. Blood 2006;108:799.

[23] Richardson PG, Barlogie B, Berenson J, et al. A phase 2 study of bortezomib in relapsed, refractory myeloma. N Engl J Med 2003;348:2609–17.

[24] Richardson PG, Sonneveld P, Schuster MW, et al. Bortezomib or high-dose dexamethasone for relapsed multiple myeloma [see comment]. N Engl J Med 2005;352:2487–98.

[25] Richardson PG, Chanan-Khan A, Schlossman RL, et al. Phase II trial of single agent bortezomib (VELCADE®) in patients with previously untreated multiple myeloma (MM). Blood 2004;104:100a (A336).

[26] Jagannath S, Durie BG, Wolf J, et al. Bortezomib therapy alone and in combination with dexamethasone for previously untreated symptomatic multiple myeloma. Br J Haematol 2005;129:776–83.

[27] Harousseau J, Attal M, Leleu X, et al. Bortezomib plus dexamethasone as induction treatment prior to autologous stem cell transplantation in patients with newly diagnosed multiple myeloma: results of an IFM phase II study. Haematologica 2006;91:1498–505.

[28] Harousseau J-L, Marit G, Caillot D, et al. VELCADE/dexamethasone (Vel/Dex) versus VAD as induction treatment prior to autologous stem cell transplantation (ASCT) in newly diagnosed multiple myeloma (MM): an interim analysis of the IFM 2005-01 randomized multicenter phase III trial. Blood 2006;108:56.

[29] Bruno B, Rotta M, Patriarca F, et al. A comparison of allografting with autografting for newly diagnosed myeloma. N Engl J Med 2007;356:1110–20.

[30] Berenson JR, Crowley J, Grogan TM, et al. Maintenance therapy with alternate-day prednisone improves survival in multiple myeloma patients. Blood 2002;99(9):3163–8.

[31] Attal M, Harousseau JL, Leyvraz S, et al. Maintenance therapy with thalidomide improves survival in patients with multiple myeloma. Blood 2006;108(10):3289–94.

[32] Spencer A, Prince M, Roberts AW, et al. First analysis of the Australasian Leukaemia and Lymphoma Group (ALLG) trial of thalidomide and alternate day prednisolone following autologous stem cell transplantation (ASCT) for patients with multiple myeloma (ALLG MM6). Blood 2006;108:58a.

[33] Facon T, Mary JY, Pegourie B, et al. Dexamethasone-based regimens versus melphalan-prednisone for elderly multiple myeloma patients ineligible for high-dose therapy. Blood 2006;107(4):1292–8.

[34] Palumbo A, Bringhen S, Petrucci MT, et al. Intermediate-dose melphalan improves survival of myeloma patients aged 50 to 70: results of a randomized controlled trial. Blood 2004;104(10):3052–7.

[35] Facon T, Mary J, Harousseau J, et al. Superiority of melphalan-prednisone (MP) + thalidomide (THAL) over MP and autologous stem cell transplantation in the treatment of newly diagnosed elderly patients with multiple myeloma. J Clin Oncol 2006;24(18S):1a.

[36] Palumbo A, Bringhen S, Caravita T, et al. Oral melphalan and prednisone chemotherapy plus thalidomide compared with melphalan and prednisone alone in elderly patients with multiple myeloma: randomised controlled trial. Lancet 2006;367:825–31.

[37] Bennet CL, Angelotta C, Yarnold PR, et al. Thalidomide and lenalidomide-associated thromboembolism among patients with cancer. JAMA 2006;296:2559–60.

[38] Mateos MV, Hernandez JM, Hernandez MT, et al. Bortezomib plus melphalan and prednisone in elderly untreated patients with multiple myeloma: results of a multicenter phase I/II study. Blood 2006;108:2165–72.

[39] Palumbo A, Falco P, Falcone A, et al. Oral revlimid plus melphalan and prednisone (R-MP) for newly diagnosed multiple myeloma: a phase I-II study. Blood 2006;108(11):800a.

[40] Jagannath S, Richardson PG, Sonneveld P, et al. Bortezomib appears to overcome the poor prognosis conferred by chromosome 13 deletion in phase 2 and 3 trials. Leukemia 2006;21:151–7.

[41] Sagaster V, Ludwig H, Kaufmann H, et al. Bortezomib in relapsed multiple myeloma: response rates and duration of response are independent of a chromosome 13q-deletion. Leukemia 2006;21:164–8.

[42] Garban F, Attal M, Michallet M, et al. Prospective comparison of autologous stem cell transplantation followed by dose-reduced allograft (IFM99-03 trial) with tandem autologous stem cell transplantation (IFM99-04 trial) in high-risk de novo multiple myeloma 10.1182/blood-2005-09-3869. Blood 2006;107:3474–80.

Hematol Oncol Clin N Am 21 (2007) 1157–1174

HEMAT●L■GY/ON●●L■GY ■LINICS
OF NORTH AMERICA

Role of Stem Cell Transplantation

Jean-Luc Harousseau, MD

Centre Hospitalier Universitaire Hôtel-Dieu, Place Alexis Ricordeau, 44093 Nantes Cedex 01, France

Hematopoietic stem cell transplantation (SCT) was introduced in the treatment of multiple myeloma (MM) in the 1980s [1,2], but almost 25 years later its role is still controversial. In the autologous setting, the use of peripheral blood stem cells instead of bone marrow has markedly improved feasibility; in newly diagnosed patients, transplant-related mortality (TRM) is 1% to 2% in fit patients who have normal renal function and are younger than 65 years of age. In this group of patients, randomized studies have shown the superiority of autologous stem cell transplantation (ASCT) compared with conventional chemotherapy (CC). ASCT is now considered the standard of care in this population of patients. It is currently challenged, however, by the introduction of novel agents, such as thalidomide, bortezomib, and lenalidomide.

In the allogeneic setting, the immunologic effect of donor's lymphoid cells, the so-called "graft-versus-myeloma" (GVM) effect, explains some long remissions and possible cures. The major issue, however, is TRM, mostly related to conditioning regimen toxicity and to graft-versus-host disease (GVHD). Reduced-intensity conditioning (RIC) allogeneic SCT was developed with the goal of reducing TRM while harnessing the GVM effect. There is a close relationship between GVM and GVHD, however, and regimens that induce less GVHD are associated with more relapses. The role of allogeneic SCT therefore remains controversial.

AUTOLOGOUS STEM CELL TRANSPLANTATION
Randomized Studies Comparing Conventional Chemotherapy and Autologous Stem Cell Transplantation

The Intergroupe Francophone du Myélome (IFM) was the first to conduct a randomized trial showing the superiority of high-dose therapy (HDT) with ASCT compared with CC. In this IFM 90 trial, HDT significantly improved the response rate, event-free survival (EFS), and overall survival (OS) [3]. Similar results were published 7 years later by the British Medical Research

E-mail address: jean-luc.harousseau@univ-nantes.fr

0889-8588/07/$ – see front matter
doi:10.1016/j.hoc.2007.08.001

Council [4]. As a consequence of these two studies, ASCT has been proposed worldwide as part of frontline therapy. Two other randomized studies showed a longer EFS and time without symptoms, treatment, and treatment toxicity in the ASCT compared with the CC arm, but no benefit in OS [5,6].

Another important finding from the IFM 90 trial was the strong relationship between quality of response and OS. Patients achieving complete remission (CR) or at least very good partial remission (VGPR) had a longer OS than patients who had only partial remission (PR) [3]. This finding led to two important changes in the management of patients who had MM.

> CR (or at least VGPR) achievement is now considered an objective of any treatment.
> Response criteria have been redefined to introduce CR and VGPR that were rarely obtained previously with CC [7,8].

Two more recent studies raised concerns because of the lack of significant survival benefit from ASCT compared with CC [9,10]. In the first study from Spain, only patients whose disease responded to initial chemotherapy were randomized to undergo ASCT or further chemotherapy [9]. Although the CR rate was higher in the ASCT arm (30% versus 11%) no difference was seen in EFS and OS. Compared with other studies in which randomization occurred at diagnosis, the design of this trial introduced a selection bias, and only 75% of the patients entering the study were randomized. This fact is important, because ASCT is a useful salvage treatment for patients who have primary refractory MM [11,12]. In the US Intergroup study, there was also a possible selection bias [10]. Because randomization occurred after induction chemotherapy, only 516 of 813 registered patients were randomized and only 424 actually underwent the assigned therapy. No difference in response rate, EFS, and OS was seen between the two arms. Although results achieved with ASCT are quite comparable to those achieved in the IFM 90 trial, results of chemotherapy were much better (Table 1). Of special interest is the CR rate achieved with CC, which was much better that in the French trial and almost identical to that achieved with ASCT.

The following conclusions can be drawn from these randomized studies.

> ASCT should not be offered only to patients responding to their initial chemotherapy but also to patients who have primary refractory multiple myeloma.

Table 1
Comparison of the Intergroupe Francophone du Myélome 90 trial and the US Intergroup S9321 trial

	CR rate		7-year EFS		7-year OS	
	CC (%)	ASCT (%)	CC (%)	ASCT (%)	CC (%)	ASCT (%)
IFM 90	5	22	8	16	27	43
S9321	17	17	16	17	42	37

> ASCT improves the outcome mostly by increasing the CR + VGPR rate.
> ASCT is generally superior to standard CC; when results of CC improve, the benefit of ASCT may be less significant.

Comparing CC with ASCT is no longer a relevant question, however, because results of ASCT have already improved compared with those achieved in the 1990s. Two different approaches have contributed to this improvement in the past few years: further dose intensification and introduction of novel agents.

Double Autologous Stem Cell Transplantation

The first step in improving results of ASCT was the introduction of double-intensive therapy with the objective of increasing the CR rate [13]. The Little Rock Group developed a double ASCT program, which yielded encouraging median EFS and OS of 43 months and 68 months, respectively, in newly diagnosed patients [14].

The IFM was again the first to conduct a randomized trial comparing single and double ASCT in 599 patients up to 60 years of age [15]. On an intent-to-treat basis, the 7-year EFS and OS were significantly improved in the double ASCT arm (20% versus 10% and 42% versus 21% respectively). Available results of three other randomized studies also show a significantly better EFS with double-intensive ASCT, but do not confirm OS benefit [16–18].

Although the IFM 94 trial confirmed the feasibility of double ASCT because 75% of patients underwent the second ASCT and the toxic death rate was less than 5%, many investigators considered the benefit of this approach to be marginal and were concerned by the cost and morbidity. Defining which patients benefited more from this aggressive management therefore seemed important. In the IFM 94 trial, the only parameter to define patients who did not benefit from double ASCT was response to the first ASCT. Patients who had less than 90% reduction of their M-component after one ASCT had a longer OS in the double ASCT arm, whereas patients experiencing CR or VGPR after the first ASCT had the same OS with or without the second ASCT.

Two groups tried to improve results of double ASCT by further dose intensification. In the Arkansas Total Therapy 2 program, including intensified induction, double ASCT, and consolidation, patients were randomized to either receive or not receive thalidomide from initiation of treatment [19]. Comparison of 345 patients in the no-thalidomide arm and 231 patients previously treated in the less-intensive double ASCT Total Therapy 1 program showed that the CR rates were identical (43% versus 41%), but the 5-year EFS (43% versus 28%; $P<.1$) was superior in the Total Therapy 2 program. This finding translated into a trend for improved OS (62% versus 57%; $P=.11$). Although not randomized, this comparison favors the more intensive regimen, and particularly post-ASCT consolidation. The IFM also proposed a more intensive regimen in the IFM 99 trial, but only for patients who had poor risk factors (high $\beta2$ microglobulin level and del 13 using fluorescence in situ hybridization [FISH] analysis) [20]. This subgroup of 219 patients underwent double ASCT with an increased dose of melphalan (220 mg/m^2) before the second procedure.

The CR + VGPR rate increased from 34% after one ASCT to 51% after two ASCTs, which translated into encouraging median EFS and OS (30 and 41 months), respectively. These results seemed to be superior to those achieved previously in high-risk patients.

In the absence of randomized trials, however, there is no convincing evidence that further dose intensification is superior to double ASCT.

Novel Agents in Combination with Autologous Stem Cell Transplantation

Another possibility to improve results of ASCT is to use the three novel agents that have been introduced in the past few years in the anti-myeloma armamentarium (thalidomide, bortezomib and lenalidomide). Novel agents have been evaluated either before or after ASCT.

Novel Agents as Induction Treatment Before Autologous Stem Cell Transplantation

The primary objective of novel agents given in this context is to increase the CR rate, not only before but also after ASCT. The increased CR rate could be converted into longer EFS and OS. Another interest would be to reduce the proportion of patients needing a second ASCT because of achieving less than VGPR after the first. Thalidomide was the first novel agent to be used in this setting, either in combination with dexamethasone (TD) compared with dexamethasone alone or to vincristine, adriamycin, dexamthasone (VAD) or in combination with adriamycin and dexamethasone and compared with VAD. The results of these comparisons are in Table 2 [21–24].

In all studies, TD or thalidomide, adriamycin, dexamethasone (TAD) was superior to dexamethasone alone or VAD in response rate. The thalidomide-based regimens did not increase the CR rate before ASCT or, until now, after

Table 2
Thalidomide-based regimens before autologous stem cell transplantation

	TD versus D[a]	TD versus VAD[b]	TAD versus VAD[a]	TD versus VAD[a]
Author	Rajkumar et al [21]	Cavo et al [22]	Goldschmidt et al [23]	Macro et al [24]
N	201	200	406	204
Response	RR: 69% versus 51%	RR: 76% versus 52%	RR: 73% versus 60%	VGPR 35% versus 17%
Before ASCT	No ≠ce in CR rate	No ≠ce in CR rate	No ≠ce in CR rate	
Response after ASCT	—	—	CR 19% versus 13%	VGPR 44% versus 42%
DVT	17% versus 3%	15% versus 2%	8% versus 4%[c]	23% versus 7.5%

Abbreviations: ≠ce, difference; A, Adriamycin; CR, complete remission; D, dexamethasone; DVT, deep vein thrombosis; RR, response rate; T, thalidomide; V, vincristine; VGPR, very good partial remission.
[a]Randomized studies.
[b]Historic control.
[c]Low molecular weight heparin prophylaxis.

ASCT. Moreover, these combinations with thalidomide induced a high incidence of deep vein thrombosis.

Bortezomib has more recently been evaluated as induction treatment before ASCT. Several nonrandomized studies have been performed with bortezomib combined with dexamethasone or included into multiagent combinations (Table 3) [25–28]. The preliminary results show very high response rates

Table 3
Bortezomib-based combinations before autologous stem cell transplantation

Author	Treatment	Number of patients	Response before ASCT	Response after ASCT	Peripheral neuropathy
Jagannath et al [25]	1.3 mg/m^2 D1, 4, 8, 11	32	RR = 88%	—	31%
	Dex 40 mg D 1–2, 4–5, 8–9		CR = 6%		Grade 36%
	<PR on cycle 2 or <CR or cycle 4		nCR = 19%		
Oakervee et al [26]	B 1.3 mg/m^2 D1, 4, 8, 11	21	RR = 95%	CR = 43%	48% grade
	A escalating doses 0, 4.5, or 9 mg/m^2		CR = 24%	CR + nCR = 57%	35%
	D1–4		nCR = 5%	CR + nCR = VGR = 81%	
	Dex 40 mg D1–4, D8–11 and 15–18 cycle 1, D1–4 cycles 2–4		VGPR = 33%		
Popat et al [27]	B 1 mg/m^2 D 1, 4, 8, 11	19	RR = 89%	RR = 100%	16% grade
	A Dex as in 9 mg/m^2 D1–4		CR = 11%	CR + nCR = 54%	30%
			Ncr = 5% VGPR = 26%		
Harousseau and Attal [28]	B 1.3 mg/m^2 D 1, 4, 8, 11	48	RR = 66%	RR = 40%	30% grade
	Dex 40 mg D1–4, 8–11 On cycle 1–2, D1–4 m cycles 3–4		CR + nCR = 21% VGPR = 10%	CR + VGPR = 54%	6%

Abbreviations: A, Adriamycin; B, bortezomib; CR, complete remission (immunofixations negative); Dex, dexamethasone; n-CR, near complete remission (immunofixations positive); RR, response rate; VGPR, very good partial remission.

(66%–95%) and an apparent increase in the CR + VGPR rate before ASCT (31%–64%). These CR + VGPR rates are comparable to those achieved with single ASCT, and could be converted to even higher CR + VGPR rates (54%–81%) after ASCT. Only randomized trials could demonstrate the superiority of bortezomib-containing regimens compared with dexamethasone alone or VAD and are currently ongoing. With the usual dose of 1.3 mg/m^2 of bortezomib, the incidence of peripheral neuropathy is 30% to 48%, but grade 3 neuropathy is rare. Combinations of bortezomib and thalidomide with either dexamethasone or chemotherapy induce rapid responses [29,30]. With these regimens, novel agents can be used at lower doses or for shorter duration to reduce the risk for toxicity, in particular of peripheral neuropathy.

Lenalidomide plus dexamethasone is currently being evaluated as primary treatment of MM. In patients who are candidates for ASCT, this combination seems very active also, and does not preclude stem cell collection [31].

Novel Agents as Maintenance After Autologous Stem Cell Transplantation

In the IFM 99-02 trial, thalidomide was evaluated as maintenance therapy after double ASCT in patients younger than 65 years who had standard prognosis (0 or 1 adverse prognostic factors defined as b2-microglobulin >3 mg/L or del 13 using FISH analysis) [32]. In this three-arm study, 597 patients experiencing response to double ASCT were randomly assigned to no further treatment or pamidronate or pamidronate plus thalidomide.

The 3-year EFS was 52% in the thalidomide arm versus 36% in the control arm and 37% in the pamidronate arm (P<.003), and the 4-year OS was 87% in the thalidomide arm versus 77% and 74% in the other 2 arms (P<.01). Although deep vein thrombosis was rare (2%) because thalidomide was used alone, peripheral neuropathy was noted in 68% of patients, and was the main reason for drug discontinuation. The median dose of thalidomide in this study was 200 mg/d, and the median duration of treatment was 15 months.

These results were recently confirmed by an Australian cooperative randomized study comparing thalidomide plus prednisone versus prednisone [33]. The preliminary results also show a benefit of the thalidomide arm in CR (24% versus 15%; P<.01), 2-year EFS (66% versus 40%; $P = .0005$), and 2-year OS (91% versus 80%; $P = .02$).

In the Total Therapy 2 program, 323 patients were randomly assigned to receive thalidomide from the onset until disease progression or adverse event, and were compared with 345 patients who did not receive thalidomide [34]. The thalidomide arm showed a significantly superior CR (62% versus 43%; P<.001) and a better 5-year EFS rate (56% versus 41%; $P = .01$); however, no difference was seen in the 5-year OS (65% in both groups) because of a shorter survival after relapse (median 1.1 versus 2.7 years; $P = .001$). Relapses in the thalidomide arm seemed to be more resistant than those in the control arm. Moreover, the combination of chemotherapy and thalidomide during induction treatment induced a high incidence of deep vein thrombosis (30%), and a peripheral neuropathy of grade greater than 2 was observed in 27% of patients.

These results raise the question of the optimal dose and duration of thalidomide in this setting. In the IFM 95-02 and in the Australian studies, thalidomide was given only after ASCT, whereas in the Arkansas study thalidomide was also given before ASCT. In the Australian study, the daily dose of thalidomide was 200 mg. In the American and French studies, the initial dose was 400 mg/d.

The benefit from thalidomide maintenance in the IFM 99-02 trial was significant only in patients who were not in CR or VGPR after the second ASCT, and was therefore mostly caused by an increase of the CR + VGPR (from 50% after two ASCTs to 68%). This observation could mean that post-ASCT thalidomide is mostly useful by increasing the CR rate. If confirmed by other studies, this could encourage use of thalidomide as a post-ASCT consolidation treatment for a limited period of time because responses to thalidomide are usually rapid.

Ongoing studies are evaluating the impact of bortezomib and lenalidomide in this setting.

Which Patients Benefit From Autologous Stem Cell Transplantation

Randomized studies showing the superiority of ASCT compared with CC have been performed in patients aged 65 years or less who had normal renal function. Although ASCT is feasible in selected patients older than 65 years of age [35], the usual preparative regimen (melphalan 200 mg/m^2) may be too toxic, especially for patients older than age 70 [36].

Palumbo and colleagues [37] showed that two to three courses of melphalan 100 mg/m^2 supported by ASCT were feasible in patients up to 75 years of age and were superior to CC, using the classic regimen melphalan-prednisone (MP) [38]. The IFM group failed to confirm this finding, however [39]. In the three-arm randomized IFM 9906 trial for patients aged 65 to 75, this regimen gave a higher CR rate than MP, but PFS and OS were not significantly superior. The combination of MP plus thalidomide was significantly superior. Results of this IFM study do not support the use of ASCT in older patients outside the context of a clinical trial.

Although ASCT is feasible in patients who have renal failure, the preparative regimen is more toxic and no randomized trial has evaluated the impact of ASCT compared with CC [40–42]. ASCT should therefore not be performed in patients who have end-stage renal failure outside the setting of a clinical trial.

Several prognostic factors have been defined in the context of ASCT, including biologic characteristics and cytogenetic abnormalities [14,43]. Although patients who have a low β2 microglobulin level but no deletion 13 have prolonged EFS [44–46], patients who have a high β2 microglobulin level and unfavorable cytogenetics (deletion 13 or hypodiploidy) have a poor outcome, even with double ASCT [44,47].

Prognostic impact of cytogenetic abnormalities in the context of ASCT has been recently reevaluated. Besides chromosome 13 deletion/monosomy, two other frequent abnormalities are associated with a poor prognosis: t (4; 14) and del (17p), which have been identified in 14% to 15% and 10% to 11% of cases, respectively. Patients who have these abnormalities have significantly shorter EFS and OS, despite HDT and ASCT [48–51]. Interestingly t (4; 14) and del (17 p) are often associated with del [13], and it seems that most of the negative impact of del [13] is related to t (4; 14) and del (17 p) [52]. In multivariate analysis of the IFM 99 trials (with double transplantation for all patients) del [13] was not found to be an independent prognostic factor, and in patients who did not have t (4; 14) and del (17 p) there was no statistically significant difference between patients who had or did not have del [13].

Finally, the combination of β2 microglobulin level or International Strategy System and assessment of t (4; 14) and del (17 p) seemed to be the most important prognostic factor [52].

Patients who had a high β2 microglobulin level and one of these abnormalities had a very poor outcome, even with double ASCT. In these patients, novel approaches are clearly needed and the role of bortezomib and lenalidomide is currently being evaluated in this subgroup of patients.

Are Novel Agents Going to Replace Autologous Stem Cell Transplant?

The IFM and the Italian group have compared MP with the same combination plus thalidomide in patients older than 65 years of age [39,53]. In both studies the response rate (including CR rate) and EFS were superior in the thalidomide arm. The OS was also longer in the thalidomide arm, although the difference was not yet significant at the time of publication in the Italian study. The logical consequence of these studies is that MP should no longer be considered the standard of care for older patients. These results also question the value of ASCT, because MP-thalidomide used in older patients yielded CR and EFS rates that are comparable to those achieved in younger patients who had HDT plus ASCT.

Other combinations with bortezomib (MPV) or with lenalidomide (MPR or revlimid dexamethasone [RD]) also yield high CR rates and encouraging short-term EFS (Table 4) [54–56].

Although these results are interesting, they do not indicate an end of ASCT for several reasons:

In the past, the arguments against ASCT were morbidity and cost. Because the combinations using novel agents have been given for at least 9 months, they have induced toxicities (peripheral neuropathy, infections, thrombosis) and are expensive.

Quality of life is an important aspect of modern treatments. Although ASCT, as a "single short" treatment, induces a severe impairment of quality of life during the short period following HDT, prolonged treatment with novel agents could also induce a delayed quality-of-life impairment.

Results of combinations including novel agents are generally compared with results achieved in the 1990s with single ASCT. But results of ASCT have recently improved, especially with double ASCT and with introduction of novel agents (Table 5).

Table 4
Combinations including novel agents as primary treatment

Author	Regimen	Number of patients	Age	CR	CR + VGPR	CR + PR	EFS
Facon et al [39]	MPT	125	65–75	16%	50%	81%	Median 28 mo
Palumbo et al [53]	MPT	129	60–85	16%	36%	76%	54% at 2 y
Mateos et al [54]	MPV	60	>65	32%	43%	89%	82% at 16 mo
Palumbo et al [55]	MPR	54	Median 71	24%	48%	81%	87% at 16 mo
Lacy et al [56]	RD	34	Median 34	18%	56%	91%	59% at 2 y

Abbreviations: CR, complete remission; EFS, event-free survival; M, melphalan; P, prednisone; PR, partial remission; R, Revlimid; T, thalidomide; V, Velcade; VGPR, very good partial remission.

Rather than comparing ASCT with novel agents, therefore, it is more useful to combine ASCT with novel agents to further increase the CR rate, to reduce the need for a second ASCT, and to prolong remission duration. Another possibility could be to compare novel agents plus early versus late ASCT.

ALLOGENEIC STEM CELL TRANSPLANTATION
Myeloablative Conditioning Regimens
Allogeneic SCT following myeloablative preparative regimens can induce molecular remissions [57], and about one third of the patients remain free of disease 6 years later [58]. Allogeneic SCT seems to be the only available therapy with a potential for cure or long-term disease control in at least some patients. Toxicity is excessively high, however, with TRM of up to 50% in some studies of previously treated patients [58–60]. Mortality is mostly related to infections and to GVHD-related complications. As a consequence of this toxicity, allogeneic SCT is not proposed for patients older than 50 to 55

Table 5
Comparison of results achieved with melphalan, prednisone, and thalidomide and with autologous stem cell transplantation

	MPT Palumbo [38]	MPT Facon [39]	IFM 99 trials (unpublished data)	TT Barlogie [36] (thalidomide arm)
CR	16%	16%	32%[a]	62%
EFS	54% at 2 y	Median 28 mo	Median 39 mo	56% at 5 y
OS	80% at 3 y	NR at 56 mo	62% at 5 y	65% at 5 y

[a] CR + n CR.

years. Because the median age at diagnosis is older than 65 years, only a small minority of younger patients who have an HLA-identical sibling are eligible for this approach. Moreover, because toxic deaths occurred mostly during the first year, short term comparisons of allogeneic SCT and ASCT are in favor of ASCT [61,62].

An improvement of outcome was observed when allogeneic SCT was proposed at earlier stages. A retrospective survey of the European Blood and Marrow Transplantation (EBMT) registry showed that survival was significantly better in patients transplanted between 1994 and 1998, compared with patients transplanted before 1994 [63]. This result was attributable to a lower toxic death rate, but was not explained by a change in the source of hematopoietic stem cells (peripheral blood versus marrow) or by the use of T-cell depletion. The only explanation for a reduced TRM was a better selection of patients, with earlier transplantations, in less heavily pretreated patients. Even in newly diagnosed patients toxicity was considered too high, however. In the US Intergroup trial comparing ASCT and CC, patients up to the age of 55 and having a matched sibling were offered an allogeneic transplantation with myeloablative conditioning. This arm was prematurely closed after 36 patients were treated, because of a TRM rate of 53% [10].

Another way to decrease TRM could have been T-cell depletion, because many toxic deaths were related to GVHD. Unfortunately, a Dutch prospective study using variable levels of T-cell depletion showed very poor results with a high toxic death rate and a high early relapse rate [64].

Allogeneic bone marrow transplantation after myeloablative conditioning regimen is therefore considered too risky by a large majority of investigators and is currently almost abandoned.

Reduced Intensity Conditioning Regimens

Much of the clinical impact of allogeneic SCT has been attributed to the immunologic effect of donor lymphoid cells, the GVM effect. Proof of the GVM effect was obtained by the occurrence of remissions following donor lymphocyte infusions in patients relapsing after allogeneic SCT [65–67]. The GVM effect was actually often associated with GVHD [68,69]. This antitumor effect of donor immunocompetent cells is the basis of the introduction of RIC allogeneic SCT in a variety of hematologic malignancies, including MM. The principle of RIC allogeneic transplantation is to reduce transplant-related toxicity while harnessing GVM effect. RIC allotransplantation therefore represents a new hope in MM. Several pilot studies have been performed and are summarized in Table 6 [70–76]. These studies confirm the feasibility of RIC allogeneic transplantation in MM. When the information was available, full chimerism was obtained in virtually all patients. Overall TRM was usually in the range of 15% to 20%. The rate of a GVHD (grade II–IV) was between 25% and 46%, and overall GVHD occurred in 27% to 70%. The CR rate varied from 10% to 35%, and short-term OS (usually 2-year) ranged from 30% to 71%.

Table 6
Reduced intensity conditioning allogeneic transplantation in multiple myeloma

Author	Number of patients (unrelated donors)	Conditioning regimen	GVHD prophylaxis	Acute GVHD (%) (II–IV)	Chronic GVHD (%)	TRM (%)	CR (%)	OS (%) (at year)
Giralt et al [70]	22 (9)	Flu Mel	Tacro MTX	46	27	41	32	30 (2)
Einsele et al [71]	22 (15)	TBI Flu C	CSA MMF	38	32	20	35	58 (2)
Peggs et al [72]	20 (8)	TBI Flu Campath	CSA MMF	25	—	15	10[a]	71 (2)
Perez-Simon et al [73]	29	Flu Mel	CSA MTX	41	51	21	28[b]	60 (2)
Mohty et al [74]	41 (0)	Bu Flu ATG	CSA MTX	36	41	17	27	62 (2)
Gerall et al [75]	52 (20)	TBI Flu	CSA MMF	37	70	17	27	4 (1.5)

Abbreviations: ATG, antithymocyte globulin; Bu, busulfan; C, cyclophosphamide; CR, complete remission; CSA, cyclosporine; Flu, fludarabine; GVHD: graft versus host disease; Mel, melphalan; MMF, mycopheno-late mofetil; MTX, methotrexate; OS, overall survival; PFS, progression-free survival; SCT, stem cell transplantation; TBI, total body irradiation; TRM, transplant-related mortality.
[a]14 received DLi for residual/progressive disease.
[b]37% with acute GVHD versus 13% without.

This preliminary experience also confirmed that RIC allogeneic SCT was possible in older patients (older than 60 years of age) and with matched unrelated donors [75,76]. Relapses were frequent, however, when RIC allotransplants were used in relapsed or refractory patients and the overall outcome was related to the status of the disease at time of transplantation. A retrospective analysis of 229 patients who received an RIC allograft for MM in 33 EBMT centers helps to define prognostic factors [77]. The outcome was not affected by either the type of conditioning regimen or by GVHD prophylaxis, although PFS was decreased in patients receiving alemtuzumab. Although 3-year PFS and OS were significantly better when RIC allotransplant was performed in first remission (34% and 67%, respectively), decreased OS was associated with chemoresistant disease and with more than one prior ASCT. Another retrospective study from the EBMT group comparing RIC and myeloablative allogeneic SCT confirmed that TRM was decreased with RIC allogeneic SCT (24% versus 37% at 2 years $P = .002$) [78]. The reduction in TRM was offset by an increase in the relapse risk, however. As a consequence, the 3-year PFS was 19% with RIC and 34.5% with myeloablative allogeneic SCT ($P = .001$); the 3-year OS was 38% versus 51%, respectively. These results suggest that the allogeneic GVM effect is not sufficient, and that there remains some benefit from HDT to reduce tumor burden. Moreover, RIC should not be proposed to patients who have advanced MM.

Tandem Autologous/Reduced-Intensity Conditioning Allogeneic Transplants

RIC allotransplantation is now mostly used after tumor burden reduction with HDT followed by ASCT. The feasibility of this approach has been shown by the Little Rock group [79]. Two groups reported their preliminary results with a planned tandem autologous RIC/allogeneic SCT approach [80,81]. Before ASCT, they used high-dose melphalan (200 g/m^2), which yields a high response rate with a low toxicity rate. Before allogeneic SCT, the Seattle group used low-dose total body irradiation (200 cGy), which had been associated with a high rate of engraftment in the canine model. The German group used an immunosuppressive regimen combining fludarabine, antithymocyte globulin, and melphalan. In both studies, the CR rate achieved after RIC allotransplantation was superior to 50%, and the early mortality rate was inferior to 10%. The 2-year PFS was 55% and the 2-year OS was 75%. Although the follow-up time was short, these results justified prospective trials comparing tandem autologous/RIC allogeneic approach with double ASCT.

Large prospective trials have been performed in the United States and in Europe but results are not yet available. Until now, only two trials have been published [82,83], and the approaches of these two studies were different. Although in the Italian study all patients who had an HLA-identical sibling were to proceed to RIC allogeneic transplantation after autologous SCT, in the French study patients were candidates to this approach only if they had two adverse prognostic factors (high β2 microglobulin level and chromosome 13 deletion by FISH analysis). Moreover, in the Italian study the conditioning regimen was based on low-dose total body irradiation, whereas in the IFM study it was based on fludarabine and antithymocyte globulin. In the two studies, the TRM was low (10% and 11%), but the overall outcome is different.

In the IFM study, the outcome of high-risk patients was not improved by the use of RIC ASCT [82]. In the updated analysis with a median follow-up of 38 months, EFS was similar in the RIC allogeneic and the double ASCT group on intention-to-treat basis (median EFS 18 months versus 22 months) and in patients who actually received the planned treatment (median EFS 21 months versus 25 months) [84]. OS was significantly longer in the double autologous SCT group because of a longer survival after relapse (59 months versus 35 months $P = .016$).

In the Italian study, the CR rate was significantly higher in the tandem autologous/RIC allogeneic group (55% versus 26%). As a consequence, at a median follow-up of 66 months the median EFS was 43 versus 33 months ($P = .07$), and the median OS has not been reached in the autologous RIC allogeneic group, whereas it is 58 months in the double ASCT group ($P = .03$). This superiority of autologous RIC is attributable to a lower rate of disease-related mortality (7% versus 43% $P<.001$), whereas the TRM was not significantly different.

There are some methodologic concerns in the Italian study, because the number of patients who did or did not have an HLA-identical sibling [79] was almost identical [83]. Moreover, the results of double ASCT are lower than expected. Nonetheless these results achieved with tandem autologous/RIC allogeneic are indeed very encouraging and justify further clinical evaluation.

Question to Be Addressed in the Near Future

The modalities of conditioning and GVHD prophylaxis are important parameters to consider to enhance GVM effect. GVM effect is closely related to GVHD, however, and efforts to reduce the risk for GVHD may increase the relapse rate.

In the Italian study, only 21 of 58 patients were still in CR after a median follow-up of 38 months. Is it possible to further improve these results? One way could be the use of donor lymphocyte infusions, but again with the risk for inducing GVHD. This method should be used early after allogeneic SCT in patients who have persistent disease without acute GVHD; after confirmed relapse the chance of achieving CR is low.

Another possibility to improve efficacy is to use novel agents after RIC allogeneic transplantation. Indeed, remissions have been achieved with thalidomide or bortezomib in patients who had residual or progressive disease after RIC allogeneic transplantation [85–88]. These agents could also be used to maintain remission after RIC allogeneic SCT [89].

RIC allogeneic SCT should probably not be offered to all patients as frontline therapy. The risks for toxicity remain too high for patients who have favorable prognostic factors. Even though TRM is reduced with RIC allogeneic SCT compared with standard myeloablative regimens, it remains at 10% to 15% for newly diagnosed patients, with an incidence of 35% to 50% chronic GVHD. In this subgroup, the very good results achieved with single or tandem ASCT could be further improved by the addition of novel therapies; therefore RIC allotransplantation should be proposed only for second-line treatment after effective tumor burden reduction.

Patients who have a poor prognosis with ASCT or CC do not have a better outcome with RIC allogeneic SCT [84]. In the German experience, patients who have 13q deletion have a lower 2-year EFS and OS than patients who do not have this abnormality [90]. In patients who have standard-risk MM, there is no available comparison of RIC allogeneic SCT with other treatments. It is hoped that results of two large prospective studies in Europe and in the United States will clarify the role of tandem autologous/RIC allogeneic SCT.

SUMMARY

The introduction of novel therapies (thalidomide, bortezomib, lenalidomide) is changing the transplantation paradigm. Prospective studies are needed to evaluate the impact of autologous and allogeneic SCT in this new era.

References

[1] Osserman EF, Dire LB, Dire J, et al. Identical twin marrow transplantation in multiple myeloma. Acta Haematol 1982;68:215–23.

[2] Barlogie B, Alexanian R, Dicke KA, et al. High-dose chemoradiotherapy and autologous bone marrow transplantation for resistant multiple myeloma. Blood 1987;70:869–72.

[3] Attal M, Harousseau JL, Stoppa AM, et al. for the Intergroupe Français du Myélome. A prospective, randomized trial of autologous bone marrow transplantation and chemotherapy in multiple myeloma. N Engl J Med 1996;335:91–7.

[4] Child JA, Morgan GJ, Davies FE, et al. Medical research Council Adult Leukemia Working Party. High-dose chemotherapy with hematopoietic stem-cell rescue for multiple myeloma. N Engl J Med 2003;348:1875–83.

[5] Fermand JP, Ravaud P, Chevret S, et al. High-dose therapy and autologous peripheral blood stem cell transplantation in multiple myeloma: up-front or rescue treatment? Results of a multicenter sequential randomized trial. Blood 1998;92:3131–6.

[6] Fermand JP, Katsahian S, Divine M, et al. High-dose therapy and autologous blood stem-cell transplantation compared with conventional treatment in myeloma patients aged 55 to 65 years: long-term results of a randomized control trial from the Groupe Myelome-Autogreffe. J Clin Oncol 2005;23:9227–33.

[7] Blade J, Samson D, Reece D, et al. Criteria for evaluating disease response and progression in patients with multiple myeloma treated by high-dose therapy and haematopoietic stem cell transplantation. Myeloma Subcommittee of the EBMT. European Group for Blood and Marrow Transplant. Br J Haematol 1998;102:1115–23.

[8] Durie BG, Harousseau JL, Miguel JS, et al. International uniform response criteria for multiple myeloma. Leukemia 2006;20:1467–73.

[9] Blade J, Rosinol L, Sureda A, et al. High-dose therapy intensification compared with continued standard chemotherapy in multiple myeloma patients responding to the initial chemotherapy: long-term results from a prospective randomized trial from the Spanish cooperative group PETHEMA. Blood 2005;106:3755–9.

[10] Barlogie B, Kyle RA, Anderson KC, et al. Standard chemotherapy compared with high-dose chemoradiotherapy for multiple myeloma: final results of phase III US Intergroup Trial S9321. J Clin Oncol 2006;24:929–36.

[11] Alexanian R, Dimopoulos MA, Hester J, et al. Early myeloablative therapy for multiple myeloma. Blood 1994;84:4278–82.

[12] Kumar S, Lacy MQ, Dispenzieri A, et al. High-dose therapy and autologous stem cell transplantation for multiple myeloma poorly responsive to initial therapy. Bone Marrow Transplant 2004;34:161–7.

[13] Harousseau JL, Milpied N, Laporte JP, et al. Double-intensive therapy in high-risk multiple myeloma. Blood 1992;79:3131–6.

[14] Barlogie B, Jagannath S, Desikan KR, et al. Total therapy with tandem transplants for newly diagnosed multiple myeloma. Blood 1999;93:55–65.

[15] Attal M, Harousseau JL, Facon T, et al. Intergroupe Francophone du Myélome: single versus double autologous stem cell transplantation for multiple myeloma. N Engl J Med 2003;349:2495–502.

[16] Sonneveld P, Van Der Holt B, Segeren CM, et al. Intensive versus double intensive therapy in untreated multiple myeloma. Updated analysis of the prospective phase III study Hovon 24-MM. Haematologica 2005;90(Suppl 1):37–8 [abstract].

[17] Cavo M, Zamagni E, Cellini C, et al. Single versus tandem autologous transplants in multiple myeloma: Italian experience. Haematologica 2005;90(Suppl 1):39–40 [abstract].

[18] Goldschmidt H. Single versus double high dose therapy in multiple myeloma: second analysis of the trial GMMG-HD2. Haematologica 2005;90(Suppl 1):38 [abstract].

[19] Barlogie B, Tricot G, Rabmussen E, et al. Total therapy 2 without thalidomide in comparison with total therapy 1: role of intensified induction and post-transplantation consolidation therapies. Blood 2006;107:2633–8.

[20] Moreau P, Hullin C, Garban F, et al. Tandem autologous stem cell transplantation in high-risk de novo multiple myeloma: final results of the prospective and randomized IFM 99-04 protocol. Blood 2006;107:397–403.

[21] Rajkumar V, Blaad E, Vesole D, et al. Phase III clinical trial of thalidomide plus dexamethasone compared with dexamethasone alone in newly diagnosed multiple myeloma: a clinical trial coordinated by the Eastern Cooperative Oncology Group. J Clin Oncol 2006;24: 431–6.

[22] Cavo M, Zamagni E, Tosi P, et al. Superiority of thalidomide and dexamethasone over vincristine-doxorubicin-dexamethasone (VAD) as primary therapy in preparation for autologous transplantation for multiple myeloma. Blood 2005;106:35–9.

[23] Goldschmidt H, Sonneveld P, Breitkreuz I, et al. HOVON 50/GMMG-HD3 trial: Phase III study on the effect of thalidomide combined with high-dose melphalan in myeloma patients up to 65 years. Blood 2005;106:128 [abstract].

[24] Macro M, Divine M, Uzunban Y, et al. Dexamethasone + thalidomide compared to VAD as pre-transplant treatment in newly diagnosed multiple myeloma: a randomized trial. Blood 2006;108:22 [abstract].

[25] Jagannath S, Durie B, Wolf J, et al. Bortezomib therapy alone and in combination with dexamethasone for previously untreated symptomatic multiple myeloma. Br J Haematol 2005;129:776–83.

[26] Oakervee HE, Pollat R, Curry N, et al. PAD combination therapy (PS341, doxorubicin and dexamethasone) for untreated multiple myeloma. Br J Haematol 2005;29:755–62.

[27] Popat R, Oakervee HE, Curry N, et al. Reduced dose PAD (PS 341, Adriamycin and dexamethasone) for previously untreated patients with multiple myeloma. Blood 2005;106:717 [abstract].

[28] Harousseau JL, Attal M. Bortezomib plus dexamethasone as induction treatment prior to autologous stem cell transplantation in patients with newly diagnosed multiple myeloma. Haematologica 2006;91:1498–505.

[29] Barlogie B, Tricot G, Rasmussen E, et al. Total therapy incorporating Velcade into upfront management of multiple myeloma: comparison with TT2 + Thalidomide. Blood 2005;106:337 [abstract].

[30] Wang M, Delaballe K, Giralt S, et al. Rapid control of previously untreated multiple myeloma with bortezomib-thalidomide-dexamethasone followed by early intensive therapy. Blood 2005;106:231 [abstract].

[31] Rajkumar SV, Hayman SR, Lacy MQ, et al. Combination therapy with lenalidomide plus dexamethasone for newly diagnosed myeloma. Blood 2005;106:4050–3.

[32] Attal M, Harousseau JL, Leyvras S, et al. Maintenance therapy with thalidomide improves survival in multiple myeloma patients. Blood 2006;15:3289–94.

[33] Spencer A, Prince M, Roberts AW, et al. First analysis of the Australian leukaemia and lymphoma group trial of thalidomide and alternate day prednisone following autologous stem cell transplantation for patients with multiple myeloma. Blood 2006;108:22 [abstract].

[34] Barlogie B, Tricot G, Anaissie E, et al. Thalidomide and hematopoietic cell transplantation for multiple myeloma. N Engl J Med 2006;354:1021–30.

[35] Siegel DS, Desikan KR, Nehta J, et al. Age is not a prognostic variable with autotransplants for multiple myeloma. Blood 1999;93:51–4.

[36] Badros A, Barlogie B, Siegel E, et al. Autologous stem cell transplantation in elderly multiple myeloma patients over the age of 70 years. Br J Haematol 2001;114:600–7.

[37] Palumbo A, Triolo S, Argentin C. Dose intensive melphalan with stem-cell support is superior to standard treatment in elderly myeloma patients. Blood 1999;94:1248–53.

[38] Palumbo A, Bringhen S, Petrucci MT, et al. Intermediate-dose melphalan improves survival of myeloma patients aged 50-70: results of a randomized controlled trial. Blood 2004;104: 3052–7.

[39] Facon T, Mary JY, Harousseau JL. Superiority of melphalan and prednisone plus thalidomide over melphalan and prednisone alone or autologous stem cell transplantation in the

treatment of newly diagnosed elderly patients with multiple myeloma. J Clin Oncol 2006;24:1s [abstract].

[40] Badros A, Barlogie B, Siegel E, et al. Results of autologous stem cell transplant in multiple myeloma patients with renal failure. Br J Haematol 2001;114:822–9.

[41] Tosi P, Zamagni E, Ronconi S, et al. Safety of autologous hematopoietic stem cell transplantation in patients with multiple myeloma and renal failure. Leukemia 2000;14:1310–3.

[42] San Miguel J, Lahuerta JJ, Garcia-Sanz R, et al. Are myeloma patients with renal failure candidate for autologous stem cell transplantation. Hematol J 2000;1:28–36.

[43] Vesole D, Tricot G, Jagannath S, et al. Autotransplant in multiple myeloma: what have we learned? Blood 1996;88:838–47.

[44] Facon T, Avet-Loiseau H, Guillerm G, et al. Chromosome 13 abnormalities identified by Fish analysis and serum b2 microglobulin produce powerful myeloma staging system for patients receiving high-dose therapy. Blood 2001;97:1566–71.

[45] Tricot G, Spencer T, Sawyer J, et al. Predicting long-term ($\geq$ 5 years) event-free survival in multiple myeloma patients following planned tandem autotransplant. Br J Haematol 2002;116:211–7.

[46] Shaughnessy J, Jacobson J, Sawyer J, et al. Continuous absence of metaphase-defined cytogenetic abnormalities especially of chromosome 13 and hypodiploidy ensures long-term survival in multiple myeloma treated with Total Therapy I: interpretation in the context of global gene expression. Blood 2003;101:3849–56.

[47] Fassas AT, Spencer T, Sawyer J, et al. Both hypodiploidy and deletion of chromosome 13 independently confer poor prognosis in multiple myeloma. Br J Haematol 2002;118:1041–7.

[48] Chang H, Sloan S, Li D, et al. The t(4;14) is associated with poor prognosis in myeloma patients undergoing autologous stem cell transplant. Br J Haematol 2004;125:64–8.

[49] Gertz M, Lacy MQ, Dispenzieri A, et al. Clinical implications of t(11;14) (q13;q32), t(4;14) (p16.3;q32), and -17p13 in myeloma patients treated with high-dose therapy. Blood 2005;106:2837–40.

[50] Jaksic W, Trudel S, Chang H, et al. Clinical outcomes in t(4;14) multiple myeloma: a chemotherapy-sensitive disease characterized by rapid relapse and alkylating agent resistance. J Clin Oncol 2005;23:7069–73.

[51] Chang H, Qi C, Yi QL, et al. p53 gene deletion detected by fluorescence in situ hybridisation is an adverse prognostic factor for patients with multiple myeloma following autologous stem cell transplantation. Blood 2005;105:358–60.

[52] Avet-Loiseau H, Attal M, Moreau P, et al. Genetic abnormalities and survival in multiple myeloma: the experience of the Intergroupe Francophone du Myélome. Blood 2007;109:3489–95.

[53] Palumbo A, Bringhen S, Caravita T, et al. Oral Melphalan and prednisone chemotherapy plus thalidomide compared with melphalan and prednisone alone in elderly patients with multiple myeloma: randomised controlled trial. Lancet 2006;367:825–31.

[54] Mateos MV, Hernandez JM, Gutierrez WC, et al. Bortezomib plus melphalan and prednisone in elderly untreated patients with multiple myeloma: results of a multicenter phase I/II study. Blood 2006;108:2165–72.

[55] Palumbo A, Falco P, Falcone A, et al. Oral Revlimid plus melphalan and prednisone for newly diagnosed multiple myeloma: results of a multicenter phase I/II study. Blood 2006; [online].

[56] Lacy M, Gertz M, Dispenzieri A, et al. Lenalidomide plus dexamethasone in newly diagnosed myeloma: response to therapy, time to progression and survival. Blood 2006;108:230 [abstract].

[57] Corradini P, Voena C, Tarella C, et al. Molecular and clinical remissions in multiple myeloma: role of autologous and allogeneic transplantation of hematopoietic cells. J Clin Oncol 1999;17:208–15.

[58] Gahrton G, Tura S, Ljungman P, et al. Prognostic factors in allogeneic bone marrow transplantation for multiple myeloma. J Clin Oncol 1995;13:1312–22.

[59] Bensinger WI, Buckner CD, Anasetti C, et al. Allogeneic marrow transplantation for multiple myeloma: an analysis of risk factors on outcome. Blood 1996;88:2787–93.

[60] Mehta J, Allogeneic hematopoietic stem cell transplantation in myeloma. In: Myeloma editions J Mehta, S Singhal. Martin Dunitz London 2002; p. 349–65.

[61] Bjorkstrand BB, Ljungman P, Svensson H, et al. Allogeneic bone marrow transplantation versus autologous stem cell transplantation in multiple myeloma: a retrospective case-matched study from the European Group for Blood and Marrow Transplantation. Blood 1996;88:4711-1718.

[62] Couban S, Stewart AK, Loach D, et al. Autologous and allogeneic transplantation for multiple myeloma. Bone Marrow Transplant 1997;19:783–9.

[63] Gahrton G, Svensson H, Cavo M, et al. Progress in allogeneic bone marrow and peripheral blood stem cell transplantation for multiple myeloma: a comparison between transplants performed 1983-93 and 1994-98 at European Group for Blood and Marrow Transplantation Centres. Br J Haematol 2001;113:209–16.

[64] Lokhorst HM, Segeren CM, Verdonck LF, et al. Partially T-cell depleted allogeneic stem-cell transplantation for first-line treatment of multiple myeloma: a prospective evaluation of patients treated in the phase III study Hovon 24 MM. J Clin Oncol 2003;21:1728–33.

[65] Tricot G, Vesole DH, Jagannath S, et al. Graft-versus myeloma effect: proof of principle. Blood 1996;87:1196–8.

[66] Verdonck L, Lokhorst H, Dekker A, et al. Graft versus myeloma effect in two cases. Lancet 1996;347:800–1.

[67] Aschan J, Lonnquist B, Ringden O, et al. Graft-versus myeloma effect. Lancet 1996;348:346.

[68] Collins RH, Shpilberg O, Drobyski WR, et al. Donor lymphocyte infusions in 140 patients with relapsed malignancies after allogeneic bone marrow transplantation. J Clin Oncol 1997;22:835–43.

[69] Lokhorst HM, Wu K, Verdonck LF, et al. The occurrence of graft versus host disease is the major predictive factor for response to donor lymphocyte infusions in multiple myeloma. Blood 2004;103:4362–4.

[70] Giralt S, Aleman A, Anagnostopoulos A, et al. Fludarabine/melphalan conditioning for allogeneic transplantation in patients with multiple myeloma. Bone Marrow Transplant 2002;30:367–73.

[71] Einsele H, Schafer HJ, Hebart H, et al. Follow-up of patients with progressive multiple myeloma undergoing allografts after reduced-intensity conditioning. Br J Haematol 2003;121:411–8.

[72] Peggs KS, Mackinnon S, Williams CD, et al. Reduced-intensity transplantation with in vivo T-cell depletion and adjuvant dose-escalating donor lymphocyte infusions for chemotherapy-sensitive myeloma: limited efficacy of graft-versus tumor activity. Biol Blood Marrow Transplant 2003;9:257–65.

[73] Perez-Simon JA, Martino R, Alegre A, et al. Chronic but not acute graft versus host disease improves outcome in multiple myeloma patients after non-myeloablative allogeneic transplantation. Br J Haematol 2003;121:104–8.

[74] Mohty M, Boiron JM, Damaj G, et al. Graft-versus myeloma effect following antithymocyte globulin-based reduced intensity conditioning allogeneic stem cell transplantation. Bone Marrow Transplant 2004;34:77–87.

[75] Gerull S, Goerner M, Benner A. Long-term outcome of non myeloablative allogeneic transplantation in patients with high-risk multiple myeloma. Bone Marrow Transplant 2005;36:963–9.

[76] Kroger N, Sayer HG, Schwerdtfeger R, et al. Unrelated stem cell transplantation in reduced-intensity conditioning with pretransplantation antithymocyte globulin is highly effective with low transplantation-related mortality. Blood 2002;100:3919–24.

[77] Crawley C, Lalancette M, Szydlo R, et al. Outcomes of reduced-intensity allogeneic transplantation for multiple myeloma: an analysis of prognostic factors from the Chronic Leukemia Working Party of the EBMT. Blood 2005;105:4532–9.

[78] Crawley C, Iacobelli S, Björkstrand B, et al. Reduced-intensity conditioning for myeloma: lower nonrelapse mortality but higher relapse rates compared with myeloablative conditioning. Blood 2007;109:3588–94.

[79] Badros A, Barlogie B, Siegel E, et al. Improved outcome of allogeneic transplantation in high-risk multiple myeloma patients after non-myeloablative conditioning. J Clin Oncol 2002;20:1295–303.

[80] Kroger N, Schwerdtfeger R, Kiehl M, et al. Autologous stem cell transplantation followed by a dose-reduced allograft induces high complete remission rate in multiple myeloma. Blood 2002;100:755–60.

[81] Maloney D, Molina A, Sahebi F, et al. Allografting with nonmyeloablative conditioning following cytoreductive autografts for the treatment of patients with multiple myeloma. Blood 2003;101:3447–54.

[82] Garban F, Attal M, Michallet M, et al. Prospective comparison of autologous stem cell transplantation followed by dose-reduced allograft (IFM 99-03 trial) with tandem autologous stem cell transplantation (IFM 99-04 trial) in high-risk de novo multiple myeloma. Blood 2006;107:3474–80.

[83] Bruno B, Rotta M, Patriarca F, et al. A comparison of allografting with autografting for newly diagnosed myeloma. N Engl J Med 2007;356:1110–20.

[84] Moreau P, Garban F, Facon T, et al. Long-term and updated results of the IFM9903 and IFM9904 protocols comparing autologous followed by RIC-allogeneic transplantation and double transplant in high-risk de novo multiple myeloma. Bone Marrow Transplant 39(Suppl 1):S24–5 [abstract].

[85] Kroger N, Shimoni A, Zagrivnaja M, et al. Low-dose thalidomide and donor lymphocyte infusions as adoptive immunotherapy after allogeneic stem cell transplantation in patients with multiple myeloma. Blood 2004;104:3361–3.

[86] Bruno B, Patriarca F, Sorasio R, et al. Bortezomib with or without dexamethasone in relapsed multiple myeloma following allogeneic hematopoietic cell transplantation. Haematologica 2006;91:837–9.

[87] Tosi P, Zamagni E, Cangini B, et al. Complete remission upon bortezomib-dexamethasone therapy in three heavily pretreated multiple myeloma patients relapsing after allogeneic stem cell transplantation. Ann Hematol 2006;85:549–58.

[88] Van de Donk NW, Kroger N, Hegenbart U, et al. Remarkable activity of novel agents bortezomib and thalidomide in patients not responding to donor lymphocyte infusions following nonmyeloablative allogeneic stem cell transplantation in multiple myeloma. Blood 2006;107:3415–6.

[89] Kroger N, Zabelina T, Ayuk F, et al. Bortezomib after dose-reduced allogeneic stem cell transplantation for multiple myeloma to enhance or maintain remission status. Exp Hematol 2006;34:770–5.

[90] Kroger N, Schilling G, Einsele H, et al. Deletion of chromosome 13q14 detected by fluorescence in situ hybridization as prognostic factor following allogeneic dose-reduced stem cell transplantation in patients with multiple myeloma. Blood 2006;103:4056–61.

Hematol Oncol Clin N Am 21 (2007) 1175–1215

HEMATOLOGY/ONCOLOGY CLINICS
OF NORTH AMERICA

Management of Relapsed and Relapsed Refractory Myeloma

Efstathios Kastritis, MD[a,1],
Constantine S. Mitsiades, MD, PhD[b,1],
Meletios A. Dimopoulos, MD[a,*], Paul G. Richardson, MD[b]

[a]Department of Clinical Therapeutics, University of Athens,
School of Medicine, 227 Kifissias Avenue, 14561 Kifissia, Athens, Greece
[b]Jerome Lipper Myeloma Center, Department of Medical Oncology, Dana-Farber Cancer Institute,
Harvard Medical School, 44 Binney Street, Boston, MA 02115, USA

Multiple myeloma (MM) has been traditionally treated with combinations of chemotherapeutic agents and glucocorticoids. Barlogie and colleagues [1] showed that the dose of melphalan could be escalated considerably and that total-body irradiation (TBI) could be added provided that previously collected autologous bone marrow cells were to be reinfused to the patient. With this approach a significant number of patients could achieve deeper responses, including complete responses [2,3]. Since then multiple studies have shown that high-dose therapy is a useful approach for many patients who have MM. Primary or secondary resistance to conventional or intensive anti-MM treatment is inevitable, however. Some patients do not respond to frontline anti-MM treatment and have been rated as having primary refractory disease. Almost all responding patients relapse, usually within 10 years of treatment initiation. When such patients experience disease progression while they are not receiving salvage anti-MM treatment or are on maintenance they are considered to have relapsed disease. Other patients respond initially to primary treatment, relapse and receive another treatment, but then progress again. Such patients who have secondary resistance are considered to have relapsed and refractory disease. For the purpose of this article, we use the term "relapsed myeloma" for patients who have initially responded and then have disease progression. In those patients, their MM may be potentially sensitive to a reinitiation of their last treatment. Patients who have primary or secondary resistance while on treatment with an active regimen (or within 60 days of completion of their last treatment) [4] are classified as having either "relapsed and refractory" or "refractory" myeloma. Over the last decade

[1]These authors contributed equally to this article.

*Corresponding author. E-mail address: mdimop@med.uoa.gr (M.A. Dimopoulos).

0889-8588/07/$ – see front matter
doi:10.1016/j.hoc.2007.08.014

the management of relapsed and refractory MM has changed considerably. This change is primarily because of the introduction in the clinical practice of three novel agents: thalidomide, bortezomib, and lenalidomide. These drugs have been administered, initially as single agents and subsequently as combinations with other anti-MM agents, to many thousands of patients who have MM refractory to standard chemotherapy with or without high-dose therapy.

CONVENTIONAL TREATMENT APPROACHES
High-Dose Dexamethasone
Dexamethasone (Dex) at pulsed high doses is used in the management of patients who have relapsed or refractory MM, but mainly for patients who are not candidates for more aggressive treatments or chemotherapy combinations. Dex doses of 40 mg per day for 4-day courses on days 1, 9, and 17 over 28-day cycles result in response rates ranging from 18% to 27% [5–8]. A phase II study by Alexanian and colleagues [5] reported that intermittent high-dose Dex in refractory MM resulted in response rates of 27% and 21% in patients unresponsive to previous treatments versus responsive ones, respectively. High-dose Dex has been the standard comparator in several recent randomized studies in relapsed/refractory MM, yielding responses rates of 18% to 21% [6–8]. Notably, the 95% confidence intervals (95% CIs) of response rates in the high-dose Dex arms of these more recent trials overlap with 95% CIs from results of earlier nonrandomized studies of high-dose Dex (P.G. Richardson and C.S. Mitsiades, unpublished observation). This finding indicates that patients in the high-dose Dex arm of contemporary trials respond to this regimen comparably to the historical experience from early trials. Intravenous pulsed methylprednisolone, 2 g three times a week, is an alternative to pulsed high-dose Dex [9].

Doxorubicin, Vincristine, and Dexamethasone
The combination of infusional doxorubicin, vincristine, and pulsed high-dose Dex (VAD) has been a widely used regimen for pretreated and untreated patients. In the initial report of this regimen, Barlogie and colleagues [10] treated 29 patients who had advanced, refractory MM. VAD treatment resulted in rapid and marked (>75%) tumor reduction in 14 of 20 patients who had disease resistant to alkylating agents and in 3 of 9 patients who had additional resistance to doxorubicin. Responses were associated with improved survival and further studies confirmed the initial results [11–16]. In a retrospective comparison, VAD was more effective than high-dose Dex alone in relapsed patients (65% versus 21%), whereas the responses were similar for refractory patients who were unresponsive to previous treatment [5]. The backbone of the regimen, doxorubicin and high-dose Dex, has been used in combinations with other chemotherapy regimens, including doxorubicin, carmustine, cyclophosphamide, and melphalan [17]; vincristine, melphalan, cyclophosphamide, prednisone, vincristine, carmustine, doxorubicin, and prednisone (VMPC/VBAP) [18]; doxorubicin, vincristine, Dex, etoposide, and cyclophosphamide (CEVAD) [19]; and

Dex, thalidomide, cisplatin, doxorubicin, cyclophosphamide, and etoposide (DT-PACE) [20]. Doxorubicin administration requires central venous access and is associated with increased risk for development of cardiomyopathy. Pegylated liposomal doxorubicin is associated with lower frequency of cardiotoxicity and less alopecia and does not require central venous access. This pegylated formulation of doxorubicin has been included in anthracycline-based combinations as an alternative to standard formulation of doxorubicin. Its safety and activity have been confirmed in the context of combination with novel agents, including thalidomide [21–23], lenalidomide [24], or bortezomib [25,26]. Conversely, its activity when combined with steroids alone has been modest. Importantly, the results of a recent international, multicenter, randomized, phase III trial comparing bortezomib with versus without pegylated liposomal doxorubicin in patients who had relapsed/refractory MM [27] led to United States Food and Drug Administration (FDA) approval of this combination regimen for the treatment of patients who have MM who have not previously received bortezomib and have received at least one prior therapy.

High-Dose Melphalan

Pioneering work from Barlogie and his colleagues [1] in the mid-1980s showed that the relationship of the clinical response to melphalan as a function of its administered dose exhibits a steep increase in responses at myeloablative doses and that such high-dose melphalan regimens are not only feasible with appropriate hematopoietic stem cell support but could also overcome resistance to conventional doses of chemotherapy in patients who have refractory MM. In their first report, 23 refractory patients received melphalan at a dose of 80 to 100 mg/m^2 (16 patients) or 140 mg/m^2 and autologous bone marrow infusion (7 patients). Although 4 patients died of complications of the procedure, 14 patients (61%) responded, albeit with short-lasting remissions in most patients. A more intensive conditioning regimen that included high-dose melphalan and TBI supported by autologous bone marrow transplantation was given in 7 patients who had refractory MM [2]. Very rapid and deep responses were achieved in 6 patients, regardless of prior chemotherapy responsiveness or bone marrow plasmacytosis. Median progression-free survival (PFS) was 15 months, and 5 patients remained alive without further cytotoxic therapy 2 to 21 months after the procedure, although 3 had early relapse and 2 died of complications. In another report Dimopoulos and colleagues [28] used thiotepa, busulfan, and cyclophosphamide as a conditioning regimen followed by autologous bone marrow or blood stem cell support. Seven of 15 patients who had primary refractory MM responded, including 1 complete response (CR) and 6 partial responses (PRs), whereas 6 did not respond and 2 died of transplant-related complications. Four of 8 patients who had relapsed refractory MM achieved a PR, 2 did not respond, and 2 died of treatment-related complications. The remissions were short (median duration of 4 months) and the median survival after transplant was only 4 months.

In a cohort of 135 patients who had refractory MM treated with high-dose therapy regimens, mortality was high in patients who received TBI or did not have ASCT. Patients who received melphalan 200 mg/m^2 with ASCT and had low β2-microglobulin levels had better outcome, with a median event-free survival (EFS) of 37 months and projected overall survival (OS) of 43 months or more. Further analysis that excluded treatment as a variable identified high β2-microglobulin and resistant relapse as the two major adverse prognostic factors. In a phase II trial conducted by the Southwest Oncology Group (SWOG) patients up to age 70 years who had refractory MM who did not have previous stem cell collection were primed with high-dose cyclophosphamide (6 g/m^2) and received high-dose therapy consisting of melphalan 200 mg/m^2 [2] with ASCT. Of the 66 assessable patients, 56 did go on to receive the transplant procedure. Thirty-seven patients received cyclophosphamide: 3 had a CR and 5 had PR. Fifty-four patients received high-dose melphalan and 16 had CR (30%) and 19 had PR (35%). The median PFS and OS were 11 months and 19 months, respectively, and 3-year actuarial PFS and OS rates were 25% and 31%, respectively.

Patients who have primary resistant disease can benefit from early myeloablative therapy [29]. The median EFS and OS of 27 patients who had primary resistant disease who received a transplant during the first year following the initiation of therapy were 3.5 and 6 years, respectively. For patients who have longstanding resistant disease high-dose melphalan may not offer any advantage [30]. In a randomized trial exploring the optimal time for high-dose therapy and autologous SCT [31], patients who received high-dose therapy up front had OS similar to that of those who received high-dose therapy as salvage. Among patients who received salvage high-dose therapy, 2-year survival rates since the beginning of up-front therapy were 59% versus 57% for those who had relapsing disease versus those who had primary refractory disease, respectively. In another comparison, patients refractory to induction therapy may achieve a good response to high-dose therapy, although with lower overall response rate (ORR) than chemosensitive patients (99% versus 90%, $P = .02$) and borderline difference in CR rates (20% versus 35%, $P = .06$). Even patients who have relapse after one or tandem autotransplantations may benefit from high dose therapy (HDT), although the depth and durability of responses are modest [32,33].

High-dose therapy with allogeneic stem cell transplantation is another option for selected patients who have an HLA-matched donor. Compared retrospectively, allogeneic transplantation may offer better PFS and OS compared with ASCT, but is associated with significantly higher treatment-related complications and mortality [33]. Nonmyeloablative approaches may have fewer complications, whereas graft-versus-MM effect may lead even to longstanding remission, although myeloablative regimens may be associated with lower relapse rates [34]. Sequential HDM with ASCT followed by nonmyeloablative allotransplants from HLA-identical siblings was encouraging when administered in mainly VAD-pretreated relapsed or refractory patients, although only a minority (8%) of patients had received prior thalidomide [35]. Donor-lymphocyte infusion at the time of relapse after allotransplant may induce durable responses, mainly in patients who experience graft-versus-host disease [36]. Patients relapsing after ASCT are often noneligible because of comorbidities, age-related limitations, or lack of an HLA-matched sibling. Prior HDT is a poor prognostic factor for treatment-related mortality in patients receiving allogeneic transplants [37].

NOVEL AGENTS

Thalidomide

Thalidomide (Thal) was first used to treat MM because of the hypothesis that its antiangiogenic properties (as identified in other disease settings, Ref. [38]) could lead to antitumor activity in MM, given the increased microvascular density in bone marrow biopsy samples of MM patients with active disease versus monoclonal gammopathy of undetermined significance [39]. The increasing understanding of the interactions of MM cells and their microenvironment allowed us to understand the mechanism of action of Thal and its immuno-modulatory analogs (IMiDs) [40,41]. These drugs, aside from their proposed antiangiogenic effects, also activate caspase-8–mediated apoptosis of MM cells; suppress production of IL-6 in the context of MM cell interactions with bone marrow stromal cells (BMSCs); sensitize MM cells to therapeutic agents that operate, at least in part, by way of caspase-9–mediated pathways (eg, Dex or bortezomib); and augment immunologic responses by activating T cells and NK cells [42–44]. Thal and IMiDs have substantial degree of overlap in their biologic and clinical functions, but also have distinct differences in potency (eg, lenalidomide is more potent than Thal) and side-effect profiles.

Single-agent thalidomide

The first clinical trial of Thal in MM was reported by Singhal and colleagues [45]: 84 patients who had relapsed/refractory MM, most of whom had relapsed after stem cell transplantation, were treated at doses ranging from 200 to 800 mg/day. Treatment resulted in a 32% response rate, including 2 patients who had complete response (CR). Responses in most of responding patients were apparent within 2 months. Updated results on 169 patients [46] were comparable with the initial report and reported a 2-year EFS and OS of 26% and 48%, respectively. Multiple trials further explored and confirmed the activity of Thal in the relapsed/refractory setting (Table 1) [46–62] with response rates ranging from 14% to 48%, whereas 28% to 66% had at least 25% decrease of their paraprotein, most within 1 to 4 months after the initiation of treatment. Deep venous thrombosis (DVT) rates in monotherapy studies were less than 5% [46,53,56]. Low plasma cell labeling index, normal cytogenetics [45,46,64], age younger than 65 years [52,62], normal levels of C-reactive protein [45,52] or LDH [45,52], and high serum albumin [63] have been reported to correlate with response to Thal.

Table 1
Studies with single-agent thalidomide in refractory relapsed multiple myeloma

Reference	Number of patients	Thal dose (mg/d)	≥PR rate (%)
Barlogie et al, [46]	169	200–800	30
Hus et al, [50]	53	200–400	36
Tosi et al, [58]	65	100–800	28
Yakoub-Agha et al, [62]	83	50–800	48
Neben et al, [53]	83	100–400	19
Grosbois et al, [63]	120	200–800	15
Mileshkin et al, [52]	75	200–1000	28
Waage et al, [59]	65	100–800	20
Schey et al, [56]	69	100–600	26
Wu et al, [61]	122	100–400	38

An optimal dose for Thal that would be applicable to all patients who have MM has not been defined, perhaps because of variable tolerability of the drug. In most early studies, Thal was started at 200 mg/d with a stepwise increase to 800 mg/d; however, only a minority of patients could tolerate such doses [45]. Higher cumulative doses of Thal (eg, >32 g to 42 g at 3 months) correlated with improved response rates in some studies [46,53,62], but not others [59], and dose escalation beyond 400 mg/d did not improve response rates but led to more frequent side effects [63]. Serum Thal levels do not seem to correlated with response [59] perhaps because Thal activity is mainly mediated by its metabolites; thus assessment of optimal dosing is difficult by means of pharmacokinetics. Yakoub-Agha and colleagues [65] randomized patients who had relapsed or refractory disease in two doses: 100 mg/d versus 400 mg/d. Dex was added to patients who had not responded after 3 months of Thal treatment. Although Dex was added more frequently in the 100 mg/d arm, overall survival at 1 year was not different between the two dosing schedules, whereas toxicity was significantly increased in the 400 mg/d group, although DVT rates were not different among the two groups.

Thalidomide-Dex (Thal-Dex) combination
The combination of Thal and Dex, two active and nonmyelosuppressive anti-MM agents, has shown potent activity in relapsed or refractory MM. In vitro data indicate that Thal enhances anti-MM activity of Dex on MM cells [43]. Weber and colleagues [66] initially reported that the combination was active in about 45% of patients who had refractory or relapsing MM, including 30% response rate in patients unresponsive to a single agent. These results were subsequently confirmed by several studies [67–69]. Dimopoulos and colleagues [68] treated with Thal (at 200 mg/d, with dose escalation to 400 mg) plus pulsed Dex 44 patients who had refractory MM (of which 100% and 77% were chemo- and Dex-resistant, respectively, whereas 32% had previously received high-dose therapy) and observed a 55% PR rate (median time to response of 1.3 months). Palumbo and colleagues [70] compared, retrospectively,

the activity of Thal-Dex to that of conventional chemotherapy in patients who relapsed after one or two lines of chemotherapy. Thal-Dex significantly improved PFS and projected OS outcome in patients who received the combination after one line of chemotherapy, but the outcome was similar for patients receiving Thal-Dex or chemotherapy after two or more lines of chemotherapy. The same group reported that Thal-Dex was as effective as second autologous transplantation in response rate and PFS but also improved OS after first relapse compared with second autologous transplantation [71,72]. Both therapies were superior to conventional chemotherapy for PFS and OS. A recently reported randomized study from France [73] compared Thal-Dex to Dex in relapsed patients: response rates (65% versus 28%) and 1-year PFS (46.5% versus 31%) were significantly better in the Thal-Dex arm, with a median tolerated Thal dose of 150 mg/d, albeit with a higher DVT rate in the Thal-Dex group.

In summary, addition of Dex to Thal increases the response rate by about 20%, achieving a PR rate up to 57%. In a systematic review of Thal-based regimens by Glasmacher and colleagues [74], Thal-Dex regimens were reported to have response rates of 51% (95% CI 45%–57%) compared with 29% (95% CI 27%–32%) for single-agent Thal. The authors concluded that because the 95% CIs for these response rates do not overlap, Thal-Dex is superior to single-agent Thal. Moreover, the combination shortens the median time to response to 1 month or less, whereas with the addition of Dex, no more than 200 mg/d of Thal are needed [69]. This treatment results in less neurotoxicity, whereas Dex reduces sedation, somnolence, or even constipation. Thal-Dex carries a higher risk for DVT, however, as evidenced by its reported DVT rate up to 10% [47,68,69]. Skin toxicity also seems to be increased in some reports and can occasionally evolve to epidermolysis [75,76].

Combining thalidomide and chemotherapy
Given the minimal, if any, myelosuppressive effect of single-agent Thal, several regimens combining Thal with chemotherapeutic agents have been studied with the goal of achieving higher response rates. Tables 2–4 summarize the results of different combinations of Thal with chemotherapy. Response rates with such regimens in relapsed or refractory patients range from 32% to 76%, but have also been associated with increased frequency of adverse events, mainly myelosuppression and higher DVT risk, especially when doxorubicin is added. In the largest series of patients receiving a chemotherapy–Thal combination, 236 previously treated patients [20] received the DTPACE regimen which consists of infusional cisplatin, doxorubicin, cyclophosphamide, and etoposide in combination with Thal-Dex. None of the patients in that study had previously received HDT and most of them had poor risk features, including chromosome 13 deletion, high plasma cell labeling index, and high β2-microglobulin and levels. After the second cycle, 7% had a CR, 9% an near complete response (nCR), 16% had at least 75% reduction from baseline serum M-protein and 54% had greater than 50% reduction in serum paraprotein

Table 2
Combination of thalidomide with intravenous chemotherapy for refractory relapsed disease

Reference	Treatment schema	
Moehler et al, [77]	T-CED	Thal 400 mg daily Cyclophosphamide 400 mg/m^2/d IV Etoposide 40 mg/m^2/d IV, both as continuous infusion days 1–4; Dex 40 mg po days 1–4; repeat every 28 d
Lee et al, [20]	DTPACE	Dex 40 mg po daily × 4 d Thal 400 mg po at night Cisplatin 10 mg/m^2/ d × 4 d, CIV Doxorubicin 10 mg/m^2/ d × 4 d, CIV Cyclophosphamide 400 mg/m^2/d × 4 d, CIV Etoposide 40 mg/m^2/ d × 4 d, CIV
Offidani et al, [78]	Liposomal doxorubicin Thal Dex	Liposomal doxorubicin 40 mg/m^2 on day 1 every 28 d, Dex 40 mg po on days 1–4 and 9–12, and Thal 100 mg each evening continuously

Abbreviations: CIV, continuous intravenous; IV, intravenous.

or bone marrow plasmacytosis. Extensive experience has also been accumulated with the oral combination of cyclophosphamide, Thal, and Dex (see Table 3). This regimen resulted in high response rates [79,81]. Dimopoulos [80] used a different Thal schedule with intermittent dosing: 53 previously treated patients received oral cyclophosphamide 150 mg/m^2 twice daily on days 1 to 5, Thal 400 mg on days 1 to 5 and 14 to 18, and Dex on days 1 to 5 and 14 to 18 (CTD regimen). This regimen led to a 60% PR rate with a median time to response of 1.5 months. Importantly, toxicities were manageable and the cumulative incidence of DVT and peripheral neuropathy were 4% and 2%, respectively.

Bortezomib

Bortezomib (Velcade; Millennium Pharmaceuticals, Inc., Cambridge, Massachusetts, and Johnson & Johnson Pharmaceuticals Research and Development, L.L.C., Raritan, New Jersey) received full approval in 2005 for the treatment of patients who have received at least one prior therapy [84–86]. Bortezomib is a novel, first-in-class proteasome inhibitor that has antiproliferative, proapoptotic, antiangiogenic, and antitumor activity through inhibition of proteasomal

Table 3
Oral combination of thalidomide with chemotherapy for refractory/relapsed disease

Reference	Regimen	No. of patients	≥PR rate (%)	CR rate (%)
Garcia-Sanz et al, [79]	Thal (200–800 mg/d), po cyclophosphamide (50 mg/d) Dex (40 mg/d × 4 d) every 3 weeks	71	57	2
Dimopoulos et al, [80]	Thal 400 mg po on days 1–5 and 14–18 Cyclophosphamide 150 mg/m^2 po every 12 h days 1–5 Dex 20 mg/m^2 on days 1–5 and 14–18 (CTD) repeated every 28 d	53	60	5
Kyriakou et al, [81]	Thal daily escalating doses to a maximum of 300 mg/d Oral cyclophosphamide (300 mg/m^2 po once weekly) Pulsed Dex (40 mg/d for 4 d po once monthly)	52	79	17

degradation of numerous regulatory proteins [87–93]. In preclinical studies, bortezomib has demonstrated synergistic or additive antitumor activity with agents commonly used in the treatment of MM, including doxorubicin, melphalan, Dex, and IMiDs, along with activity in MM cells resistant to these agents [94–97].

Bortezomib in relapsed and/or refractory multiple myeloma
Bortezomib, with or without Dex, was shown to be active in two phase II studies in patients who had relapsed/refractory MM (SUMMIT [4] and CREST [98] Tables 4 and 5). The international, randomized phase II Assessment of Proteasome Inhibition for EXtending Remissions (APEX) trial enrolled patients who had relapsed MM who had received one to three prior lines of therapy. The trial showed that single-agent bortezomib provides significantly longer time to progression (TTP), higher response rate, and improved survival compared with high-dose Dex [7]. At the moment, bortezomib is the only single agent that has been shown to provide a survival benefit in the relapsed setting. An updated analysis of APEX after extended follow-up (median 22 months) revealed a median OS of 29.8 months with bortezomib versus 23.7 months with Dex. This 6-month benefit was seen despite that most (62%) patients in the Dex arm crossed over to receive bortezomib [100]. The ORR (43%) and CR/nCR rate (15%) with bortezomib were also higher in the updated analysis than at initial analysis [100]. Results from the APEX trial also indicate that bortezomib is more active when used earlier in the relapsed setting, with TTP, duration of response (DOR), and OS appearing longer and response rate higher among patients who had only one prior therapy compared with those who had two or three prior therapies [7].

Table 4
Clinical trials of bortezomib in patients who have relapsed or refractory multiple myeloma

Author	Agents	Regimen	N (enrolled/evaluable)	Response rate (CR + PR)	Time-to-event data	Key toxicities
Richardson et al, [4,99]	Bortezomib ± Dex	Bortezomib 1.3 mg/m^2 on days 1, 4, 8, and 11 for up to eight 3-wk cycles Dex 20 mg may be added on day of/day after bortezomib for suboptimal response	202/193	27% CR/nCR: 10% (bortezomib alone)	DOR: 13 mo (bortezomib alone) TTP: 7 mo OS: 17 mo	Grade 3/4: thrombocytopenia 28%/3%; peripheral neuropathy 12%/0%; fatigue 12%/0%; neutropenia 11%/3%
Jagannath et al, [98]	Bortezomib ± Dex	Bortezomib 1.0 mg/m^2 on days 1, 4, 8, and 11 for up to eight 3-wk cycles Dex 20 mg may be added on day of/day after bortezomib for suboptimal response	28/27	30% CR/nCR: 11% ±Dex: 37% CR/nCR: 19%	DOR: 9.5 months TTP: 7 months OS: 26.7 months	Grade 3/4: thrombocytopenia 29%/0%; neutropenia 11%/0%; lymphopenia 11%/0%; hyponatraemia 11%/0%; pain in limb 11%/0%; peripheral neuropathy 4%/4%
		Bortezomib 1.3 mg/m^2 on days 1, 4, 8, and 11 for up to eight 3-wk cycles Dex 20 mg may be added on day of/day after bortezomib for suboptimal response	26/26	38% CR/nCR: 4% ±Dex: 50% CR/nCR: 4%	DOR: 13.7 months TTP: 11 months OS: Not reached	Grade 3/4: neutropenia 23%/0%; thrombocytopenia 19%/4%; peripheral neuropathy 15%/0%; pneumonia 15%/0%; lymphopenia 12%/0%; weakness 12%/0%

Richardson et al, [7,100]	Single-agent bortezomib versus high-dose Dex	Bortezomib 1.3 mg/m² days 1, 4, 8, and 11 for up to eight 3-wk cycles followed by treatment on days 1, 8, 15, and 22 for up to three 5-wk cycles	333/315	43% CR/nCR: 15%	DOR: 7.8 months TTP: 6.2 months OS: 29.8 months	Grade 3/4: thrombocytopenia 26%/4%; neutropenia 12%/2%; anemia 9/1%; peripheral neuropathy 7%/1%
Kropff et al, [101]	Bortezomib + Dex	Bortezomib 1.3 mg/m² on days 1, 4, 8, and 11 for up to eight 3-wk cycles Dex 20 mg on day of/day after bortezomib	15/15	73% CR/nCR: 7%	EFS: not reached OS: not reached	Grade 3/4: thrombocytopenia 0%/47% (no bleeding); neutropenia 27%/7%; fatigue 20%/0%; anemia 13%/7%; peripheral neuropathy 7%/0%
Kropff et al, [102][a]	Bortezomib + cyclophosphamide + Dex	Bortezomib 1.3 mg/m² days 1, 4, 8, and 11 for up to eight 3-wk cycles followed by bortezomib 1.3 mg/m² days 1, 8, 15, and 22 for up to three 5-wk cycles Dex 20 mg on day of/day after bortezomib Cyclophosphamide 50 mg daily	50/50	82% CR/nCR: 12%	EFS: 12 months OS: not reached	Dose-limiting grade 3/4: thrombocytopenia 0%/19%; infection 25%/0%; peripheral neuropathy 19%/0%; herpes zoster 17%/0%; fatigue 15%/0%; cardiovascular 9%/0%; diarrhea 8%/0%; orthostatic hypotension 6%/0%

(continued on next page)

Table 4
(continued)

Author	Agents	Regimen	N (enrolled/ evaluable)	Response rate (CR + PR)	Time-to-event data	Key toxicities
Reece et al, [103][a]	Bortezomib + cyclophosphamide + prednisone	Bortezomib 0.7–1.5 mg/ m² on days 1, 8, and 15, or days 1, 4, 8, and 11 Cyclophosphamide 150/ 300 mg/m² days 1, 8, 15, 22 Prednisone 100 mg every other day 28-d cycles	21/20	45% CR/nCR: 15%		Grade 3/4 (cycles 2–8 only): hyperglycemia 29%/0%; neutropenia 24%/5%; hypophosphatemia 19%/10%; thrombocytopenia 14/5%
Suvannasankha et al, [104][a]	Bortezomib ± methylprednisolone	Bortezomib 1.3 mg/m² and methylprednisolone 500–2000 mg on days 1, 8, 15, and 22 of a 28-d cycle	30/28 (4 received bortezomib alone)	60% CR/nCR: 7%	TTP: 6.5 months OS: 11.1 months	Grade 3: peripheral neuropathy (7%)
Orlowski et al, [26][a]	Bortezomib + pegylated liposomal doxorubicin (Doxil)	Bortezomib 0.9–1.5 mg/m² on days 1, 4, 8, and 11 Doxil 30 mg/m² on day 4 Up to 11 3-wk cycles	24/22	73% CR/nCR: 36%	TTP: 9.3 months	Grade ≥3: thrombocytopenia 43%; lymphopenia 40%; neutropenia 17%; fatigue 14%; pneumonia 14%; peripheral neuropathy 12%; febrile neutropenia 10%; diarrhea 10%
Biehn et al, [25][b]					OS: 38.3 months	

Study	Regimen	Dosing	No.	Response	Survival	Toxicity
Friedman et al, [105]c; Jakubowiak et al, [106]	Bortezomib + Doxil + Dex	Bortezomib 1.3 mg/m² on days 1, 4, 8, 11 Doxil 30 mg/m² on day 4 Dex 40 mg on days 1–4, then 20 mg on day of/day after bortezomib Six 3-wk cycles	23/23	65% CR/nCR: 22%		Grade 3/4 include fatigue, thrombocytopenia, infections, neutropenia, diarrhea, neuropathy, and DVT/PE
Berenson et al, [107]	Bortezomib + melphalan	Bortezomib 0.7–1.0 mg/m² on days 1, 4, 8, and 11 Melphalan 0.025–0.25 mg/kg on days 1–4 Up to eight 4-wk cycles	35/34	47% CR/nCR: 15%	PFS: 8 months	Grade 3/4: neutropenia 34%/6%; thrombocytopenia 37%/3%; anemia 23%/6%
Popat et al, [108]a	Bortezomib + melphalan + Dex	Bortezomib 1.3 mg/m² on days 1, 4, 8, and 11 Melphalan 2.5–10 mg/m² on day 2 Up to eight 4-week cycles Dex added after two to four cycles for PD or SD, respectively	22/21	52% CR/nCR: 5%	TTP: 6.8 months OS: not reached	Grade ≥3: thrombocytopenia 45%; neutropenia 27%; peripheral neuropathy 18%
Chari et al, [109]	Bortezomib + Doxil + melphalan	Bortezomib 0.7–1.0 mg/m² on days 1, 4, 8, 11 Doxil 10–20 mg/m² on day 1 Melphalan 5–10 mg/m² on day 1 Up to six 4-wk cycles	5/4	25% CR/nCR: 25%		Grade 3 neutropenia in one patient

(continued on next page)

Table 4
(*continued*)

Author	Agents	Regimen	N (enrolled/ evaluable)	Response rate (CR + PR)	Time-to-event data	Key toxicities
Hrusovsky et al, [110]	Bortezomib + bendamustine + Dex	Bortezomib 1.0–1.3 mg/m^2 on days 1, 4, 8, and 11 Bendamustine 60 mg/m^2 on days 1 and 8 Dex 24 mg on days 1–3 and 8–10 Ondansetrone 8 mg on days 1, 4, 8, and 11 3-wk cycles	17/17	71%[d] CR/nCR: 12%	DOR: >6 months	No significant toxicities reported
Berenson et al, [111][c]	Bortezomib + arsenic trioxide + ascorbic acid	Bortezomib 0.7–1.3 mg/m^2 on days 1, 4, 8, and 11 Arsenic trioxide 0.125–0.25 mg/kg on days 1, 4, 8, and 11 Ascorbic acid 1000 mg on days 1, 4, 8, and 11 Up to eight 3-wk cycles	22/21	19% CR/nCR: 10%		Grade 4 thrombocytopenia 5%

Yeh et al, [112]	Bortezomib + ^{153}Sm-lexidronam	Bortezomib 1.0–1.3 mg/m² on days 1, 4, 8, and 11 153Sm-lexidronam 0.25–1.0 mCi/kg on day 3 8-wk cycle	12/12	17% CR/nCR: 8%	Grade ≥3 include headache (17%), leg cramps (8%), neutropenia (8%), and thrombocytopenia (8%)
Chanan-Khan et al, [113]b	Bortezomib + KOS-953	Bortezomib 0.7–1.3 mg/m² and KOS-953 100–220 mg/m² on days 1, 4, 8, and 11 3-wk cycles	28/21	19% CR/nCR: 10%	Grade 4 hepatotoxicity (5%), grade 3 pancreatitis (5%); grade 3/4: thrombocytopenia 5%, thrombophlebitis 5%

Abbreviations: CR, complete response; DOR, duration of response; EFS, event-free survival; OS, overall survival; PD, progressive disease; PFS, progression-free survival; PR, partial response; SD, stable disease; TTP, time to progression.
aPreliminary data presented at the American Society of Hematology Annual Meeting.
bPreliminary data presented at the American Society of Clinical Oncology Annual Meeting.
cPreliminary data presented at the European Haematology Society Annual Meeting.
dSWOG criteria.

Table 5
Clinical trials of combination regimens including both bortezomib and thalidomide or lenalidomide in patients with relapsed or refractory multiple myeloma

Author	Agents	Regimen	N (enrolled/evaluable)	Response ryate (CR + PR)	Time-to-event data	Key toxicities
Padmanabhan et al, [114][a]	Bortezomib + Doxil + Thal	Bortezomib 1.3 mg/m^2 on days 1, 4, 15, and 18 Doxil 20 mg/m^2 on days 1 and 15 Thal 200 mg/d Up to six 4-wk cycles	23/17	65%[b] CR/nCR: 23%	PFS: 11 mo OS: 16 mo	No grade 3/4 nonhematologic toxicities
Zangari et al, [115][c]	Bortezomib + Thal + Dex	Bortezomib 1.0–1.3 mg/m^2 on days 1, 4, 8, 11 Thal 50–200 mg/d from cycle two Dex 20 mg on day of/day after bortezomib for suboptimal response after three cycles Up to eight 3-wk cycles	85/85	55% CR/nCR: 16%	EFS: 9 mo OS: 22 mo	Most common grade 3/4 toxicities were thrombocytopenia and neutropenia
Teoh et al, [116][d]	Bortezomib + Thal + Dex + zoledronic acid	Bortezomib 1.3 mg/m^2 on days 1, 4, 8, 11 Thal 50 mg/d Dex 20 mg days 1–4, 8–11, 15–18 Zoledronic acid 4 mg on day 1 Up to 11 3-wk cycles	14/14	93% CR/nCR: 64%	—	Painful grade 3 peripheral neuropathy in 14%, transient grade 3 thrombocytopenia in 36%, rash 21%

Study	Regimen	Dosing	No.	Response	Survival	Toxicity
Leoni et al, [117]a	Bortezomib + liposomal doxorubicin (Myocet) + Thal + Dex	Bortezomib 1.0 mg/m² on days 1, 4, 8, and 11 Myocet 50 mg/m² on day 4 Thal 100 mg/d Dex 24 mg on day of/day after bortezomib Up to four 4-wk cycles	27/27	74% CR/nCR: 33%	TTP: NR OS: NR	Grade 4 hematologic toxicity in 18%
	Bortezomib + Thal + Dex	As above, minus Myocet	18/18			NR
Hollmig et al, [118]c	Bortezomib + doxorubicin + Thal + Dex	Bortezomib 0.8–1.3 mg/m² on days 1, 4, 8, 11 Doxorubicin 2.5–5 mg/m² on days 1–4 and 9–12 Thal 50–100 mg/d on days 1–12 Dex 20–40 mg on days 1–4 and 9–12	20/16	50% CR/nCR:17% 63%e CR/nCR: 25%	TTP: 8 mo OS: 13 mo 89% survival at 6 mo	Grade 3 thrombocytopenia in 40%e
Palumbo et al, [119]	Bortezomib + melphalan + prednisone + Thal	Bortezomib 1–1.6 mg/m² on days 1, 4, 15, 22 Melphalan 6 mg/m² and prednisone 60 mg/m² on days 1–5 Thal 100 mg continuously Six 5-wk cycles	30/30	67% CR/nCR: 17%	—	Grade 3/4 include thrombocytopenia, febrile neutropenia, fatigue, anemia, pneumonia, vasculitis, infections, and sensory neuropathy
Terpos et al, [120]	Bortezomib + melphalan + Dex + Thal	Bortezomib 1.0 mg/m² on days 1, 4, 8, and 11 Melphalan 0.15 mg/kg days 1–4 Dex 12 mg/m² days 1–4 and 17–20 Thal 100 mg/d For four 4-wk cycles	62/62	66% CR/VGPR: 13%/27%	PFS: 8.4 mo	Grade ≥3 include thrombocytopenia 20%, neutropenia 8%, anemia 7%, and peripheral neuropathy 6%

(continued on next page)

Table 5
(continued)

Author	Agents	Regimen	N (enrolled/evaluable)	Response ryate (CR + PR)	Time-to-event data	Key toxicities
Richardson et al, [83][c]	Bortezomib + lenalidomide ± Dex	Bortezomib 1.0–1.3 mg/m² on days 1, 4, 8, 11 Lenalidomide 5–20 mg on days 1–14 Dex 20 mg on day of/day after bortezomib for PD Up to eight 3-wk cycles	24/21	52% CR/nCR: 10%	—	Grade 3/4 include thrombocytopenia, neutropenia, and hyponatremia. No significant fatigue or peripheral neuropathy.
Musto et al, [121]	Bortezomib + intermediate-dose melphalan + Thal + Dex + stem cell support	Bortezomib 1.3 mg/m² and melphalan 50 mg/m² on days 6 and 3 Thal 200 mg and Dex 20 mg on days 6 to 3 Hematopoietic stem cell support on day 0	26/26	65% CR/nCR: 15%	PFS: 6 mo	Grade 3/4: thrombocytopenia 46%/54%; anemia 42%/38%, neutropenia 0%/100%; pneumonia 35%/0%; febrile neutropenia 12%/0%

Abbreviations: CR, complete response; EFS, event-free survival; NR, not reached; OS, overall survival; PD, progressive disease; PFS, progression-free survival; PR, partial response; TTP, time to progression; VGPR, very good partial response.

[a]Preliminary data presented at the European Haematology Society Annual Meeting.
[b]SWOG criteria.
[c]Preliminary data presented at the American Society of Hematology Annual Meeting.
[d]Preliminary data presented at the American Society of Clinical Oncology Annual Meeting.
[e]PR defined as ≥75% reduction in serum/urine M-protein, response rate, and toxicity reported after one cycle of treatment.

The most common adverse events associated with bortezomib treatment include fatigue, gastrointestinal events, and peripheral neuropathy. The most commonly reported grade 3 or greater side effects are peripheral neuropathy, thrombocytopenia, neutropenia, and anemia. Bortezomib-related peripheral neuropathy is an important side effect, and based on the results of the SUMMIT and CREST trials, specific management guidelines were proposed [125] and tested in the APEX study. Bortezomib-related peripheral neuropathy was shown to be reversible in most patients in the APEX trial [126]. Similarly, bortezomib-emergent neuropathy in the SUMMIT and CREST trials resolved or improved in 71% of patients who had grade 3 or greater peripheral neuropathy or neuropathy requiring discontinuation [125]. Comparable results were observed in the frontline setting [83,127,128]. The hematologic adverse events associated with bortezomib are also predictable and manageable. Bortezomib-related thrombocytopenia and neutropenia are transient and cyclical; in patients experiencing thrombocytopenia with bortezomib treatment, platelet counts decrease and recover predictably during each treatment cycle, without any evidence of cumulative toxicity [126,129]. Patients who have low baseline platelet count ($<70 \times 10^9$/L) are at increased risk for grade 3 or greater thrombocytopenia [129]. Although in the APEX trial a higher incidence of grade 3 or greater thrombocytopenia was observed in the bortezomib arm versus the comparator Dex arm, the incidence of clinically significant bleeding events (including grade 3 or greater bleeding events, serious bleeding, and cerebral hemorrhage) was similar between the two arms [130]. Finally, in an extension study of the SUMMIT and CREST trials, no new or cumulative toxicities were reported [131].

Combinations of bortezomib with conventional anti–multiple myeloma agents
Bortezomib-based combinations containing anthracyclines. Bortezomib has shown substantial activity when combined with commonly used anti-MM agents. For instance, combination regimens including bortezomib and doxorubicin or liposomal doxorubicin provide high ORR and CR/nCR rates, with promising OS and time-to-event data [25,26,105,106,114,117,118]. In a phase I trial of bortezomib plus liposomal doxorubicin in patients who had advanced hematologic malignancies, the response rate among 22 evaluable patients was 73%, including 36% CR/nCR [26]. An updated analysis after extended follow-up showed that the regimen provided substantial increases compared with patients' last prior regimen in median TTP (9.3 versus 3.8 months), and median time from start of therapy to start of subsequent therapy (24.2 versus 5.9 months). Median OS was 38.3 months [25]. Importantly, among patients who had progressive disease (PD), stable disease (SD), or an initial response followed by PD or SD with a previous anthracycline-based regimen, responses were seen in 8 of 13 after their treatment with the bortezomib plus anthracycline combination [26]. These results are consistent with prior preclinical studies that suggested that bortezomib can sensitize MM cells to conventional chemotherapeutics to which a patient has previously become resistant [95,97].

Following the remarkably positive results of a large phase III trial comparing Velcade and pegylated liposomal doxorubicin with Velcade monotherapy, the FDA approved the use of this combination in May 2007 for patients who have not previously received Velcade and who have received at least one prior therapy [132].

In further support of this concept, clinical responses (with ORR of 65%, including 23% CR/nCR according to SWOG criteria) to the combination of bortezomib, liposomal doxorubicin, and Thal have been observed in patients resistant to regimens containing bortezomib, doxorubicin, or Thal [114]. Similarly, a response rate of 63%, including 25% CR/nCR, was seen with a regimen composed of bortezomib, doxorubicin, Thal, and Dex, even though these agents had been previously administered in the course of the disease in these patients [118]. The addition of liposomal doxorubicin to bortezomib, Thal, and Dex has also been shown to produce an increased response rate (81% versus 55%; CR/nCR: 33% versus 17%) and longer median TTP and OS compared with the triplet regimen [117]. Responses were seen despite patients having previously received bortezomib, doxorubicin, Thal, and Dex [117].

Bortezomib-based combinations containing anthracyclines. Combinations of bortezomib with alkylating agents have also been shown to be active in advanced MM [107,108,119,120]. In a dose-escalation study of bortezomib with oral melphalan, the response rate was 47% (including 15% CR/nCR), with responses seen in five of six (83%) patients at the maximum tolerated dose [107]. A dose-escalation study of bortezomib with low-dose intravenous melphalan showed a 43% response rate, which increases to 52% with addition of Dex for patients who had suboptimal response [108]. Activity seemed greatest in patients receiving the highest melphalan dose [108]. The addition of Thal, along with Dex or prednisone, seems to increase the activity of the combination, with response rates of 66% (37% CR/nCR) [120] and 67% (17% CR/nCR) [119] for the Dex- and prednisone-containing regimens, respectively.

Bortezomib-thalidomide regimens
Bortezomib has shown activity in relapsed/refractory disease, even in patients refractory to Thal [4,7]. By acting through different molecular mechanisms than conventional chemotherapy or steroids, bortezomib has the potential to act synergistically with either of them and with other novel agents, including Thal and IMiDs [42,43]. A significant initial concern about combinations of Thal with bortezomib was the possibility of cumulative neurotoxicity. Clinical trials have shown that the neuropathy associated with this combination can be manageable, however. Zangari and colleagues [115] enrolled 85 refractory patients in a phase I/II trial of bortezomib, Thal, and Dex combination (VTD regimen). Most patients had abnormal cytogenetics (including deletion of chromosome 13 in approximately half of the patients), had one or two prior autotransplants, and had previously received Thal, but none had received prior bortezomib. Bortezomib was started at 1 mg/m^2 and daily Thal was added at the second cycle at dose increments of 50 mg up to 200 mg. Bortezomib dose

was increased to 1.3 mg/m^2 in the absence of neuropathy after the Thal dose reached 200 mg and Dex was added if PR or better was not achieved. Fifty-five percent of patients treated with this VTD regimen achieved a PR (including a 16% CR or nCR rate), and an additional 15% had a MR. Median EFS and OS were 9 months and 22 months, respectively. The dose of Thal (>100 mg/d versus <100 mg/d) did not affect EFS or OS. Instead, cytogenetic abnormalities were associated with shorter EFS ($P = .01$) and OS ($P = .03$). Prior Thal treatment was also associated with inferior EFS (26% versus 63%, $P = .03$), suggesting that the combination should perhaps be considered in advance of other Thal-containing regimens. A final dose of bortezomib 1.0 mg/m^2, Thal 200 mg/d, and Dex 40 mg was proposed for further investigation and combination with chemotherapy. Palumbo [119] used a four-drug combination regimen: Thal daily at 50 mg plus bortezomib, melphalan, and prednisone to treat 30 patients who had relapsed or refractory MM. Sixty-seven percent of patients achieved a PR, including 43% who achieved at least a VGPR. The 1-year PFS was 61% and the 1-year survival from study entry was 84%. Terpos and colleagues [133] reported the combination of bortezomib, oral melphalan, intermittent Thal (100 mg/d for 4 days), and pulsed Dex (12 mg/m^2). Patients who did not have evidence of progressive disease continued for up to eight cycles. Thirty-one pretreated patients were enrolled, including 20 patients who had refractory relapse, and 56% achieved an objective response (CR 8% and PR 48%); 8% had a MR with a median time to response of 30 days.

Lenalidomide

Lenalidomide (CC-5013) is the first member of the new class of immunomodulatory Thal derivatives (IMiDs) that has been approved by the FDA for the treatment of patients who have MM after at least one line of prior therapy. In a phase I dose-escalation study [122], lenalidomide was administered at doses of 5 to 50 mg/d in 27 relapsed and refractory MM patients. This patient population was a heavily pretreated, with a median number of prior therapies of three (range two to six), whereas 15 patients had previously received HDT and 16 had prior Thal treatment. Most clinical responses were observed at the dose levels of 25 mg/d and 50 mg/d. Myelosuppression was the dose-limiting toxicity in this study and a dose of 25 mg/d was suggested for subsequent clinical trials. MR or better was seen in 71% of the patients, with 7 (29%) patients achieving at least a PR. Moreover, among patients who had previously received Thal therapy, 11 of 16 responded to lenalidomide. Compared with Thal, the profile of adverse events of lenalidomide is favorable: no significant somnolence, constipation, or neuropathy was observed in any dose cohort of the phase I study. A second phase I study by Zangari and colleagues [134] in 15 patients who had advanced MM confirmed a maximum tolerated dose of 25 mg/d.

A subsequent multicenter phase II trial evaluated two different schedules of lenalidomide (30 mg once daily or 15 mg twice daily for 21 days every 28 days) in 102 patients who had relapsed/refractory MM (median number of prior treatments 4, range 1 to 13) [124]. A prespecified interim analysis after the enrollment of the first 70 patients showed shorter time to development of myelosuppression and higher rate of clinically significant myelosuppressive events in the twice-daily arm, thereby supporting the selection of the daily dosing of lenalidomide for further evaluation in a subsequent cohort of 32 patients. Overall in that trial, 102 evaluable patients were enrolled: 17% achieved PR or better response (including 6% CR rate of patients in the once-daily treatment arm), whereas 5% and 8% in the twice- and once-daily treatment groups, respectively, achieved PR. In addition, 9% of patients had MR and 42% had stable disease. Subsequently, Dex was added to those patients who after two cycles of single-agent lenalidomide had either stable disease or progressed: 67% had Dex added for an ORR of 29% and 21% had stabilization of their disease. There were no significant differences in response rates between the daily versus twice-daily regimens. More importantly, prior Thal or bortezomib treatment did not affect the response rates to single-agent lenalidomide or to its combination with Dex. The median overall survival among patients in the twice-daily and once-daily arms was 27 and 28 months, respectively (27 months for both arms combined). The median PFS was 3.9 months (95% CI 2.8–7.5), 7.7 months (95% CI 3.8–11.5), and 4.6 months for the twice-daily, once-daily, and both arms combined, respectively. The median PFS for lenalidomide, censoring for addition of Dex, was 4.1 months for both arms combined, and median PFS for lenalidomide, considering the addition of Dex as an event, was 3 months for both arms combined. No significant differences were found between arms in overall survival ($P = .8$), PFS ($P = .17$), or PFS for lenalidomide either with ($P = .7$) or without the addition of Dex ($P = .4$). The most common grade 3 to 4 toxicity during therapy was myelosuppression. Peripheral neuropathy was reported in 23% and 10% and constipation in 31% and 25% of the twice-and once-daily arms, respectively. Thromboembolic events occurred in 3 patients but only after Dex was added to lenalidomide treatment.

In another study conducted in the University of Arkansas [64], 55 patients who had relapsed or refractory MM were treated with single-agent lenalidomide in two dosing schedules. Patients either received lenalidomide in a dose of 25 mg daily for 21 days every 28 days, or 50 mg daily for 10 days every 28 days. Because of increased frequency of thrombocytopenia in the 50-mg arm, the schedule was changed to 50 mg every other day for 10 days. Dex was added in the regimen after two cycles with lenalidomide monotherapy. Among the patients enrolled in the study, 93% had previously received Thal and 47% had prior HDT. Forty percent of patients receiving lenalidomide 25 mg had at least a 50% decrease in paraprotein levels compared with 14% in the 50-mg arm patients. Similarly, 44% of patients in the 25 mg/d arm had a reduction of 25% or greater versus 21% of patients in the 50-mg arm. The study also showed that cytogenetic profile did not affect event-free and overall survival.

Two large phase III randomized double-blind multicenter trials conducted in the United States, Canada, Australia, and Europe compared lenalidomide plus high-dose Dex to high-dose Dex alone in previously treated patients who had MM, including more than 700 patients who had relapsed/refractory MM. (Table 6) Patients resistant to Dex were excluded from these studies. In both studies patients were treated with high-dose Dex and were randomized to receive either lenalidomide 25 mg daily orally on days 1 to 21 every 28 days or placebo. In both trials patients were stratified with respect to β2-microglobulin (2.5 versus >2.5 mg/mL), prior stem cell transplant (none versus one), and number of prior regimens (1 versus >1). Preplanned, protocol-specified, interim analyses determined statistically significant benefit in TTP for the lenalidomide/Dex arms of both trials and therefore the Independent Data Monitoring Committee recommended that Dex arm patients could cross over to lenalidomide-Dex treatment. These trials provided the basis for FDA approval of the combination of lenalidomide and Dex in patients who had MM who had received at least one prior therapy.

In the 2005 American Society of Hematology (ASH) Meeting, Dimopoulos [6] reported the results of the first trial (MM-010) from centers in Europe, Israel, and Australia, which enrolled 351 patients. After a median follow-up of 18 months, the median TTP for patients treated with the combination of lenalidomide/Dex was 13.3 months compared with 5.1 months for patients treated with Dex alone ($P < .000001$). The ORR was higher in the lenalidomide/Dex versus Dex-only arm (58% versus 22%; $P < .001$). Grade 3 or 4 neutropenia was more frequent in the combination therapy arm than in patients treated with Dex alone (16.5% versus 1.2%). The frequency of grade 3 or 4 infections was similar in the two arms, however. Thromboembolic events occurred in 8.5% of patients in the lenalidomide/Dex group and in 4.5% of patients in the Dex-alone group. Otherwise, the safety profile of lenalidomide/Dex was similar to that of Dex alone. In the 2006 Weber and colleagues [8] reported results from the second trial (MM-009), which included 354 patients. The ORR was again higher in the lenalidomide/Dex arm compared with Dex/placebo (59.4% versus 21.1%; $P < .001$). CR was achieved in 12.9% of lenalidomide/Dex-treated patients and in only 0.6% of patients treated with Dex/placebo. Median TTP was 11.1 months versus 4.7 months in lenalidomide/Dex and Dex/placebo arms, respectively ($P < .000001$). The median OS was not reached in the lenalidomide/Dex arm, but was 24 months in the Dex/placebo group (hazard ratio [HR] = 1.76, $P = .0125$). Grade 3 to 4 neutropenias were more frequent in the lenalidomide/Dex arm, but the frequency of grade 3 infections was similar in both groups. Thromboembolic events occurred in 15% and 3.5% of patients in the lenalidomide/Dex and Dex/placebo arms, respectively. Atrial fibrillation and CHF occurred in 8 and 4 patients, respectively, treated with lenalidomide/Dex. Subsequent analysis of these trials, reported in latest ASH meetings, showed that lenalidomide/Dex was significantly more effective than Dex in patients treated at first relapse. Among 248 patients who had only

Table 6
Clinical trials of lenalidomide in patients with relapsed or refractory multiple myeloma

Author	Agents	Regimen	N (enrolled/evaluable)	Response rate (CR + PR)	Time-to-event data	Key toxicities
Richardson et al, [122]	Lenalidomide	Lenalidomide 5–50 mg/d	27/24	29%	NR	Grade 3/4: neutropenia 60%, thrombocytopenia 20%
Richardson et al, [123]	Lenalidomide	Lenalidomide 30 mg on days 1–21 4-wk cycles	222/212	25%	TTP: 5.2 mo	Upper respiratory tract infection, neutropenia, thrombocytopenia
Richardson et al, [124]	Lenalidomide	Lenalidomide 30 mg once daily or 15 mg twice daily, days 1–21 Dex 40 mg for 4 d every 14 d for suboptimal response 4-wk cycles	67 (once daily) 35 (twice daily)	18% CR/nCR: 6% (Once daily) 14% CR/nCR: 0% (Twice daily)	DOR: 19 mo (once daily), 23 months (twice daily) PFS: 4.6 mo (combined) OS: 27 mo (combined)	Grade 3/4 (once daily): neutropenia 49%/12%, thrombocytopenia 15%/16%, leukopenia 36%/2%, lymphopenia 31%/6%, anemia 15%/2% Grade 3/4 (twice daily): neutropenia 57%/11%, thrombocytopenia 26%/17%, leukopenia 34%/0%, lymphopenia 31%/9%, anemia 11%/3%

Study	Regimen	Treatment	N	Response	Outcome	Toxicity
Weber et al, [8]ᵃ	Lenalidomide + Dex	Lenalidomide 25 mg on days 1–21 Dex 40 mg on days 1–4, 9–12, 17–20 (days 1–4 only from cycle 5) 4-wk cycles	170	59% CR/nCR: 13%	TTP: 11.1 mo OS: 29.6 mo	Grade ≥3: neutropenia 24%, thrombocytopenia 12%, peripheral neuropathy 12%, pneumonia >10% DVT/PE 18%
Dimopoulos et al, [6,54,169]ᵇ,ᶜ	Lenalidomide + Dex	As above	176	59% CR/nCR: 15%	TTP: 11.3 mo OS: NR	Grade ≥3: neutropenia 27%, thrombocytopenia 10%, anemia 8%, DVT 5%, PE 4%
Knop et al, [82]	Lenalidomide + doxorubicin + Dex	Lenalidomide 10/15 mg on days 1–21 Doxorubicin 4/6/9 mg/m² on days 1–4 Dex 40 mg on days 1–4 and 17–20 Three to six 4-wk cycles	69/56 (23 in phase I)	All patients responded ORR 78%, CR 22%, nCR 52%	NR	Well tolerated at first two dose levels DVT: 7.5% with aspirin prophylaxis 100 mg/d High neutropenia rates and infections requires G-CSF prophylaxis

(continued on next page)

Table 6
(continued)

Author	Agents	Regimen	N (enrolled/ evaluable)	Response rate (CR + PR)	Time-to-event data	Key toxicities
Baz et al, [24]	Lenalidomide + liposomal doxorubicin + vincristine + Dex	Lenalidomide ≥10 mg on days 1–21 Liposomal doxorubicin 40 mg/m^2 on day 1 Vincristine 2 mg on day 1 Dex 40 mg on days 1–4 4-wk cycles	62/62	75%[d] CR/nCR: 29%[d]	PFS: 12 mo OS: NR	Grade ≥3: neutropenia 32%, thrombocytopenia 13%, infectious 13%, DVT/PE 9%

Abbreviations: DVT, deep venous thrombosis; EFS, event-free survival; NR, not reached; OS, overall survival; PE, pulmonary embolism; PFS, progression-free survival; TTP, time to progression.

[a]Preliminary data presented at the American Society of Clinical Oncology Annual Meeting.
[b]Preliminary data presented at the European Haematology Society Annual Meeting.
[c]Preliminary data presented at the American Society of Hematology Annual Meeting.
[d]SWOG criteria.

one prior line of therapy, lenalidomide/Dex treatment led to higher response rates (CR + PR, 65% versus 26% for those treated with Dex alone) and longer TTP (71 versus 20 weeks). Among patients who had more than one prior therapy, lenalidomide/Dex was again more active than Dex alone (ORR 58% versus 20% and TTP of 41 versus 20 weeks). Patients who received lenalidomide/Dex as their second-line therapy, however, had higher ORR and longer TTP than those receiving the combination latter in the course of their disease [135]. Importantly, lenalidomide was active even in patients who had prior Thal treatment: 43% of Thal-resistant patients responded to lenalidomide/ Dex, but this was significantly lower than in Thal-sensitive patients (ORR 63%, $P < .05$) [136]. Data from MM-009 and MM-010 also showed that patients who had renal impairment (creatinine clearance <50 mL/min) could receive lenalidomide, although they developed thrombocytopenia more frequently than patients who had creatinine clearance greater than 50 mL/min [137]. Another report of patients who received lenalidomide with or without corticosteroids showed that patients who had renal impairment had similar response rates to patients who had normal renal function, again at the expense of thrombocytopenia rates [138]. Interestingly, in both reports neutropenia rates were not different between patients with or without normal renal function. At the moment, lenalidomide is not recommended for patients who have serum creatinine greater than 2.5 mg/dL.

Lenalidomide combinations with chemotherapy
The combination of lenalidomide with liposomal doxorubicin, vincristine, and reduced-frequency Dex was studied in a phase I/II trial in 62 patients who had relapsed or refractory MM [24] (see Table 6). The maximum tolerated dose of lenalidomide in the combination was 10 mg, and nonneutropenic sepsis was the dose-limiting toxicity. The median number of prior treatments was three (range one to seven). Most patients (66%) in that study had been previously treated with Thal, 26% had prior treatment with bortezomib, and 18% had prior HDT. In 52 patients evaluable for response, an impressive 75% ORR was noted, and 29% of patients achieved CR or near CR. Thirty-five patients received maintenance therapy with lenalidomide at a dose of 10 mg/d for 21 days and prednisone 50 mg every other day for a median of 7 months (range 1–19). After a median follow-up of 7.5 months, the median PFS was 12 months, whereas the median overall survival had not been reached yet. In a second report from a dose-escalation study [82], pretreated patients who had a maximum of three previous treatment lines were treated with the combination of lenalidomide, infusional doxorubicin, and Dex. Maximum tolerated dose of lenalidomide was 25 mg on days 1 to 21 of each cycle, which is consistent with the daily dosing regimen identified through the initial lenalidomide monotherapy trials. Of 31 evaluable patients (out of 41 enrolled), the ORR was 84% (including one confirmed CR), whereas 3 patients had SD and 2 progressed. Notably, 8 of 10 patients who had chromosome 13 deletion on cytogenetic analysis responded to the treatment. Toxicity of the combination was manageable.

Combinations of lenalidomide and bortezomib

A key advantage of lenalidomide is that it is less neurotoxic than Thal. The combinations of lenalidomide with bortezomib, a known neurotoxic agent, were therefore expected to have a better toxicity profile compared with combinations of Thal with bortezomib. On the other hand, however, lenalidomide and bortezomib can lead to hematologic adverse effects and thus their combination is associated with increased rates of myelosuppression. Preclinical studies showed that lenalidomide sensitizes MM cells to bortezomib and Dex [43,44], thus suggesting that combination therapy may enhance clinical activity. In a phase I study of lenalidomide and bortezomib combination in patients who have refractory MM, including patients who have had prior lenalidomide, bortezomib, Thal, and HDT, the maximum tolerated dose of lenalidomide was 15 mg/d for 21 days and for bortezomib 1.0 mg/m^2 on days 1, 4, 8, and 11. No significant peripheral neuropathy was reported and no anticoagulant prophylaxis was given (only one patient had a DVT while on lenalidomide alone). Among 36 evaluable patients, an ORR (CR + PR + MR) of 58% (90% CI: 46%, 75%) was reported, including 6% CR/nCR after a median of six cycles (range: 4–17). Responses were durable (median 6 months, range: 1–26), and 11 patients remained on therapy beyond 1 year. Subsequently, Dex was added in 14 patients who had PD, resulting in PR/MR/SD in 10 (71%) [83]. The dosing of lenalidomide 15 mg and bortezomib 1.0 mg/m^2 has been selected for ongoing Phase 2 studies in newly diagnosed and relapsed/refractory MM, with dose escalation in the upfront setting being also planned.

Rational design of combinations of novel agents

The design of clinical combinations of bortezomib with lenalidomide was based on the results of preclinical studies that had evaluated the mechanisms of anti-MM action of these agents: bortezomib triggers apoptosis of MM cells in a dual caspase-8 and -9–mediated manner [96]. Regarding the direct anti-MM activity of lenalidomide and other IMiDs, this is mediated by activation of caspase-8. Although bortezomib and Thal/IMiDs can suppress the transcriptional activity of nuclear factor (NF)–κB in MM cells, each of these classes of drugs achieves this effect by likely acting at different levels of the molecular mechanisms that regulate the NF-κB activity: bortezomib leads to accumulation of IκB, an inhibitor of NF-κB activity, whereas IMiDs are proposed to act at more upstream molecular levels of this cascade. The concept that these two classes of anti-MM agents operate at these different functional levels (Fig. 1) suggested that the exposure of MM cells to a combination of these agents could mutually enhance the anti-MM activity of each one of them. This hypothesis was first validated in preclinical in vitro studies involving the combination of a proteasome inhibitor, such as bortezomib, with lenalidomide or CC-4047 (Actimid) [44], and was then followed by the initiation of clinical trials of bortezomib in combination with lenalidomide (or lenalidomide plus Dex).

Another key conceptual framework for the design of combination regimens involves the pairing of drug classes in which one of them serves to neutralize

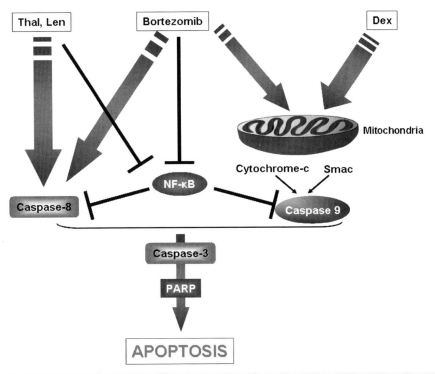

Fig. 1. Main caspase-mediated pathways and NF-κB inhibitory effects for the direct anti-MM effect of proteasome inhibitors, immunomodulatory thalidomide derivatives (IMiDs) and Dex.

a molecular pathway that can confer resistance to the other agent or agents of the combination. An example of that approach is the combination of proteasome inhibitors, such as bortezomib, with hsp90 inhibitors, such as 17-AAG. MM cells exposed to the proteasome inhibitor bortezomib up-regulate the expression of heat shock proteins, including hsp90 [139], as a stress response to counteract the intracellular accumulation of misfolded proteins. This finding suggested that small molecule hsp90 inhibitors may be able to sensitize MM cells to the proapoptotic effects of bortezomib. This hypothesis, which was first confirmed in preclinical MM models [96,139], provided the basis for ongoing clinical trials of tanespimycin (17-AAG in the KOS-953 cremophor-based formulation) either as a single agent [140] or in combination with bortezomib [141] in patients who had relapsed or refractory MM. In these trials, tanespimycin has exhibited a manageable profile of side effects (without significant cardiotoxicity, peripheral neuropathy, or DVT), durable disease stabilization, and minor responses with single-agent treatment in relapsed and refractory MM patients, along with encouraging anti-MM activity by the combination of tanespimycin with bortezomib. These results, coupled with the absence of major additive toxicity or pharmacokinetic interactions of the bortezomib plus tanespimycin combination, have provided a platform for future phase III trials of this regimen.

The Role of Bortezomib, Thalidomide, and IMiD Treatment in Patients who have Renal Dysfunction

Renal impairment is one of the main pathophysiologic manifestations of MM. It is estimated that 30% of patients who have MM have underlying renal dysfunction (serum creatinine levels ≥ 1.5 mg/dL) already at presentation [142,143], with conceivably higher probability of at least some degree of renal dysfunction in more or less heavily pretreated patients who have relapsed and refractory disease. Consequently, it is important to evaluate for any novel anti-MM agent, such as bortezomib, whether it can be safely administered in patients who have renal dysfunction in a manner that does not compromise the clinical activity of the drug. An analysis of the subset of SUMMIT and CREST patients who had impaired renal function indicated that renal function has little impact on response rate to bortezomib treatment and, similarly to the overall population, bortezomib-attributable adverse events are manageable in that subgroup [144,145]. Furthermore, a prospective pharmacologic trial of the NCI in adult patients who had cancer showed that bortezomib clearance is independent of renal function and that the standard bortezomib dose of 1.3 mg/m^2 is well tolerated in patients who have mild to moderate renal dysfunction. Further accrual to that trial addresses this question for patients who have more severe renal dysfunction or those requiring dialysis [146]. A retrospective multicenter analysis of 24 patients who had MM and severe renal dysfunction requiring dialysis showed high response rates (including CR rates) and durable responses with bortezomib and bortezomib-based combinations [147]. Interestingly, two studies [147,148] have shown that bortezomib-based therapy can reverse renal dysfunction in some patients, and eliminate the need for dialysis or spare patients from imminent dialysis. This finding may perhaps reflect the potent antitumor effect of bortezomib and the corresponding decrease in the levels of M-protein (or fragments thereof) or the suppression of other nephrotoxic products released from the MM clone, because currently it has not been formally studied whether bortezomib has any direct nephroprotective effect that would directly contribute to improvement of renal function in MM. Thal alone or in combination with Dex has also been shown to contribute to eventual reversal of renal dysfunction in some patients who have relapsed or refractory MM [149]. The reversibility of dialysis-dependent renal failure may be limited, however [149]. As seen with bortezomib-based regimens, the toxicity profile of Thal with or without Dex is comparable to that in patients who have normal renal function [149]. Thal treatment has been associated with a risk for severe and potentially fatal hyperkalemia, however, particularly in patients on hemodialysis [150,151]. Lenalidomide is not yet adequately studied in patients who have renal impairment, but is known to be renally excreted; therefore, the risk for increased side effects is likely. In fact, serum creatinine greater than 2.5 mg/dL was an exclusion criterion during enrollment for two phase III studies of lenalidomide plus Dex in relapsed MM, and the drug was held in those who developed renal insufficiency while on these studies [152]. Dose reduction should be considered in patients who have serum creatinine 2.5 mg/dL or greater and further data with this agent in this clinical setting are eagerly awaited.

Novel Anti–Multiple Myeloma Therapies in the Context of Elderly and High-Risk Patients who have Relapsed/Refractory Multiple Myeloma

Bortezomib alone and in combination [110,153,154], Thal plus Dex [155–162], and lenalidomide plus Dex [152] have been shown to be active and well tolerated in elderly ($\geq$65 years) patients who have MM. In a subgroup analysis of the APEX trial focused on patients 65 years or older, bortezomib resulted in longer TTP and higher response rate compared with high-dose Dex [154]. Additionally, multivariate analyses of data from the SUMMIT trial showed that age did not affect TTP, DOR, or OS [163]. In a phase 3 trial of Thal plus Dex (albeit in patients who had newly diagnosed MM) [164], no differences were detected in efficacy or safety in patients aged 65 years or older versus younger patients [155]. In relapsed/refractory MM, however, age older than 65 predicts for inferior outcome with Thal in OS and response rate [52]. In the two phase II trials of lenalidomide plus Dex versus Dex alone in patients who have relapsed or refractory MM, no differences in efficacy were observed between lenalidomide-Dex–treated patients aged 65 or older versus younger than 65 years; however, patients aged 65 years or older were more likely to experience diarrhea, fatigue, pulmonary embolism, and syncope [152].

Bortezomib is active and well tolerated in patients who have high risk factors. In subgroup analyses of the APEX trial, bortezomib offered longer TTP and higher response rate versus Dex in patients with more than one line of prior therapy, patients who had β_2-microglobulin level 2.5 mg/L or greater, or patients refractory to prior treatment [154]. Age, serum β_2-microglobulin level, and the number or type of previous therapies did not affect TTP, DOR, or OS in a multivariate analysis [163], whereas according to results of SUMMIT and APEX trials chromosome 13 deletion or translocation t(4;14) do not seem to have an adverse prognostic impact on survival and response rates to bortezomib treatment [101,165–168], although the role of 1q21 amplification as a putative marker of adverse prognosis remains to be further explored. Notably, although bortezomib is active, with comparable overall response rates in light- and heavy-chain disease, most responders who had light-chain disease achieved complete remission (compared with about 25% of responders who had heavy-chain disease) [163]. Furthermore, the association of bortezomib treatment with significant increases in bone-specific alkaline phosphatase suggests bortezomib-induced activation of osteoblasts, providing an additional reason that bortezomib may be an attractive option for the management of patients who have extensive osteolytic disease [169].

In a phase II study of Thal in relapsed/refractory MM, β_2-microglobulin level and response to previous therapy did not affect response rate; however, multivariate analysis showed that high baseline β_2-microglobulin levels were predicted for shorter PFS, but not OS [52]. A study of Thal plus Dex in the relapsed setting showed that the regimen was superior to conventional chemotherapy in median PFS and OS in patients who had received one prior line of therapy, but comparable in patients who had received two or more lines of therapy [70]. Finally, in a pooled analysis of the two phase III studies of lenalidomide plus Dex versus Dex in the relapsed setting, lenalidomide plus Dex produced a higher response rate and longer TTP and OS compared with Dex alone in patients who had received more than one prior line of therapy [135], reflecting results in the overall study populations.

SUMMARY

Studies of bortezomib, thalidomide, and lenalidomide have shown promising clinical activity in relapsed/refractory MM. Bortezomib alone and in combination with other agents is associated with high response rates, consistently high rates of CR, and a predictable and manageable profile of adverse events. Thal-based regimens have also shown substantial clinical activity, and the FDA approval of the Thal analog lenalidomide (in its combination with Dex) has been another key step in the evolution of the clinical management of MM, because lenalidomide not only seems to be more potent but also has a manageable profile of side effects that lends itself to combinations with agents such as bortezomib. The accumulating experience from ongoing trials of bortezomib/lenalidomide/Dex combinations in patients who have relapsed/refractory or newly diagnosed MM will provide critical information that will determine the possible role of this combination as the basic backbone for combination regimens for management of advanced MM.

References

[1] Barlogie B, Hall R, Zander A, et al. High-dose melphalan with autologous bone marrow transplantation for multiple myeloma. Blood 1986;67:1298.

[2] Barlogie B, Alexanian R, Dicke KA, et al. High-dose chemoradiotherapy and autologous bone marrow transplantation for resistant multiple myeloma. Blood 1987;70:869.

[3] Barlogie B, Anaissie E, Bolejack V, et al. High CR and near-CR rate with bortezomib incorporated into up-front therapy of multiple myeloma with tandem transplants. J Clin Oncol 2006;24:426S.

[4] Richardson PG, Barlogie B, Berenson J, et al. A phase 2 study of bortezomib in relapsed, refractory myeloma. N Engl J Med 2003;348:2609.

[5] Alexanian R, Barlogie B, Dixon D. High-dose glucocorticoid treatment of resistant myeloma. Ann Intern Med 1986;105:8.

[6] Dimopoulos MA, Spencer A, Attal M, et al. Study of lenalidomide plus dexamethasone versus dexamethasone alone in relapsed or refractory multiple myeloma (MM): results of a phase 3 study (MM-010). Blood 2005;106:6A.

[7] Richardson PG, Sonneveld P, Schuster MW, et al. Bortezomib or high-dose dexamethasone for relapsed multiple myeloma. N Engl J Med 2005;352:2487.

[8] Weber DM, Chen C, Niesvizky R, et al. Lenalidomide plus high-dose dexamethasone provides improved overall survival compared to high-dose dexamethasone alone for relapsed or refractory multiple myeloma (MM): results of a North American phase III study (MM-009). J Clin Oncol 2006;24:7521.

[9] Gertz MA, Garton JP, Greipp PR, et al. A phase II study of high-dose methylprednisolone in refractory or relapsed multiple myeloma. Leukemia 1995;9:2115.

[10] Barlogie B, Smith L, Alexanian R. Effective treatment of advanced multiple myeloma refractory to alkylating agents. N Engl J Med 1984;310:1353.

[11] Anderson H, Scarffe JH, Ranson M, et al. VAD chemotherapy as remission induction for multiple myeloma. Br J Cancer 1995;71:326.

[12] Anderson K, Richardson P, Chanan-Khan A, et al. Single-agent bortezomib in previously untreated multiple myeloma (MM): results of a phase II multicenter study. J Clin Oncol 2006;24:423S.

[13] Gertz MA, Kalish LA, Kyle RA, et al. Phase III study comparing vincristine, doxorubicin (Adriamycin), and dexamethasone (VAD) chemotherapy with VAD plus recombinant interferon alfa-2 in refractory or relapsed multiple myeloma. An Eastern Cooperative Oncology Group study. Am J Clin Oncol 1995;18:475.

[14] Lokhorst HM, Meuwissen OJ, Bast EJ, et al. VAD chemotherapy for refractory multiple myeloma. Br J Haematol 1989;71:25.

[15] Phillips JK, Sherlaw-Johnson C, Pearce R, et al. A randomized study of MOD versus VAD in the treatment of relapsed and resistant multiple myeloma. Leuk Lymphoma 1995;17:465.

[16] Popat R, Oakervee HE, Curry N, et al. Reduced dose PAD combination therapy (PS-341/bortezomib, adriamycin and dexamethasone) for previously untreated patients with multiple myeloma. Blood 2005;106:717A.

[17] MacLennan IC, Chapman C, Dunn J, et al. Combined chemotherapy with ABCM versus melphalan for treatment of myelomatosis. The Medical Research Council Working Party for Leukaemia in Adults. Lancet 1992;339:200.

[18] Durie BG, Dixon DO, Carter S, et al. Improved survival duration with combination chemotherapy induction for multiple myeloma: a Southwest Oncology Group Study. J Clin Oncol 1986;4:1227.

[19] Giles FJ, Wickham NR, Rapoport BL, et al. Cyclophosphamide, etoposide, vincristine, adriamycin, and dexamethasone (CEVAD) regimen in refractory multiple myeloma: an International Oncology Study Group (IOSG) phase II protocol. Am J Hematol 2000;63:125.

[20] Lee CK, Barlogie B, Munshi N, et al. DTPACE: an effective, novel combination chemotherapy with thalidomide for previously treated patients with myeloma. J Clin Oncol 2003;21:2732.

[21] Hussein MA. Modifications to therapy for multiple myeloma: pegylated liposomal Doxorubicin in combination with vincristine, reduced-dose dexamethasone, and thalidomide. Oncologist 2003;(8 Suppl 3):39–45.

[22] Hussein MA, Baz R, Srkalovic G, et al. Phase 2 study of pegylated liposomal doxorubicin, vincristine, decreased-frequency dexamethasone, and thalidomide in newly diagnosed and relapsed-refractory multiple myeloma. Mayo Clin Proc 2006;81:889.

[23] Zervas K, Dimopoulos MA, Hatzicharissi E, et al. Primary treatment of multiple myeloma with thalidomide, vincristine, liposomal doxorubicin and dexamethasone (T-VAD doxil): a phase II multicenter study. Ann Oncol 2004;15:134.

[24] Baz R, Walker E, Karam MA, et al. Lenalidomide and pegylated liposomal doxorubicin-based chemotherapy for relapsed or refractory multiple myeloma: safety and efficacy. Ann Oncol 2006;17:1766.

[25] Biehn SE, Moore DT, Voorhees PM, et al. Extended follow-up of outcome measures in multiple myeloma patients treated on a phase I study with bortezomib and pegylated liposomal doxorubicin. Ann Hematol 2007;86:211.

[26] Orlowski RZ, Voorhees PM, Garcia RA, et al. Phase 1 trial of the proteasome inhibitor bortezomib and pegylated liposomal doxorubicin in patients with advanced hematologic malignancies. Blood 2005;105:3058.

[27] Manochakian R, Miller KC, Chanan-Khan AA. Bortezomib in combination with pegylated liposomal doxorubicin for the treatment of multiple myeloma. Clin Lymphoma Myeloma 2007;7:266.

[28] Dimopoulos MA, Alexanian R, Przepiorka D, et al. Thiotepa, busulfan, and cyclophospha-mide: a new preparative regimen for autologous marrow or blood stem cell transplantation in high-risk multiple myeloma. Blood 1993;82:2324.

[29] Alexanian R, Dimopoulos MA, Hester J, et al. Early myeloablative therapy for multiple myeloma. Blood 1994;84:4278.

[30] Alexanian R, Dimopoulos M, Smith T, et al. Limited value of myeloablative therapy for late multiple myeloma. Blood 1994;83:512.

[31] Fermand JP, Ravaud P, Chevret S, et al. High-dose therapy and autologous peripheral blood stem cell transplantation in multiple myeloma: up-front or rescue treatment? Results of a multicenter sequential randomized clinical trial. Blood 1998;92:3131.

[32] Fassas AB, Barlogie B, Ward S, et al. Survival after relapse following tandem autotrans-plants in multiple myeloma patients: the University of Arkansas total therapy I experience. Br J Haematol 2003;123:484.

[33] Lee CK, Barlogie B, Zangari M, et al. Transplantation as salvage therapy for high-risk patients with myeloma in relapse. Bone Marrow Transplant 2002;30:873.

[34] Crawley C, Iacobelli S, Bjorkstrand B, et al. Reduced-intensity conditioning for myeloma: lower nonrelapse mortality but higher relapse rates compared with myeloablative condi-tioning. Blood 2007;109:3588.

[35] Maloney DG, Molina AJ, Sahebi F, et al. Allografting with nonmyeloablative conditioning following cytoreductive autografts for the treatment of patients with multiple myeloma. Blood 2003;102(9):3447–54.

[36] Huff CA, Fuchs EJ, Noga SJ, et al. Long-term follow-up of T cell-depleted allogeneic bone marrow transplantation in refractory multiple myeloma: importance of allogeneic T cells. Biol Blood Marrow Transplant 2003;9(5):312–9.

[37] Kroger N, Perez-Simon JA, Myint H, et al. Relapse to prior autograft and chronic graft-versus-host disease are the strongest prognostic factors for outcome of melphalan/ fludarabine-based dose-reduced allogeneic stem cell transplantation in patients with multiple myeloma. Biol Blood Marrow Transplant 2004;10:698.

[38] D'Amato RJ, Loughnan MS, Flynn E, et al. Thalidomide is an inhibitor of angiogenesis. Proc Natl Acad Sci U S A 1994;91:4082.

[39] Vacca A, Ribatti D, Roncali L, et al. Bone marrow angiogenesis and progression in multiple myeloma. Br J Haematol 1994;87:503.

[40] Anderson KC. Lenalidomide and thalidomide: mechanisms of action–similarities and differences. Semin Hematol 2005;42:S3.

[41] Badros A, Goloubeva AR, Ruehle K, et al. Phase I trial of bortezomib (V) in combination with "DT-PACE": toxicity, stem cell collection and engraftment in newly diagnosed multiple myeloma (MM) patients (Pts). Blood 2005;106:771A.

[42] Davies FE, Raje N, Hideshima T, et al. Thalidomide and immunomodulatory deriva-tives augment natural killer cell cytotoxicity in multiple myeloma. Blood 2001;98: 210.

[43] Hideshima T, Chauhan D, Shima Y, et al. Thalidomide and its analogs overcome drug resistance of human multiple myeloma cells to conventional therapy. Blood 2000;96: 2943.

[44] Mitsiades N, Mitsiades CS, Poulaki V, et al. Apoptotic signaling induced by immunomod-ulatory thalidomide analogs in human multiple myeloma cells: therapeutic implications. Blood 2002;99:4525.

[45] Singhal S, Mehta J, Desikan R, et al. Antitumor activity of thalidomide in refractory multiple myeloma. N Engl J Med 1999;341:1565.

[46] Barlogie B, Desikan R, Eddlemon P, et al. Extended survival in advanced and refractory multiple myeloma after single-agent thalidomide: identification of prognostic factors in a phase 2 study of 169 patients. Blood 2001;98:492.

[47] Alexanian R, Weber D, Ananostopoulos A, et al. Thalidomide with or without dexameth-asone for refractory or relapsing multiple myeloma. Semin Hematol 2003;40:3.

[48] Brenne AT, Romstad LH, Gimsing P, et al. A low serum level of soluble tumor necrosis factor receptor p55 predicts response to thalidomide in advanced multiple myeloma. Haematologica 2004;89:552.

[49] Hus I, Dmoszynska A, Manko J, et al. An evaluation of factors predicting long-term response to thalidomide in 234 patients with relapsed or resistant multiple myeloma. Br J Cancer 2004;91:1873.

[50] Hus M, Dmoszynska A, Soroka-Wojtaszko M, et al. Thalidomide treatment of resistant or relapsed multiple myeloma patients. Haematologica 2001;86:404.

[51] Kumar S, Gertz MA, Dispenzieri A, et al. Response rate, durability of response, and survival after thalidomide therapy for relapsed multiple myeloma. Mayo Clin Proc 2003;78:34.

[52] Mileshkin L, Biagi JJ, Mitchell P, et al. Multicenter phase 2 trial of thalidomide in relapsed/refractory multiple myeloma: adverse prognostic impact of advanced age. Blood 2003;102:69.

[53] Neben K, Moehler T, Benner A, et al. Dose-dependent effect of thalidomide on overall survival in relapsed multiple myeloma. Clin Cancer Res 2002;8:3377.

[54] Rajkumar SV, Fonseca R, Dispenzieri A, et al. Thalidomide in the treatment of relapsed multiple myeloma. Mayo Clin Proc 2000;75:897.

[55] Rajkumar SV, Hayman SR, Lacy MQ, et al. Combination therapy with lenalidomide plus dexamethasone (Rev/Dex) for newly diagnosed myeloma. Blood 2005;106:4050.

[56] Schey SA, Cavenagh J, Johnson R, et al. An UK myeloma forum phase II study of thalidomide; long term follow-up and recommendations for treatment. Leuk Res 2003;27:909.

[57] Tosi P, Ronconi S, Zamagni E, et al. Salvage therapy with thalidomide in multiple myeloma patients relapsing after autologous peripheral blood stem cell transplantation. Haematologica 2001;86:409.

[58] Tosi P, Zamagni E, Cellini C, et al. Salvage therapy with thalidomide in patients with advanced relapsed/refractory multiple myeloma. Haematologica 2002;87:408.

[59] Waage A, Gimsing P, Juliusson G, et al. Early response predicts thalidomide efficiency in patients with advanced multiple myeloma. Br J Haematol 2004;125:149.

[60] Wang M, Delasalle K, Giralt S, et al. Rapid control of previously untreated multiple myeloma with bortezomib-thalidomide-dexamethasone followed by early intensive therapy. Blood 2005;106:231A.

[61] Wu KL, Helgason HH, van der Holt B, et al. Analysis of efficacy and toxicity of thalidomide in 122 patients with multiple myeloma: response of soft-tissue plasmacytomas. Leukemia 2005;19:143.

[62] Yakoub-Agha I, Attal M, Dumontet C, et al. Thalidomide in patients with advanced multiple myeloma: a study of 83 patients—report of the Intergroupe Francophone du Myelome (IFM). Hematol J 2002;3:185.

[63] Grosbois B, Bellissant E, Moreau P, et al. Thalidomide (Thal) in the treatment of advanced multiple myeloma (MM). A prospective study of 120 patients. Blood 2001;98:163A.

[64] Barlogie B. Thalidomide and CC-5013 in multiple myeloma: the University of Arkansas experience. Semin Hematol 2003;40:33.

[65] Yakoub-Agha I, Doyen C, Hulin C, et al. A multicenter prospective randomized study testing non-inferiority of thalidomide 100 mg/day as compared with 400 mg/day in patients with refractory/relapsed multiple myeloma: results of the final analysis of the IFM 01-02 study. J Clin Oncol 2006;24:427S.

[66] Weber DM, Gavino M, Delasalle K, et al. Thalidomide alone or with dexamethasone for multiple myeloma. Blood 1999;94:604A.

[67] Anagnostopoulos A, Weber D, Rankin K, et al. Thalidomide and dexamethasone for resistant multiple myeloma. Br J Haematol 2003;121:768.

[68] Dimopoulos MA, Zervas K, Kouvatseas G, et al. Thalidomide and dexamethasone combination for refractory multiple myeloma. Ann Oncol 2001;12:991.

[69] Palumbo A, Giaccone L, Bertola A, et al. Low-dose thalidomide plus dexamethasone is an effective salvage therapy for advanced myeloma. Haematologica 2001;86:399.

[70] Palumbo A, Bertola A, Falco P, et al. Efficacy of low-dose thalidomide and dexamethasone as first salvage regimen in multiple myeloma. Hematol J 2004;5:318.

[71] Palumbo A, Falco P, Ambrosini MT, et al. Thalidomide plus dexamethasone is an effective salvage regimen for myeloma patients relapsing after autologous transplant. Eur J Haematol 2005;75:391.

[72] Palumbo A, Falco P, Falcone A, et al. Oral Revlimid (R) plus melphalan and prednisone (R-MP) for newly diagnosed multiple myeloma: results of a multicenter phase I/II study. Blood 2006;108:240A.

[73] Fermand JP, Jaccard A, Macro M, et al. A randomized comparison of dexamethasone plus thalidomide (Dex/Thal) vs dex plus placebo (Dex/P) in patients (pts) with relapsing multiple myeloma (MM). Blood 2006;108:1017A.

[74] Glasmacher A, Hahn C, Hoffmann F, et al. Thalidomide in relapsed or refractory patients with multiple myeloma: monotherapy or combination therapy? A report from systematic reviews. Blood 2005;106:364B.

[75] Hall VC, El-Azhary RA, Bouwhuis S, et al. Dermatologic side effects of thalidomide in patients with multiple myeloma. J Am Acad Dermatol 2003;48:548.

[76] Harousseau JL, Attal M, Coiteux V, et al. Bortezomib plus dexamethasone as induction treatment prior to autologous stem cell transplantation in patients with newly diagnosed multiple myeloma: premilinary results of an IFM phase II study. J Clin Oncol 2005;23:598S.

[77] Moehler TM, Neben K, Benner A, et al. Salvage therapy for multiple myeloma with thalidomide and CED chemotherapy. Blood 2001;98:3846.

[78] Offidani M, Corvatta L, Marconi M, et al. Low-dose thalidomide with pegylated liposomal doxorubicin and high-dose dexamethasone for relapsed/refractory multiple myeloma: a prospective, multicenter, phase II study. Haematologica 2006;91:133.

[79] Garcia-Sanz R, Gonzalez-Porras JR, Hernandez JM, et al. The oral combination of thalidomide, cyclophosphamide and dexamethasone (ThaCyDex) is effective in relapsed/refractory multiple myeloma. Leukemia 2004;18:856.

[80] Dimopoulos MA, Hamilos G, Zomas A, et al. Pulsed cyclophosphamide, thalidomide and dexamethasone: an oral regimen for previously treated patients with multiple myeloma. Hematol J 2004;5:112.

[81] Kyriakou C, Thomson K, D'Sa S, et al. Low-dose thalidomide in combination with oral weekly cyclophosphamide and pulsed dexamethasone is a well tolerated and effective regimen in patients with relapsed and refractory multiple myeloma. Br J Haematol 2005;129:763.

[82] Knop S, Gerecke C, Topp MS, et al. Lenalidomide (Revlimid (TM)), adriamycin and dexamethasone chemotherapy (RAD) is safe and effective in treatment of relapsed multiple myeloma—first results of a German multicenter phase I/II trial. Blood 2006;108:125A.

[83] Richardson PG, Jagannath S, Avigan DE, et al. Lenalidomide plus Bortezomib (Rev-Vel) in relapsed and/or refractory multiple myeloma (MM): final results of a multicenter phase 1 trial. ASH Annual Meeting Abstracts 2006;108(11):405.

[84] Bross PF, Kane R, Farrell AT, et al. Approval summary for bortezomib for injection in the treatment of multiple myeloma. Clin Cancer Res 2004;10:3954.

[85] Kane RC, Bross PF, Farrell AT, et al. Velcade: U.S. FDA approval for the treatment of multiple myeloma progressing on prior therapy. Oncologist 2003;8:508.

[86] Kane RC, Farrell AT, Sridhara R, et al. United States Food and Drug Administration approval summary: bortezomib for the treatment of progressive multiple myeloma after one prior therapy. Clin Cancer Res 2006;12:2955.

[87] Adams J. The development of proteasome inhibitors as anticancer drugs. Cancer Cell 2004;5:417.

[88] Adams J. Development of the proteasome inhibitor PS-341. Oncologist 2002;7:9.

[89] Adams J. The proteasome: a suitable antineoplastic target. Nat Rev Cancer 2004;4:349.

[90] Adams J, Behnke M, Chen S, et al. Potent and selective inhibitors of the proteasome: dipeptidyl boronic acids. Bioorg Med Chem Lett 1998;8:333.

[91] Adams J, Palombella VJ, Elliott PJ. Proteasome inhibition: a new strategy in cancer treatment. Invest New Drugs 2000;18:109.

[92] Adams J, Palombella VJ, Sausville EA, et al. Proteasome inhibitors: a novel class of potent and effective antitumor agents. Cancer Res 1999;59:2615.

[93] Voorhees PM, Dees EC, O'Neil B, et al. The proteasome as a target for cancer therapy. Clin Cancer Res 2003;9:6316.

[94] Hideshima T, Richardson P, Chauhan D, et al. The proteasome inhibitor PS-341 inhibits growth, induces apoptosis, and overcomes drug resistance in human multiple myeloma cells. Cancer Res 2001;61:3071.

[95] Ma MH, Yang HH, Parker K, et al. The proteasome inhibitor PS-341 markedly enhances sensitivity of multiple myeloma tumor cells to chemotherapeutic agents. Clin Cancer Res 2003;9:1136.

[96] Mitsiades N, Mitsiades CS, Poulaki V, et al. Molecular sequelae of proteasome inhibition in human multiple myeloma cells. Proc Natl Acad Sci U S A 2002;99:14374.

[97] Mitsiades N, Mitsiades CS, Richardson PG, et al. The proteasome inhibitor PS-341 potentiates sensitivity of multiple myeloma cells to conventional chemotherapeutic agents: therapeutic applications. Blood 2003;101:2377.

[98] Jagannath S, Barlogie B, Berenson J, et al. A phase 2 study of two doses of bortezomib in relapsed or refractory myeloma. Br J Haematol 2004;127:165.

[99] Richardson PG, Barlogie B, Berenson J, et al. Extended follow-up of a phase II trial in relapsed, refractory multiple myeloma: final time-to-event results from the SUMMIT trial. Cancer 2006;106:1316.

[100] Richardson P, Sonneveld P, Schuster M, et al. Bortezomib continues to demonstrate superior efficacy compared with high-dose dexamethasone in relapsed multiple myeloma: updated results of the APEX trial. Blood 2005;106:715A.

[101] Kropff MH, Bisping G, Wenning D, et al. Bortezomib in combination with dexamethasone for relapsed multiple myeloma. Leuk Res 2005;29:587.

[102] Kropff M, Bisping G, Liebisch P, et al. Bortezomib in combination with high-dose dexamethasone and continuous low-dose oral cyclophosphamide for relapsed multiple myeloma. Blood 2005;106:716A.

[103] Reece DE, Piza G, Trudel S, et al. A phase I-II trial of bortezomib (Veleade) (Vc) and oral cyclophosphamide (CY) plus prednisone (P) for relapsed/refractory multiple myeloma (MM). Blood 2005;106:718A.

[104] Suvannasankha A, Smith GG, Abonour R. Weekly bortezomib with or without glucocorticosteroids is effective in patients with relapsed or refractory multiple myeloma. Blood 2005;106:720A.

[105] Friedman J, Al-Zoubi A, Kaminski M, et al. A new model predicting at least a very good partial response in patients with multiple myeloma after 2 cycles of velcade-based therapy [abstract P.0741]. Haematologica 2006;91:273.

[106] Jakubowiak AJ, Brackett L, Kendall T, et al. Combination therapy with velcade, doxil, and dexamethasone (VDD) for patients with relapsed/refractory multiple myeloma (MM). Blood 2005;106:378B.

[107] Berenson JR, Yang HH, Sadler K, et al. Phase I/II trial assessing bortezomib and melphalan combination therapy for the treatment of patients with relapsed or refractory multiple myeloma. J Clin Oncol 2006;24:937.

[108] Popat R, Oakervee HE, Foot N, et al. A phase I/II study of bortezomib and low dose intravenous melphalan (BM) for relapsed multiple myeloma. Blood 2005;106:718A.

[109] Chari A, Kaplan L, Linker C, et al. Phase I/II study of bortezomib in combination with lipo-somal doxorubicin and melphalan in relapsed or refractory multiple myeloma. Blood 2005;106:379B.

[110] Hrusovsky I, Heidtmann HH. Combination therapy of bortezomib with low-dose benda-mustine in elderly patients with advanced multiple myeloma. Blood 2005;106:363B.

[111] Berenson JR, Matous JV, Ferretti D, et al. A phase I/II study of arsenic trioxide, bortezomib, and ascorbic acid in relapsed or refractory multiple myeloma. J Clin Oncol 2006;24:449S.

[112] Yeh HS, Swift RA, Ferretti D, et al. Phase I study of bortezomib and Sm-153-lexidronam combination for refractory and relapsed multiple myeloma. J Clin Oncol 2006;24:450S.

[113] Chanan-Khan AA, Richardson PG, Alsina M, et al. Phase 1 clinical trial of KOS-953+Bortezomib (BZ) in relapsed refractory multiple myeloma (MM). Blood 2005;106:109a.

[114] Padmanabhan S, Miller K, Musiel L, et al. Bortezomib (Velcade) in combination with lipo-somal doxorubicin (Doxil) and thalidomide is an active salvage regimen in patients with relpase or refractory multiple myeloma: final results of a phase II trial. Haematologica 2006;91:277.

[115] Zangari M, Barlogie B, Burns MJ, et al. Velcade (V)-thalidomide (T)-dexamethasone (D) for advanced and refractory multiple myeloma (MM): Long-term follow-up of Phase I-II trial UARK 2001-37: superior outcome in patients with normal cytogenetics and no prior T. Blood 2005;106:717A.

[116] Teoh G, Tan D, Hwang W, et al. Addition of bortezomib to thalidomide, dexamethasone and zoledronic acid (VTD-Z regimen) significantly improves response rate complete remis-sion rate in patients with relapsed/refractory multiple myeloma [abstract 17537]. J Clin Oncol 2006;24:68368s.

[117] Leoni F, Casini C, Breschi C, et al. Low dose bortezomib, dexamethasone, thalidomide plus liposomal doxorubicin in relapsed and refractory myeloma. Haematologica 2006;9:281.

[118] Hollmig K, Stover J, Talamo G, et al. Bortezomib (Velcade (TM)) plus Adriamycin (TM) plus thalidomide plus dexamethasone (VATD) as an effective regimen in patients with refractory or relapsed multiple myeloma (MM). Blood 2004;104:659A.

[119] Palumbo A, Ambrosini MT, Benevolo G, et al. Bortezomib, melphalan, prednisone, and thalidomide for relapsed multiple myeloma. Blood 2007;109(7):2767–72.

[120] Terpos E, Anagnostopoulos A, Heath D, et al. The combination of bortezomib, melphalan, dexamethasone and intermittent thalidomide (VMDT) is an effective regimen for relapsed/refractory myeloma and reduces serum levels of Dickkopf-1, RANKL, MIP-1 alpha and angiogenic cytokines. Blood 2006;108:1010A.

[121] Musto P, Avonto I, Scalzulli PR, et al. Intermediate-dose melphalan (100 mg/m^2), bortezo-mib, thalidomide, dexamethasone and stem cell support in patients with refractory or relapsed myeloma. Haematologica 2006;91:88.

[122] Richardson PG, Schlossman RL, Weller E, et al. Immunomodulatory drug CC-5013 over-comes drug resistance and is well tolerated in patients with relapsed multiple myeloma. Blood 2002;100:3063.

[123] Richardson P, Jagannath S, Hussein M, et al. A multicenter, single-arm, open-label study to evaluate the efficacy and safety of single-agent lenalidomide in patients with relapsed and refractory multiple myeloma; Prelininary results. Blood 2005;106:449A.

[124] Richardson PG, Blood E, Mitsiades CS, et al. A randomized phase 2 study of lenalidomide therapy for patients with relapsed or relapsed and refractory multiple myeloma. Blood 2006;108:3458.

[125] Richardson PG, Briemberg H, Jagannath S, et al. Frequency, characteristics, and revers-ibility of peripheral neuropathy during treatment of advanced multiple myeloma with bortezomib. J Clin Oncol 2006;24:3113.

[126] San Miguel JF, Richardson P, Sonneveld P, et al. Frequency, characteristics, and reversibil-ity of peripheral neuropathy (PN) in the APEX trial. Blood 2005;106:111A.

[127] Oakervee HE, Popat R, Curry N, et al. PAD combination therapy (PS-341/bortezomib, doxorubicin and dexamethasone) for previously untreated patients with multiple myeloma. Br J Haematol 2005;129:755.

[128] Richardson P, Schlossman R, Munshi N, et al. A phase 1 trial of lenalidomide (REVLIMID (R)) with bortezomib (VELCADE (R)) in relapsed and refractory multiple myeloma. Blood 2005;106:110A.

[129] Lonial S, Waller EK, Richardson PG, et al. Risk factors and kinetics of thrombocytopenia associated with bortezomib for relapsed, refractory multiple myeloma. Blood 2005;106:3777.

[130] Lonial S, Richardson P, Sonneveld P, et al. Hematologic profiles in the phase 3 APEX trial. Blood 2005;106:970A.

[131] Berenson JR, Jagannath S, Barlogie B, et al. Safety of prolonged therapy with bortezomib in relapsed or refractory multiple myeloma. Cancer 2005;104:2141.

[132] Orlowski RZ, Zhuang SH, Parekh T, et al. The combination of pegylated liposomal doxorubicin and bortezomib significantly improves time to progression of patients with relapsed/refractory multiple myeloma compared with bortezomib alone: results from a planned interim analysis of a randomized phase III study. Blood 2006;108:124A.

[133] Terpos E, Anagnostopoulos A, Kastritis E, et al. The combination of bortezomib, melphalan, dexamethasone and intermittent thalidomide (VMDT) is an effective treatment for relapsed/refractory myeloma: results of a phase II clinical trial. Blood 2005;106:110A.

[134] Zangari M, Tricot G, Zeldis J, et al. Results of phase I study of CC-5013 for the treatment of multiple myeloma (MM) patients who relapse after high dose chemotherapy (HDCT). Blood 2001;98:775A.

[135] Stadtmauer EA, Weber D, Dimopoulos MA, et al. Lenalidomide (Len) in combination with dexamethasone (Dex) is more effective than Dex alone at first relapse and provides better outcomes when used early rather than as later salvage therapy in relapsed multiple myeloma (MM). J Clin Oncol 2006;24:446S.

[136] Wang M, Knight R, Dimopoulos M, et al. Lenalidomide in combination with dexamethasone was more effective than dexamethasone in patients who have received prior thalidomide for relapsed or refractory multiple myeloma. Blood 2006;108:1014A.

[137] Weber D, Wang M, Chen C, et al. Lenalidomide plus high-dose dexamethasone provides improved overall survival compared to high-dose dexamethasone alone for relapsed or refractory multiple myeloma (MM): results of 2 phase III studies (MM-009, MM-010) and subgroup analysis of patients with impaired renal function. Blood 2006;108:1012A.

[138] Reece DE, Masih-Khan E, Chen C, et al. Use of lenalidomide (Revlimid (R) +/- corticosteroids in relapsed/refractory multiple myeloma patients with elevated baseline serum creatinine levels. Blood 2006;108:1013A.

[139] Mitsiades CS, Mitsiades NS, McMullan CJ, et al. Antimyeloma activity of heat shock protein-90 inhibition. Blood 2006;107:1092.

[140] Richardson PG, Chanan-Khan AA, Alsina M, et al. Safety and activity of KOS-953 in patients with relapsed refractory multiple myeloma (MM): interim results of a phase 1 trial. Blood 2005;106:10910a.

[141] Richardson P, Chanan-Khan A, Lonial S, et al. A multicenter phase 1 clinical trial of Tanespimycin (KOS-953) + Bortezomib (BZ): encouraging activity and manageable toxicity in heavily pre-treated patients with relapsed refractory multiple myeloma (MM). ASH Annual Meeting Abstracts 2006;108(11):406.

[142] Knudsen LM, Hippe E, Hjorth M, et al. Renal function in newly diagnosed multiple myeloma—a demographic study of 1353 patients. The Nordic Myeloma Study Group. Eur J Haematol 1994;53:207.

[143] Knudsen LM, Hjorth M, Hippe E. Renal failure in multiple myeloma: reversibility and impact on the prognosis. Nordic Myeloma Study Group. Eur J Haematol 2000;65:175.

[144] Jagannath S, Barlogie B, Berenson JR, et al. Bortezomib in recurrent and/or refractory multiple myeloma. Cancer 2005;103:1195.

[145] Jagannath S, Durie B, Wolf J, et al. Bortezomib therapy alone and in combination with dexamethasone for patients with previously untreated multiple myeloma. Blood 2005;106:231A.

[146] Mulkerin D, Remick S, Ramanathan R, et al. A dose-escalating and pharmacologic study of bortezomib in adult cancer patients with impaired renal function. J Clin Oncol 2006;24: 87S.

[147] Chanan-Khan AA, Richardson P, Lonial S, et al. Safety and efficacy of bortezomib in multiple myeloma patients with renal failure requiring dialysis. Blood 2005;106:716A.

[148] Mohrbacher A, Levine AM. Reversal of advanced renal dysfunction on bortezomib treatment in multiple myeloma patients. J Clin Oncol 2005;23:612S.

[149] Tosi P, Zamagni E, Cellini C, et al. Thalidomide alone or in combination with dexamethasone in patients with advanced, relapsed or refractory multiple myeloma and renal failure. Eur J Haematol 2004;73:98.

[150] Fakhouri F, Guerraoui H, Presne C, et al. Thalidomide in patients with multiple myeloma and renal failure. Br J Haematol 2004;125:96.

[151] Harris E, Behrens J, Samson D, et al. Use of thalidomide in patients with myeloma and renal failure may be associated with unexplained hyperkalaemia. Br J Haematol 2003;122:160.

[152] REVLIMID (lenalidomide) Package Insert, in. Summit, NJ, USA: Celgene Corporation, 2006.

[153] Mateos MV, Hernandez JM, Hernandez MT, et al. Bortezomib plus melphalan and prednisone in elderly untreated patients with multiple myeloma: results of a multicenter phase 1/2 study. Blood 2006;108:2165.

[154] Richardson PG, Sonneveld P, Schuster MW, et al. Safety and efficacy of bortezomib in high-risk and elderly patients with relapsed myeloma. J Clin Oncology 2005;23:568S.

[155] THALOMID (thalidomide) Product Information, in. Summit, NJ, USA: Celgene Corporation, 2006.

[156] Dingli D, Rajkumar SV, Nowakowski GS, et al. Combination therapy with thalidomide and dexamethasone in patients with newly diagnosed multiple myeloma not undergoing upfront autologous stem cell transplantation: a phase II trial. Haematologica 2005;90: 1650.

[157] Dispenzieri A, Blood E, Vesole D, et al. A phase II study of PS-341 for patients with high risk, newly diagnosed multiple myeloma: a trial of the Eastern Cooperative Oncology Group (E2A02). Blood 2005;106:715A.

[158] Facon T, Mary J, Harousseau J, et al. Superiority of melphalan-prednisone (MP) plus thalidomide (THAL) over MP and autologous stem cell transplantation in the treatment of newly diagnosed elderly patients with multiple myeloma. J Clin Oncol 2006;24:1S.

[159] Ludwig H, Drach J, Tothova E, et al. Thalidomide-dexamethasone versus melphalan-prednisolone as first line treatment in elderly patients with multiple myeloma: An interim analysis. Blood 2005;106:231A.

[160] Offidani M, Corvatta L, Piersantelli MN, et al. Thalidomide, dexamethasone, and pegylated liposomal doxorubicin (ThaDD) for patients older than 65 years with newly diagnosed multiple myeloma. Blood 2006;108:2159.

[161] Orlowski RZ, Peterson BL, Sanford B, et al. Bortezomib and pegylated liposomal doxorubicin as induction therapy for adult patients with symptomatic multiple myeloma: Cancer and Leukemia Group B study 10301. Blood 2006;108:239A.

[162] Palumbo A, Bringhen S, Caravita T, et al. Oral melphalan and prednisone chemotherapy plus thalidomide compared with melphalan and prednisone alone in elderly patients with multiple myeloma: randomised controlled trial. Lancet 2006;367:825.

[163] Richardson PG, Barlogie B, Berenson J, et al. Clinical factors predictive of outcome with bortezomib in patients with relapsed, refractory multiple myeloma. Blood 2005;106: 2977.

[164] Rajkumar SV, Blood E, Vesole D, et al. Phase III clinical trial of thalidomide plus dexamethasone compared with dexamethasone alone in newly diagnosed multiple myeloma:

a clinical trial coordinated by the Eastern Cooperative Oncology Group. J Clin Oncol 2006;24:431.

[165] Chang H, Trieu Y, Qi X, et al. Bortezomib therapy response is independent of cytogenetic abnormalities in relapsed/refractory multiple myeloma. Leuk Res 2007;31:779.

[166] Drach J, Kuenburg E, Sagaster V, et al. Short survival, despite promising response rates, after bortezomib treatment of multiple myeloma patients with a 13q-deletion. Blood 2005;106:152A.

[167] Drach J, Sagaster V, Odelga V, et al. Amplification of 1q21 is associated with poor outcome after treatment with bortezomib in relapsed/refractory multiple myeloma. Blood 2006;108:970A.

[168] Jagannath S, Richardson PG, Sonneveld P, et al. Bortezomib appears to overcome the poor prognosis conferred by chromosome 13 deletion in phase 2 and 3 trials. Leukemia 2007;21:151.

[169] Zangari M, Yaccoby S, Cavallo F, et al. Response to bortezomib and activation of osteoblasts in multiple myeloma. Clin Lymphoma Myeloma 2006;7:109.

Hematol Oncol Clin N Am 21 (2007) 1217–1230

HEMAT⬛L⬛GY/ON⬛⬛L⬛GY ⬛LINICS
OF NORTH AMERICA

ELSEVIER
SAUNDERS

Immune Therapies

Rao H. Prabhala, PhD[a,b], Nikhil C. Munshi, MD[c,*]

[a]Jerome Lipper Multiple Myeloma Center, Dana-Farber Cancer Institute, Boston, MA 02115, USA
[b]Veterans Administration Boston Healthcare System, West Roxbury, MA 02132, USA
[c]Jerome Multiple Myeloma Medical Center, Department of Medical Oncology, Dana Farber
Cancer Institute, Harvard Medical School, 44 Binney Street, Boston, MA 02115, USA

N ovel targeted therapies are achieving responses in more than 90% of patients who have newly diagnosed multiple myeloma (MM), with one third of these patients achieving complete or near-complete responses. Patients still experience disease progression, however, and curative outcomes are rare. This situation has led to evaluation of novel therapeutic interventions, including immune therapy, in MM. Allogeneic transplant has provided the rationale for development of vaccination strategies. Development of successful immune therapy in MM has been directed at two aspects: first, to develop a successful vaccine that is able to target MM cells with therapeutic efficacy; and second, to improve the immune function to allow robust responses to immune-based intervention [1].

In this article, we provide a brief summary of the status of the immune system in myeloma and a detailed account of the clinical trials performed with myeloma-related antigens, including idiotype (Id) alone or in conjugation with other proteins and pulsed with dendritic cells (DCs). Future immunotherapy strategies for the improvement of treatment of multiple myeloma and monoclonal gammopathy of undetermined significance (MGUS) are also covered.

OBSTACLES TO EFFECTIVE ANTI-MYELOMA IMMUNITY

With the advancements in immunology, there is better understanding of the interrelationships between MM cells and immune cells. To develop an effective cancer vaccine, one has to strike a balance between triggering autoimmunity and generating tumor immunity. Low-avidity autoreactive T cells are present and can be used to mount anti-tumor immunity [2]. Additionally, to generate robust immune responses even against foreign pathogenic antigens, dendritic

The National Institutes of Health and Veterans Administration support this work.

*Corresponding author. Department of Medical Oncology Dana-Farber Cancer Institute, 44 Binney Street, Boston, MA 02115. E-mail address: nikhil_munshi@dfci.harvard.edu (N.C. Munshi).

0889-8588/07/$ – see front matter
doi:10.1016/j.hoc.2007.08.011

Published by Elsevier Inc.
hemonc.theclinics.com

cells orchestrate an appropriate inflammatory cytokine milieu [3]. However, identifying tumor antigens, which are important in eliciting antitumor immunity rather than triggering autoimmunity, has been a major obstacle in developing immune therapy for MM. The approaches pursued are first to identify patient-specific self-antigens that are randomly mutated over time because of genetic instability [4]. These types of antigens do not generally induce autoimmunity and tolerance; however, this approach may be less practical for large-scale applications. The second approach involves use of shared nonmutated self-antigens, which may be prone to develop tolerance when generating antitumor immunity. In this context, telomerase reverse transcriptase has been targeted to vaccinate cancer patients to reduce tumor evasion [5,6]. Additionally, there is increased realization of the importance of microenvironmental components, including stromal cells and cytokines, in supporting the tumor cell survival and the expression of antigenic determinants that need to be considered for effective immune therapy strategies [7]. Finally, to optimize immune therapy strategies, multivariable trials evaluating immunologic endpoints along with clinical efficacy should take the place of the traditional clinical trial design for testing cytotoxic drugs [8].

INTERACTIONS BETWEEN IMMUNE CELLS AND MULTIPLE MYELOMA CELLS

Tumor vaccines have concentrated on generating CTLs (cytotoxic T lymphocytes) to kill tumor cells [9]. A growing body of literature provides convincing evidence that CD4 cells and antibody production increase the efficacy of immune therapy approaches [10–13]. Furthermore, one has to take advantage of homeostatic proliferation [14,15] in a lymphopenic host toward developing antitumor immunity. The additional role of immune regulation by Forkhead box protein 3 (FOXP3)$^+$ CD4 cells [16–23], the influence of the cytokine milieu to generate T_H17 cells [24–26], and stress-related natural killer group 2 member D ligands (MICA and MICB, MHC class I polypeptide-related sequence A and B) [27,28] in modulating immune responses in myeloma is being defined. The regulatory T cells that are positive for FOXP3 (natural, expanded, and induced) play a critical role in immune homeostasis and are capable of modulating immunity, autoimmunity, or tolerance. They predominantly express CD4 and CD25 [29] in addition to FOXP3, CTL-associated protein 4, and glucocorticoid-induced tumor necrosis factor receptor. Their functions are mediated by TGF-β (transforming growth factor β) and vitamin A derivatives [30] and are associated with other transcription factors, including nuclear factor of activated T cells, activator protein 1, runt-related transcription factor 1, and nuclear factor-κB [22,31,32]. Naïve CD4 cells can be differentiated to FOXP3$^+$ cells in the presence of TGF-β and can be differentiated into T_H17 cells in the presence of TGF-β and interleukin (IL)–6 [33,34] and IL-1β or IL-23 [24,26]. On the other hand, IL-6 suppresses the induction of FOXP3 [34,35]. Complex networks of cytokines play a crucial role in the differentiation of FOXP3 or $T_H17$cells during which antigen-specific immune responses are generated.

With reduced FOXP3$^+$ cell number and function, autoimmunity may be observed, whereas their increased activity may lead to immune suppression in instead of immunity.

IMMUNOBIOLOGY IN MYELOMA

Multiple myeloma exhibits several immune deficiencies in various compartments of the immune system. The complex nature of the network that prevents the generation of robust immune responses in patients who have myeloma is represented in Fig. 1.

Cell-Mediated Responses

Myeloma patients have hyperactive T-cell responses and deficient antibody responses mediated by B cells [1]. CD4 and CD8 T cells seem to be impaired in the expression of various surface markers and functional ability in MGUS and myeloma [36–38]; however, the basis for these deficiencies remains unclear. An impairment in the diversity of T-cell receptors by defective V-beta repertoire is observed in myeloma following high-dose chemotherapy [39]. Although specific cellular and humoral responses against viral and tumor antigens have been reported [40], protective antibody production against pneumonia-causing bacteria is lacking in more than 80% of patients who have myeloma [41,42]. In

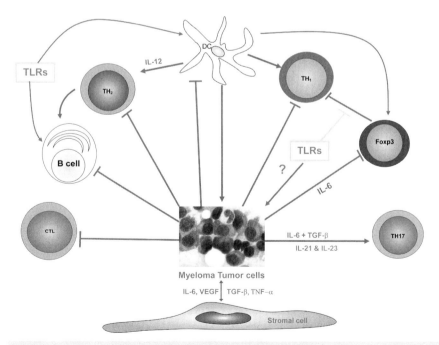

Fig. 1. Interplay between myeloma-bone marrow stromal cells microenvironment and immune responses.

addition, patients who have myeloma showed poor cytotoxic T-cell responses against viral antigens [40]. Several studies have shown that idiotype-specific responses can be generated in myeloma, following vaccination, indicating at least a partly competent immune system with the ability to generate antitumor immune responses is feasible.

Antigen-Presenting Cells

Antigen-presenting cells (APCs) are generally equipped with antigen processing, presentation, and costimulatory machinery and human leukocyte antigen (HLA) molecules, to generate specific immune responses. We and others have shown in earlier studies that APCs are functional, at least partially, in myeloma and can be used for the immune-based clinical studies [43]. In our laboratory, different classes of myeloma proteins pulsed with DCs were used in generating in vivo anti-myeloma immune responses [44]. Others have shown impaired DC function, however. For example, in one study DCs failed to up-regulate necessary CD80 expression, which may be associated with myeloma progression [37]. This failure might be because of exposure to cytokines, such as TGF-β and IL-10. $CD34^+$ DC progenitor cell development may be influenced by IL-6 in myeloma and can be corrected by the treatment with anti–IL-6 antibodies [45]. In addition, in a recent study [46] monocyte-derived DCs from patients who have myeloma expressed lower levels of important activation surface markers, including CD40, CD80, and HLA-DR, and presented recall antigens poorly to T cells. This phenomenon might be because of several cytokines elevated in the tumor microenvironment and serum, including IL-6, IL-10, TGF-β, and vascular endothelial growth factor (VEGF). It is now feasible to improve the defective DC functions in myeloma [47] by in vitro DC development techniques and by using innate immune stimulants like CpGs [48,49].

Regulatory T Cells

Dysregulation of naturally occurring $CD4^+CD25^+$ T regulatory cells in myeloma at initial diagnosis has been reported [50]. This study indicated lower numbers of $Foxp3^+$ regulatory T cells in peripheral blood mononuclear cells of patients who had myeloma compared with normal healthy volunteers, which was additionally associated with impaired inhibitory responses, Regulatory T cells contribute in establishing homeostasis following specific immunity and in keeping autoantigen-based immune responses under control or with a minimal level of pathologic consequences. High IL-6 levels in myeloma may down-regulate regulatory T cell suppressive activity [34,51]. In another study, however, a higher number of regulatory T cells were reported in myeloma in a purified $CD4^+CD25^{high}$ population, capable of suppressive activity at 1:2 ratio in a three-way mixed lymphocyte reaction following 24 hours of in vitro activation [52]. These regulatory T cells were activated away from the tumor microenvironment cytokine milieu before evaluation of their functional capacity; and under these conditions regulatory T cells may have been expanded or induced.

T$_H$17 Cells

The role of T$_H$17 cells in tumor immunity is not well established [53]; however, two cytokines, IL-6 and TGF-β, important in their development, are highly expressed in myeloma. A recent study has reported elevated levels of IL-17 in myeloma compared with normal donor sera. This particular inflammatory cytokine may promote tumor growth by way of promotion of angiogenesis [54]. Similarly, IL-21, an IL-17–associated cytokine, has been reported to increase myeloma growth and block IL-6–dependent apoptosis in myeloma cell lines [55].

Despite the abnormalities and deficiencies observed in myeloma in various compartments of the immune system, antitumor immune responses are observed in MM and an ongoing effort is to devise strategies to induce and augment specific responses that may then have clinically relevant effects.

MYELOMA CLINICAL TRIALS

As a potential target for immunotherapy, idiotype protein, the immunoglobulin produced in large quantities by myeloma cells, has been extensively studied. These antibody molecules are generated by rearrangement of variable, diversity, and joining regions of heavy and light chains. In the past decade, several studies have demonstrated that a T$_H$1 type of immunity can be generated using idiotype-pulsed DCs in an HLA-restricted fashion. These studies thus demonstrate the feasibility of developing idiotype-specific T cell–mediated anti-myeloma responses.

In vivo Experimentations

In the early 1970s, animal experiments [56] showed that immunizations with purified idiotype proteins were able to produce anti-idiotype antibodies in mice. Furthermore, when tumor cells that were producing immunized idiotype were transferred to naïve and unimmunized animals, only 11% of animals developed tumors. When tumor cells only producing light chains were transferred to naïve animals, however, such protection was not observed.

Preclinical Studies

Yi and colleagues [57] reported that T cells from myeloma patients were capable of responding to autologous idiotype in vitro. Specific idiotype-mediated interferon-gamma (IFN-γ) and IL-2 production was observed in 66% and 76% of T cells, respectively, from patients who had myeloma. Idiotype-specific proliferation was observed in 36% of the patients tested. These results indicated that the T cells against self-idiotype can be used to generate T-cell responses and provided the rationale to use the idiotype as a tumor-specific target for vaccination studies. In addition, another study by King and colleagues [58] showed that in mice immunized with DNA vaccine consisting of idiotype and fragment C of tetanus toxin, 70% of the animals survived for more than 2 months after challenge with tumor cells compared with vehicle control animals. This particular study indicated that DNA fusion vaccines could be effective in generating protective immunity against tumors. Stritzke and colleagues [59] have reported that when animals were vaccinated with tumor cells along with granulocyte-macrophage colony-stimulating factor (GM-CSF), followed by IL-2 administration, the tumor recurrence was delayed and survival improved compared with control animals. This finding indicated that NK cells and CD8 T cells were important in generating tumor-specific immunity to render the protection in these animals tested.

Idiotype-Based Vaccination Clinical Results

To vaccinate patients with a given antigen to generate immune responses, one has to have a large quantity of clinical-grade antigen that is specific to the tumor. It is easy to purify a large amount of monoclonal paraprotein or idiotype from the serum of patients who have myeloma. As shown in Table 1, several clinical trials using idiotype alone or in combination with cytokines as tumor antigen to vaccinate patients who have myeloma have been performed. Bergenbrant and colleagues [60] used myeloma paraprotein alone to repeatedly immunize 5 patients. T cells following vaccination produced higher levels of IFN-γ in response to idiotype protein. With repeated immunizations, however, T-cell responses seemed to be rare and patients did not achieve clinical responses following vaccination. Osterborg and colleagues [61] immunized 5 patients who had myeloma with autologous idiotype protein along with GM-CSF and although in vitro studies showed that CD4 and CD8 cells produced IFN-γ and IL-2 following vaccination, significant T-cell proliferative and delayed-type hypersensitivity (DTH) responses were not observed. Changes in paraprotein levels were also not reported in these immunized patients. Rasmussen and colleagues [62] have administered seven vaccinations to 6 patients who have idiotype and IL12 with or without GM-CSF. Immediately following vaccination, clonal B cells went down and most of the patients showed specific T-cell responses. After 30 weeks post-vaccination, however, T-cell responses were diminished and paraprotein levels were elevated. In another study by Bertinetti and colleagues [63], three autologous stem cell transplantation (autoSCT) patients who had myeloma were given four immunizations of idiotype with GM-CSF in addition to hepatitis B vaccine. Although partial clinical remission was observed in vaccinated patients, it did not correlate with T-cell responses and hepatitis B antibodies were not detected following vaccination. In a long-term study, Massaia and colleagues [64] and Coscia and colleagues [65] vaccinated 12 patients who had idiotype with keyhole limpet hemocyanin (KLH) and GM-CSF following high-dose chemotherapy and autoSCT in first complete response (CR). Although most of the patients (85%) showed DTH response, T-cell responses and anti-idiotype antibodies were not significantly increased following vaccinations and no clinical benefit was observed following vaccinations. In the allogeneic transplantation setting, we have vaccinated [66] HLA-matched sibling donors first with idiotype and KLH in addition to GM-CSF before bone marrow collection and transplant. The rationale for vaccinating bone marrow transplant (BMT) donors before transplantation is to transfer tumor-specific immune components with the graft. After BMT, patients

Table 1
Idiotype-based clinical trials in myeloma

Vaccine	Patients	Cellular responses		Clinical response	Author [Ref]
		T cell	B cell		
Id alone, repeated vaccines	5	3/5	+	No response	Bergenbrant et al [60]
Id + GM-CSF, 6 vaccines	5	1/5	–	Paraprotein levels unchanged	Osterborg et al [61]
Id + KLH + GM-CSF (+ IL-2), autoSCT at remission	12 T cell HD chemotherapy	2/11	–	Paraprotein levels unchanged	Massaia et al, Coscia et al [64,65]
Id + IL-12 ± GM-CSF, 7 vaccines	6	5/6	–	Paraprotein levels unchanged	Rasmussen et al [62]
Id + GM-CSF, 4 vaccines, + HepB Vac	3 AutoSCT	1/3	–	No Abs to HepB	Bertinetti et al [63]
Tumor cell + GM-CSF-K562, 8 vaccines	16 AutoSCT	3/5	+	3/16 Increase in paraprotein	Borrello et al (ASH presented)
Id + KLH +GM-CSF, 6 vaccines	5 AlloSCT	4/5	+	3/5 Stable CR	Neelapu et al [66]
Id + KLH + GM-CSF, 3 or 6 vaccines	50 AutoSCT	28/48	+	No response	Munshi et al (ASH presented)

Abbreviations: Abs, antibody; AlloSCT, allogeneic stem cell transplant; ASH, American Society of Hematology; AutoSCT, autologous stem cell transplantation; CR, complete response; GM-CSF, granulocyte-macrophage colony-stimulating factor; HD, high dose; HepB, hepatitis B vaccine; Id, idiotype; IL-12, interleukin-12; KLH, keyhole limpet hemocyanin.

received three booster vaccinations. Three of 5 patients after vaccination showed idiotype-specific T-cell responses, improved clinical response from partial remission before BMT and idiotype vaccinations to CR, and maintenance of response up to 5 to 8 years. In the autologous transplant setting, we have conducted a large study with three cohorts and a total of 50 patients who have myeloma. In this study, patients following double autotransplant received three or six vaccinations with idiotype coupled with KLH with GM-CSF in the first two cohorts. A third cohort was vaccinated before and after transplantation. The majority of the patients (58%) following vaccinations produced idiotype-specific T_H1-type responses and had an elevated proliferative response in addition to DTH responses (42%).

In summary, these studies demonstrated that patients who have myeloma do respond to vaccination and that idiotype is a weak immunogen; the responses are not robust and do not persist for prolonged periods of time, and clinically meaningful outcomes have not been observed. This situation has prompted investigation of novel approaches and antigens for immunotherapy.

IDIOTYPE-PULSED DENDRITIC CELL TRIALS IN MYELOMA

Most clinical trials conducted using idiotype-pulsed DCs showed immune response, yet significant clinical responses are lacking (Table 2). Lim and colleagues [67] showed that following three idiotype-pulsed DC vaccinations, both idiotype-specific T cell and anti-idiotypic antibody responses were observed; however, none of the vaccinated patients showed clinical improvements. Titzer and colleagues [68] vaccinated 11 patients who had myeloma with idiotype pulsed with CD34-derived DCs. T cells from only 4 out of 10

Table 2
Clinical trails using dendritic cells pulsed with idiotype of patients who have myeloma

Vaccines	Patients (no. and status)	Clinical outcome	Authors [Ref]
2-iv Id + DCs & 5- Id + KLH	12 AutoSCT high-dose chemotherapy	Stable	Reichardt et al [71,72]
3 Id + DCs	6	Progressed	Lim et al [67]
7 2-Id + DCs & 5-Id + KLH	26 High-dose chemotherapy, AutoSCT	17 Live/stable	Liso et al [69]
4 1-Id + DCs & 3-Id + GM-CSF	11	Progressed	Titzer et al [68]
3 Id + DCs + IL-2	5 High-dose chemotherapy at stable PR	4 Stable/1 relapsed	Yi et al [70]
4–7 Id + KLH + GM-CSF	4 AlloSCT	3 Progressed	Bendandi et al [73]

Abbreviations: AlloSCT, allogeneic stem cell transplant; AutoSCT, autologous stem cell transplantation; DCs, dendritic cells; GM-CSF, granulocyte-macrophage colony stimulating factor; Id, idiotype; IL-2, interleukin 2; KLH, keyhole limpet hemocyanin; PR, partial response.

patients were able to show antigen-specific production of cytokines following vaccination and clinical responses were not observed following vaccination.

Liso and colleagues [69] immunized 26 patients following high-dose chemotherapy with idiotype-pulsed DCs with or without KLH. Only 4 of the 26 patients showed specific proliferative responses; however, 17 patients are alive at 30 months post-vaccination. Yi and colleagues [70] vaccinated 5 patients at remission following high-dose chemotherapy. Three idiotype-pulsed monocyte-derived DC vaccinations were administered followed by IL-2 therapy for 5 days. Four of the 5 patients showed idiotype-specific T-cell cytokine production and 1 patient achieved partial response (PR) following vaccination. Reichardt and colleagues [71] vaccinated 12 patients post-autoSCT with idiotype-pulsed DCs. In T-cell responses, only 2 of 12 demonstrated idiotype-specific proliferation and 1 of 3 patients showed specific CTL-mediated killing. Clinical improvement was not reported following vaccinations [72]. Bendandi and colleagues [73] conducted a clinical trial using DCs loaded with idiotype in 4 patients who had myeloma following reduced intensity-conditioning allogeneic SCT. Anti-idiotype antibody responses were not seen. T-cell responses by production of T_H1 cytokines were noted in 2 out of 4 patients. Three patients in this study had transient responses and 1 patient had stable disease. Recently, 16 patients who have myeloma have been vaccinated following autoSCT with irradiated autologous myeloma plasma cells and genetically modified K562 cells to produce GM-CSF. Of the 16 patients who have completed the study, 6 showed CR and 5 showed PR after autoSCT and vaccination without noticeable toxicities. Cellular and antibody responses have been observed in addition to DTH responses.

In summary, generating antitumor immunity is feasible, yet convincing clinical efficacy is lacking in myeloma even with DC-pulsed idiotypic vaccinations. Its intravenous DC vaccinations lead to its sequestration [74,75], one can improve DC migration patterns by subcutaneous administration to generate protective T_H1-type responses [76]. Additionally, immature DCs are unstable when necessary cytokines are withdrawn [77], the use of mature DCs derived from peripheral blood monocytes would be superior in presenting antigens to T cells. Although idiotype is a weak immunogen, one can generate adequate immunity against this type of tumor-specific antigen both post-autologous transplantation and donor-vaccinated post-allogeneic stem cell transplantation.

FUTURE DIRECTIONS

Targeting a single tumor-specific antigen allows tumor cells to become resistant by mutation of a particular gene and by evading immunity. To avoid this obstacle, one must use approaches directed at multiple antigenic targets. One example is pulsing DCs with whole-cell myeloma lysates or fusing DCs with myeloma cells. A preclinical study using animal cells and human cells has confirmed the feasibility of presenting a wide array of myeloma-related antigens by fusing myeloma cells with DCs for the development of effective CTLs [78]. A clinical study of MM/DC fusion cell vaccination with GM-CSF is ongoing. Eleven patients have been enrolled in this study and demonstrated that adequate numbers of functional MM/DC fusion cells can be obtained to vaccinate patients three or more times without toxicity. Most of the patients were stabilized with tumor-specific T-cell responses as demonstrated by increased production of IFN-γ following vaccination.

Because production of patient-specific vaccination is difficult, there is an ongoing effort to identify a cocktail of antigens that can be used in universally in all the patients. Several investigators have identified novel myeloma-specific antigens by screening myeloma cDNA expression libraries using the SEREX (serologic expression cloning) technique for eventual development of an antigen cocktail. With this technology, myeloma-specific antigens, such as XBP1, orofaciodigital 1, B-cell maturation receptor, and rho-associated kinase 1, are identified. Recently, immune responses directed at an embryonic stem cell marker, SOX2, expressed in the CD138- compartment in patients who have MGUS have been reported. Such responses may help in predicting clinical outcomes based on the SOX2-induced immunity [79]. Furthermore, other transmembrane proteins, including MUC1, previously reported to be expressed in glandular epithelial cells [80], have been shown to be overexpressed in myeloma cell lines and primary myeloma cells [81,82]. Malignancy-associated cancer-testis antigens, including the MAGE family: BAGE, GAGE, PRAME, NY-ESO-1, and Sperm protein17 [83], generally not expressed in normal tissues, have been shown to be expressed in myeloma. These have been targeted for active investigation for cancer immunotherapy because of their tumor-specific expression and the ability to induce tumor-specific immunity. However, the vaccinations with these cellular antigens generating significant clinical response have yet to be seen. In addition, because most of these cellular antigens are present in the late phase of myeloma and associated with only a subset of myeloma cells, using them for vaccination may not translate into clinical efficacy.

The ongoing future approach to obtain clinically effective vaccination includes methods to increase the immunogenicity of DCs, to apply methods to extend tumor immunity following vaccinations, develop approaches to improve immune status in patients, use homeostatic proliferation to generate efficient tumor immunity, establish regulatory T-cell homeostatic functions to the normal threshold level, and abrogate T_H17-mediated immunopathology. Eventually, a combination of vaccination with tumor-specific antigens and adoptive transfer of T cells cultured with immunomodulatory agents will provide robust and sustained immune responses with clinical efficacy.

References

[1] Munshi NC. Immunoregulatory mechanisms in multiple myeloma. Hematol Oncol Clin North Am 1997;11:51–69.
[2] Bouneaud C, Kourilsky P, Bousso P. Impact of negative selection on the T cell repertoire reactive to a self-peptide: a large fraction of T cell clones escapes clonal deletion. Immunity 2000;13:829–40.

[3] Banchereau J, Steinman RM. Dendritic cells and the control of immunity. Nature 1998;392: 245–52.

[4] Lengauer C, Kinzler KW, Vogelstein B. Genetic instabilities in human cancers. Nature 1998;396:643–9.

[5] Shammas MA, Shmookler Reis RJ, Li C, et al. Telomerase inhibition and cell growth arrest after telomestatin treatment in multiple myeloma. Clin Cancer Res 2004;10:770–6.

[6] Vonderheide RH, Hahn WC, Schultze JL, et al. The telomerase catalytic subunit is a widely expressed tumor-associated antigen recognized by cytotoxic T lymphocytes. Immunity 1999;10:673–9.

[7] Liotta LA, Kohn EC. The microenvironment of the tumour-host interface. Nature 2001;411: 375–9.

[8] Simon RM, Steinberg SM, Hamilton M, et al. Clinical trial designs for the early clinical development of therapeutic cancer vaccines. J Clin Oncol 2001;19:1848–54.

[9] Zeis M, Siegel S, Wagner A, et al. Generation of cytotoxic responses in mice and human individuals against hematological malignancies using survivin-RNA-transfected dendritic cells. J Immunol 2003;170:5391–7.

[10] Janssen EM, Lemmens EE, Wolfe T, et al. CD4 + T cells are required for secondary expansion and memory in CD8 + T lymphocytes. Nature 2003;421:852–6.

[11] Sun JC, Bevan MJ. Defective CD8 T cell memory following acute infection without CD4 T cell help. Science 2003;300:339–42.

[12] Shedlock DJ, Shen H. Requirement for CD4 T cell help in generating functional CD8 T cell memory. Science 2003;300:337–9.

[13] Smith CM, Wilson NS, Waithman J, et al. Cognate CD4(+) T cell licensing of dendritic cells in CD8(+) T cell immunity. Nat Immunol 2004;5:1143–8.

[14] Ernst B, Lee DS, Chang JM, et al. The peptide ligands mediating positive selection in the thymus control T cell survival and homeostatic proliferation in the periphery. Immunity 1999;11:173–81.

[15] Watanabe N, Hanabuchi S, Soumelis V, et al. Human thymic stromal lymphopoietin promotes dendritic cell-mediated CD4 + T cell homeostatic expansion. Nat Immunol 2004;5:426–34.

[16] Hori S, Nomura T, Sakaguchi S. Control of regulatory T cell development by the transcription factor Foxp3. Science 2003;299:1057–61.

[17] Pennington DJ, Silva-Santos B, Silberzahn T, et al. Early events in the thymus affect the balance of effector and regulatory T cells. Nature 2006;444:1073–7.

[18] Zheng Y, Josefowicz SZ, Kas A, et al. Genome-wide analysis of Foxp3 target genes in developing and mature regulatory T cells. Nature 2007;445:936–40.

[19] Gavin MA, Rasmussen JP, Fontenot JD, et al. Foxp3-dependent program of regulatory T-cell differentiation. Nature 2007;445:771–5.

[20] Wan YY, Flavell RA. Regulatory T-cell functions are subverted and converted owing to attenuated Foxp3 expression. Nature 2007;445:766–70.

[21] Marson A, Kretschmer K, Frampton GM, et al. Foxp3 occupancy and regulation of key target genes during T-cell stimulation. Nature 2007;445:931–5.

[22] Wu Y, Borde M, Heissmeyer V, et al. FOXP3 controls regulatory T cell function through cooperation with NFAT. Cell 2006;126:375–87.

[23] Ivanov II, McKenzie BS, Zhou L, et al. The orphan nuclear receptor RORgammat directs the differentiation program of proinflammatory IL-17 + T helper cells. Cell 2006;126: 1121–33.

[24] Acosta-Rodriguez EV, Rivino L, Geginat J, et al. Surface phenotype and antigenic specificity of human interleukin 17-producing T helper memory cells. Nat Immunol 2007;8: 639–46.

[25] Acosta-Rodriguez EV, Napolitani G, Lanzavecchia A, et al. Interleukins 1beta and 6 but not transforming growth factor-beta are essential for the differentiation of interleukin 17-producing human T helper cells. Nat Immunol 2007;8:942–9.

[26] Wilson NJ, Boniface K, Chan JR, et al. Development, cytokine profile and function of human interleukin 17-producing helper T cells. Nat Immunol 2007;8:950–9.

[27] Diefenbach A, Jensen ER, Jamieson AM, et al. Rae1 and H60 ligands of the NKG2D receptor stimulate tumour immunity. Nature 2001;413:165–71.

[28] Stern-Ginossar N, Elefant N, Zimmermann A, et al. Host immune system gene targeting by a viral miRNA. Science 2007;317:376–81.

[29] Sakaguchi S. Regulatory T cells: key controllers of immunologic self-tolerance. Cell 2000;101:455–8.

[30] Mucida D, Park Y, Kim G, et al. Reciprocal TH17 and regulatory T cell differentiation mediated by retinoic acid. Science 2007;317:256–60.

[31] Ono M, Yaguchi H, Ohkura N, et al. Foxp3 controls regulatory T-cell function by interacting with AML1/Runx1. Nature 2007;446:685–9.

[32] Ziegler SF. FOXP3: of mice and men. Annu Rev Immunol 2006;24:209–26.

[33] Veldhoen M, Hocking RJ, Atkins CJ, et al. TGFbeta in the context of an inflammatory cytokine milieu supports de novo differentiation of IL-17-producing T cells. Immunity 2006;24: 179–89.

[34] Bettelli E, Carrier Y, Gao W, et al. Reciprocal developmental pathways for the generation of pathogenic effector TH17 and regulatory T cells. Nature 2006;441:235–8.

[35] Laurence A, Tato CM, Davidson TS, et al. Interleukin-2 signaling via STAT5 constrains T helper 17 cell generation. Immunity 2007;26:371–81.

[36] Massaia M, Bianchi A, Attisano C, et al. Detection of hyperreactive T cells in multiple myeloma by multivalent cross-linking of the CD3/TCR complex. Blood 1991;78:1770–80.

[37] Brown RD, Pope B, Murray A, et al. Dendritic cells from patients with myeloma are numerically normal but functionally defective as they fail to up-regulate CD80 (B7-1) expression after huCD40LT stimulation because of inhibition by transforming growth factor-beta1 and interleukin-10. Blood 2001;98:2992–8.

[38] Xie J, Wang Y, Freeman ME 3rd, et al. Beta 2-microglobulin as a negative regulator of the immune system: high concentrations of the protein inhibit in vitro generation of functional dendritic cells. Blood 2003;101:4005–12.

[39] Mariani S, Coscia M, Even J, et al. Severe and long-lasting disruption of T-cell receptor diversity in human myeloma after high-dose chemotherapy and autologous peripheral blood progenitor cell infusion. Br J Haematol 2001;113:1051–9.

[40] Maecker B, Anderson KS, von Bergwelt-Baildon MS, et al. Viral antigen-specific CD8 + T-cell responses are impaired in multiple myeloma. Br J Haematol 2003;121:842–8.

[41] Zinneman HH, Hall WH. Recurrent pneumonia in multiple myeloma and some observations on immunologic response. Ann Intern Med 1954;41:1152–63.

[42] Robertson JD, Nagesh K, Jowitt SN, et al. Immunogenicity of vaccination against influenza, Streptococcus pneumoniae and Haemophilus influenzae type B in patients with multiple myeloma. Br J Cancer 2000;82:1261–5.

[43] Raje N, Gong J, Chauhan D, et al. Bone marrow and peripheral blood dendritic cells from patients with multiple myeloma are phenotypically and functionally normal despite the detection of Kaposi's sarcoma herpesvirus gene sequences. Blood 1999;93:1487–95.

[44] Butch AW, Kelly KA, Munshi NC. Dendritic cells derived from multiple myeloma patients efficiently internalize different classes of myeloma protein. Exp Hematol 2001;29:85–92.

[45] Ratta M, Fagnoni F, Curti A, et al. Dendritic cells are functionally defective in multiple myeloma: the role of interleukin-6. Blood 2002;100:230–7.

[46] Wang S, Hong S, Yang J, et al. Optimizing immunotherapy in multiple myeloma: Restoring the function of patients' monocyte-derived dendritic cells by inhibiting p38 or activating MEK/ERK MAPK and neutralizing interleukin-6 in progenitor cells. Blood 2006;108: 4071–7.

[47] Dauer M, Obermaier B, Herten J, et al. Mature dendritic cells derived from human monocytes within 48 hours: a novel strategy for dendritic cell differentiation from blood precursors. J Immunol 2003;170:4069–76.

[48] West MA, Wallin RP, Matthews SP, et al. Enhanced dendritic cell antigen capture via toll-like receptor-induced actin remodeling. Science 2004;305:1153–7.

[49] Hermans IF, Silk JD, Gileadi U, et al. Dendritic cell function can be modulated through co-operative actions of TLR ligands and invariant NKT cells. J Immunol 2007;178:2721–9.

[50] Prabhala RH, Neri P, Bae JE, et al. Dysfunctional T regulatory cells in multiple myeloma. Blood 2006;107:301–4.

[51] Pasare C, Medzhitov R. Toll pathway-dependent blockade of CD4 + CD25 + T cell-mediated suppression by dendritic cells. Science 2003;299:1033–6.

[52] Beyer M, Kochanek M, Giese T, et al. In vivo peripheral expansion of naive CD4 + CD25high FoxP3+ regulatory T cells in patients with multiple myeloma. Blood 2006;107:3940–9.

[53] Steinman L. A brief history of T(H)17, the first major revision in the T(H)1/T(H)2 hypothesis of T cell-mediated tissue damage. Nat Med 2007;13:139–45.

[54] Alexandrakis MG, Pappa CA, Miyakis S, et al. Serum interleukin-17 and its relationship to angiogenic factors in multiple myeloma. Eur J Intern Med 2006;17:412–6.

[55] Brenne AT, Ro TB, Waage A, et al. Interleukin-21 is a growth and survival factor for human myeloma cells. Blood 2002;99:3756–62.

[56] Lynch RG, Graff RJ, Sirisinha S, et al. Myeloma proteins as tumor-specific transplantation antigens. Proc Natl Acad Sci U S A 1972;69:1540–4.

[57] Yi Q, Osterborg A, Bergenbrant S, et al. Idiotype-reactive T-cell subsets and tumor load in monoclonal gammopathies. Blood 1995;86:3043–9.

[58] King CA, Spellerberg MB, Zhu D, et al. DNA vaccines with single-chain Fv fused to fragment C of tetanus toxin induce protective immunity against lymphoma and myeloma. Nat Med 1998;4:1281–6.

[59] Stritzke J, Zunkel T, Steinmann J, et al. Therapeutic effects of idiotype vaccination can be enhanced by the combination of granulocyte-macrophage colony-stimulating factor and interleukin 2 in a myeloma model. Br J Haematol 2003;120:27–35.

[60] Bergenbrant S, Yi Q, Osterborg A, et al. Modulation of anti-idiotypic immune response by immunization with the autologous M-component protein in multiple myeloma patients. Br J Haematol 1996;92:840–6.

[61] Osterborg A, Yi Q, Henriksson L, et al. Idiotype immunization combined with granulocyte-macrophage colony-stimulating factor in myeloma patients induced type I, major histocompatibility complex-restricted, CD8- and CD4-specific T-cell responses. Blood 1998;91:2459–66.

[62] Rasmussen T, Hansson L, Osterborg A, et al. Idiotype vaccination in multiple myeloma induced a reduction of circulating clonal tumor B cells. Blood 2003;101:4607–10.

[63] Bertinetti C, Zirlik K, Heining-Mikesch K, et al. Phase I trial of a novel intradermal idiotype vaccine in patients with advanced B-cell lymphoma: specific immune responses despite profound immunosuppression. Cancer Res 2006;66:4496–502.

[64] Massaia M, Borrione P, Battaglio S, et al. Idiotype vaccination in human myeloma: generation of tumor-specific immune responses after high-dose chemotherapy. Blood 1999;94:673–83.

[65] Coscia M, Mariani S, Battaglio S, et al. Long-term follow-up of idiotype vaccination in human myeloma as a maintenance therapy after high-dose chemotherapy. Leukemia 2004;18:139–45.

[66] Neelapu SS, Munshi NC, Jagannath S, et al. Tumor antigen immunization of sibling stem cell transplant donors in multiple myeloma. Bone Marrow Transplant 2005;36:315–23.

[67] Lim SH, Bailey-Wood R. Idiotypic protein-pulsed dendritic cell vaccination in multiple myeloma. Int J Cancer 1999;83:215–22.

[68] Titzer S, Christensen O, Manzke O, et al. Vaccination of multiple myeloma patients with idiotype-pulsed dendritic cells: immunological and clinical aspects. Br J Haematol 2000;108:805–16.

[69] Liso A, Stockerl-Goldstein KE, Auffermann-Gretzinger S, et al. Idiotype vaccination using dendritic cells after autologous peripheral blood progenitor cell transplantation for multiple myeloma. Biol Blood Marrow Transplant 2000;6:621–7.

[70] Yi Q, Desikan R, Barlogie B, et al. Optimizing dendritic cell-based immunotherapy in multiple myeloma. Br J Haematol 2002;117:297–305.

[71] Reichardt VL, Okada CY, Liso A, et al. Idiotype vaccination using dendritic cells after autologous peripheral blood stem cell transplantation for multiple myeloma—a feasibility study. Blood 1999;93:2411–9.

[72] Reichardt VL, Milazzo C, Brugger W, et al. Idiotype vaccination of multiple myeloma patients using monocyte-derived dendritic cells. Haematologica 2003;88:1139–49.

[73] Bendandi M, Rodriguez-Calvillo M, Inoges S, et al. Combined vaccination with idiotype-pulsed allogeneic dendritic cells and soluble protein idiotype for multiple myeloma patients relapsing after reduced-intensity conditioning allogeneic stem cell transplantation. Leuk Lymphoma 2006;47:29–37.

[74] Eggert AA, Schreurs MW, Boerman OC, et al. Biodistribution and vaccine efficiency of murine dendritic cells are dependent on the route of administration. Cancer Res 1999;59:3340–5.

[75] Morse MA, Coleman RE, Akabani G, et al. Migration of human dendritic cells after injection in patients with metastatic malignancies. Cancer Res 1999;59:56–8.

[76] Fong L, Brockstedt D, Benike C, et al. Dendritic cells injected via different routes induce immunity in cancer patients. J Immunol 2001;166:4254–9.

[77] Palucka KA, Taquet N, Sanchez-Chapuis F, et al. Dendritic cells as the terminal stage of monocyte differentiation. J Immunol 1998;160:4587–95.

[78] Gong J, Koido S, Chen D, et al. Immunization against murine multiple myeloma with fusions of dendritic and plasmacytoma cells is potentiated by interleukin 12. Blood 2002;99:2512–7.

[79] Spisek R, Kukreja A, Chen LC, et al. Frequent and specific immunity to the embryonal stem cell-associated antigen SOX2 in patients with monoclonal gammopathy. J Exp Med 2007;204:831–40.

[80] Ho SB, Niehans GA, Lyftogt C, et al. Heterogeneity of mucin gene expression in normal and neoplastic tissues. Cancer Res 1993;53:641–51.

[81] Treon SP, Maimonis P, Bua D, et al. Elevated soluble MUC1 levels and decreased anti-MUC1 antibody levels in patients with multiple myeloma. Blood 2000;96:3147–53.

[82] Takahashi T, Makiguchi Y, Hinoda Y, et al. Expression of MUC1 on myeloma cells and induction of HLA-unrestricted CTL against MUC1 from a multiple myeloma patient. J Immunol 1994;153:2102–9.

[83] Zendman AJ, Ruiter DJ, Van Muijen GN. Cancer/testis-associated genes: identification, expression profile, and putative function. J Cell Physiol 2003;194:272–88.

Hematol Oncol Clin N Am 21 (2007) 1231–1246

HEMATOLOGY/ONCOLOGY CLINICS
OF NORTH AMERICA

ELSEVIER
SAUNDERS

Complications of Multiple Myeloma

Joan Bladé, MD*, Laura Rosiñol, MD, PhD

Institute of Hematology and Oncology, Postgraduate School of Hematology Farreras-Valentí,
Institut d'Investigacions Biomèdiques August Pi i Sunyer, Hospital Clínic, Barcelona, Spain

RENAL INSUFFICIENCY

Frequency

Between 20% and 25% of patients with multiple myeloma (MM) have a serum creatinine equal to or higher than 2 mg/dL at the time of diagnosis [1,2]. The degree of renal failure is usually moderate, with a serum creatinine lower than 4 mg/dL. However, in series from tertiary hospitals the proportion of patients with newly diagnosed MM and renal failure requiring dialysis may be as high as 10%. In contrast, in large reference centers the proportion of patients requiring dialysis is very low [3]. The causes of renal failure in monoclonal gammopathies are:

- Light chain excretion
  Myeloma kidney (cast nephropathy)
- Immunoglobulin tissue deposition
  Systemic amyloidosis (AL)
  Immunoglobulin deposition disease (MIDD)
- Tubular dysfunction
  Fanconi syndrome

Pathogenesis of Renal Failure

Light chain excretion

The main cause of renal failure in patients with MM is the so-called "myeloma kidney," consisting of light chain tubular damage. Light chains are filtered through the glomerulus and catabolized by proximal tubular renal cells. The characteristic feature of myeloma kidney is the presence of myeloma casts, characterized by eosinophilic material composed of light chains within renal tubule lumens, surrounded by multinucleated giant cells of foreign body type in the distal tubules and collecting ducts [4,5]. There is a correlation between the degree of cast formation and the severity of renal failure [6]; however, there are patients with a very high light chain urine protein excretion who never develop renal failure [7]. One important aspect is that patients with MM and renal

*Corresponding author. *E-mail address*: jblade@clinic.ub.es (J. Bladé).

0889-8588/07/$ – see front matter
doi:10.1016/j.hoc.2007.08.006

failure are usually diagnosed simultaneously with both conditions. This indicates that when a light chain is nephrotoxic, it causes renal failure from the beginning, even before other manifestations of myeloma become apparent [2,8].

Light chain kidney deposition

Light chain tissue deposition consists of glomerular deposits of immunoglobulins that usually results in nephrotic syndrome. The amyloid deposits consist of fibrillar structures composed of light chains showing a positive staining with Congo red. Amyloid deposition is found in mesangial or glomerular basement membranes. The frequency of associated AL in MM varies according to the M-protein type. Thus, in a series from the Mayo Clinic including 1705 subjects with MM, the incidence of amyloidosis was 2% in IgA, 5% in IgG, 13% in light chain, and 19% in IgD myeloma [9].

The light-chain deposition disease is characterized by the deposition of non-fibrillar material (Congo red negative) [10]. Given the fact that in some patients the tissue deposits may also be composed of immunoglobulin heavy chain fragments, this condition has recently been termed as "monoclonal immunoglobulin deposition disease" (MIDD) [11]. In MIDD the light chain is usually of kappa type. The most characteristic feature of MIDD is nephrotic syndrome caused by glomerular involvement. Renal function may rapidly deteriorate, resembling glomerulonephritis. Patients with MIDD may also have heart, liver, or other organ involvement [11]. Nodular glomerulosclerosis resembling diabetic lesions or membranoproliferative glomerulonephritis is the most characteristic pathological feature of MIDD. Interstitial fibrosis is also a constant finding.

Tubular dysfunction

The acquired Fanconi syndrome is an uncommon condition characterized by the lack of reabsorption capacity of the proximal renal tubules, resulting in glucosuria, aminoaciduria, hypouricemia, and hypophosphatemia [12]. The renal damage is caused by incomplete digested light chains that result in crystaline inclusions within the proximal tubular cells that interfere with membrane transporters. The light chain is almost always of kappa type. The majority of patients are asymptomatic and the findings of glycosuria, hypokaliemia, unexplained hypouricemia, or renal tubular acidosis are the diagnostic key. Mild renal insufficiency and bone pain from osteoporosis are the most usual complications [12]. The transformation to MM is unusual.

Reversibility of Renal Insufficiency

The reversibility of renal failure in patients with MM is highly variable (20%–60%) [1,2,13–15]. About 50% of patients with serum creatinine lower than 4 mg/dL recover a normal renal function [1,2]. In contrast, in patients with a serum creatinine higher than 4 mg/dL the recovery rate is lower than 10% [2]. The factors associated with renal function recovery are: a serum creatinine level lower than 4 mg/dL, a 24-hour urine protein excretion lower than 1 gram per 24 hours, and a serum calcium level higher than 11.5 mg/dL (Box 1) [2].

Box 1: Predictors of reversibility of renal failure in multiple myeloma

Serum creatinine < 4 mg/dL

Serum calcium ≥ 11.5 mg/dL

Urine protein excretion < 1 g/24 h

Data from Bladé J, Fernández-Lama P, Bosch F, et al. Renal failure in multiple myeloma. Presenting features and predictors of outcome in a series of 94 patients. Arch Intern Med 1998;158:1889–93.

Treatment Approaches

Conventional chemotherapy

In patients with MM and renal failure, the response rate to chemotherapy ranges from 40% to 50% [2,16,17] and treatment with melphalan and prednisone should not be employed because of the need for dose ajustments of melphalan to avoid excessive myelosuppression, leading to suboptimal treatment. On the other hand, combination chemotherapy could produce a faster response. In this regard, the 4-day infusion of adriamycin and vincristine, plus high-dose dexamethasone, VAD (vincristine, doxorubicin, and desamethasone), or cyclophosphamide/dexamethasone is the treatment of choice in patients with MM and renal failure. The use of bortezomib/dexamethasone is an attractive approach. In fact, a high response rate to bortezomib has been reported in patients with relapsed or refractory MM and severe renal failure on dialysis [18].

High-dose therapy or autologous transplantation

Badros and colleagues [19] reported the results of high-dose therapy/autologous stem cell transplantation (HDT/SCT) with melphalan 200 mg/m^2 (MEL-200) or melphalan 140 mg/m^2 (MEL-140) in 81 patients with renal failure at the time of transplantation. The transplant related mortality was 6% and 13% after a single or double transplant, respectively. It is of note that nonhematologic toxicity, particularly in dialysis-dependent patients who were given MEL-200, was high (serious bacterial infections, atrial arrhythmias, and encephalopathy). The frequency of complications was significantly higher with MEL-200 than with MEL-140. Chemoresistant disease, low serum albumin, and older age were associated with a poorer outcome. It is the authors' view that in patients with renal failure HDT/SCT, the high-dose regimen should be MEL-140 and the procedure should be restricted to younger patients (less than 60 years) with chemosensitive disease and good performance status. In patients with no overt myeloma in whom the plasma cell mass is low and the organ impairment is the result of tissue deposition (AL, MIDD, polyneuropathy, organomegaly, endocrinopathy, monoclonal gammopathy syndrome), the likelihood of response to high-dose therapy is higher because the tumor burden at transplantation is low. That is, it would be a similar situation to that of patients with MM with chemosensitive disease in whom the M-protein at the time of transplant is low. Furthermore, in the above-mentioned conditions there is no need for tumor reduction before stem cell mobilization and high-dose therapy.

Supportive Measures
Plasma exchange
The removal of nephrotoxic light chains with plasma exchange could theoretically prevent irreversible renal failure by avoiding further renal damage [20,21]. In a small randomized trial, the Mayo Clinic group compared forced diuresis and chemotherapy versus forced diuresis, chemotherapy, and plasma exchange [6]. Only a statistical trend in favor of plasma exchange was found. In the authors' experience, patients with renal failure requiring dialysis do not benefit from plasma exchange [8]. This is in agreement with the findings by Johnson and colleagues [6] and others who identified the severity of myeloma cast formation as the major factor associated with nonreversible renal failure, even in patients undergoing plasma exchange [22]. However, the authors strongly believe that in nonoliguric patients not requiring dialysis, an early plasma exchange program along with forced diuresis and chemotherapy is likely to benefit. Finally, a large randomized controlled trial showed no conclusive evidence that plasma exchange improves the outcome of patients with MM and acute renal failure [23].

Renal replacement with dialysis
The response rate to chemotherapy in patients with MM on long-term dialysis programs ranges from 40% to 60% [8,16,17]. Renal failure does not have a negative impact on the response to chemotherapy, per se. In patients requiring dialysis, the reversibility rate of renal failure is usually less than 10% [6,8,16,17] and the recovery rate is rarely observed after 4 months on dialysis. The mortality rate in patients with MM and severe renal failure during the first 2 months from diagnosis is about 30% [2,8]. When considering patients not dying within the first 2 months on dialysis, the median survival is about 2 years, with one-third of patients surviving for more than 3 years [11]. Thus, long-term dialysis is a worthwhile treatment for patients with myeloma and severe nonreversible renal failure. Supportive measures for patients with renal failure in multiple myeloma are plasma exchange and dialysis. Those most likely to benefit from plasma exchange are patients with severe nonoliguric renal failure. Those for whom it has limited or no efficacy are patients with severe myeloma kidney (patients already on dialysis). For patients with renal failure in multiple myeloma, dialysis is a worthwhile palliative measure.

HEMATOLOGIC COMPLICATIONS
Anemia
Anemia is the most common hematologic complication in patients with MM. About 10% and 35% of patients have a hemoglobin (Hb) level lower that 8 g/dL and 9 g/dL, respectively [24,25]. Anemia is associated with a loss in quality of life and is a poor prognostic factor. In addition to those patients

presenting with anemia at diagnosis, many others will develop severe anemia later in the course of the disease because of progressive myeloma.

The cause of anemia is multifactorial [26] and can be a result of bone marrow replacement by plasma cells, relative erytheropoietin (EPO) deficiency, renal failure, chemotherapy or radiation therapy, disregulated cell apoptosis, or other factors, such as B_{12} or folate deficiency or haemolytic anutoinmne (rare). Bone marrow replacement by plasma cells is usually the main cause. However, some patients with severe anemia have only a discrete increase in bone marrow plasma cells. Patients with cancer do not respond to anemia through the common increase in EPO production. Thus, Berguin and colleagues [27] found a decreased EPO level, even in patients with no extensive bone marrow involvement by plasma cells. Patients with very high serum levels of IgG and IgA have a higher degree of anemia as a result of hemodilution. This must be taken into account in patients with smoldering myeloma, in whom a moderate degree of anemia should not be an indication for initiation of treatment with chemotherapy. Occasionally, folate or B_{12} vitamin deficiency can occur. In patients heavily pretreated with alkylating agents, particularly with melphalan, the development of an "unexplained" anemia may be the first feature of myelodysplasia. Usually, the response to chemotherapy results in a significant and quick increase in the Hb level.

Apart from packed red cell transfusions, the beneficial effect of recombinant human EPO (rHuEPO) and darbepoietin alfa has been confirmed in a number of trials. Patients responding to rHuEPO have a significant increase in Hb level, decrease in transfusion requirement, and improvement in quality of life. A practical issue is that the greatest quality of life improvement is found when the Hb level increases from 11 g/dL to 12 g/dL. There are several critical factors in the use of EPO: (1) dose or schedule and type of EPO, (2) importance of baseline erytropoietin level, (3) predictors of response, and (4) role of iron repletion. The American Societies of Hematology and Clinical Oncology have provided evidence-based guidelines for the use of rHuEPO in patients with cancer (Box 2) [28,29]. These recommendations should be carefully followed to ensure the correct use of rHuEPO. The most common causes of failure to respond or loss of rHuEPO efficacy are functional iron deficiency, infection, surgery, and advanced disease with extensive plasma-cell bone marrow involvement. The major cause is functional iron defficiency. The indications for iron repletion are suspected iron deficiency (ie, serum ferritin less than 100 mg/L in anemia chronic disorders) and functional iron deficiency (soluble transferrin receptor ⇑). Iron can be administered orally (with limited efficacy) or intravenously with iron saccharate (100 mg/wk–300 mg/wk). It seems that the intravenous administration of 100 mg to 300 mg of iron saccharate is the best iron supplemental therapy.

Bone Marrow Failure

Severe granulocytopenia and thrombocytopenia at the time of diagnosis are very unusual. Moderate degrees of granulocytopenia and thrombocytopenia have been reported in about 10% of patients with bone marrow failure

Box 2: Recommendations for rHuEPO therapy in patients with cancer

Hb level < 10 g/dL

Restricted to certain clinical circumstances if Hb is between 10 g/dL and 12 g/dL

Discontinue therapy if there is no response at 8 weeks (Hb ↑↑; 1–2 g/dL)

Dose tritiation to maintain Hb around 12 g/dL

   If Hb > 12 g/dL: reduce dose by 25%

   If Hb > 14 g/dL: discontinue EPO and restart at reduced dose if it falls < 12 g/dL

Iron repletion

Data from Ludwig H, Roi K, Blade J, et al. Management of disease-related anemia in patients with multiple myeloma or chronic lymphocytic leukemia: epoetin treatment recommendations. Hematol J 2002;3(3):121–30; and Rizzo JD, Lichtin AE, Woolf SH, et al. Use of epoetin in patients with cancer: evidence-based clinical practice guidelines of the American Society of Clinical Oncology and the American Society of Hematology. Blood 2002;100(7):2303–20.

[24,25]. Platelet counts lower than $20 \times 10E9/L$ with risk of severe bleeding are very unusual.

The development of an unexplained pancytopenia in a patient who has been treated with melphalan is suspicious of myelodysplasia or acute leukemia (MDS/AL) [30]. If this occurs, a bone marrow aspirate in the search of dyshemopoietic features, ring-sideroblasts, and cytogenetic abnormalities must be done. Although the development of AL might be part of the natural history of plasma cell dyscrasias, the exposure to alkylating agents is crucial. Thus, the expected incidence of MDS/AL in patients with MM treated with alkylating agents is 100 to 230 higher than that expected in a normal population [31,32]. Melphalan is much more leukemogenic than cyclophosphamide [33]. In patients undergoing HDT/SCT, the standard dose of alkylating agents before transplant is the cause of MDS/AL, rather than the myeloablative therapy with high-dose melphalan [34].

Hyperviscosity Syndrome and Bleeding Disorders

The hyperviscosity syndrome is a characteristic feature of Waldenström's macroglobulinemia (WM). However, symptomatic hyperviscosity requering plasma exchange is extremely rare in patients with MM.

Significant bleeding is uncommon in patients with MM, except in late phases of the disease when bone marrow replacement by plasma cells and the effect of chemotherapy can lead to severe thrombocytopenia. Patients with MM associated with AL have an increased bleeding tendency because of the amyloid vascular involvement. These patients are at risk of massive hemorrhage or bleeding from unusual locations with surgical procedures. Furthermore, about 10% of patients with systemic AL have an acquired factor X deficiency as a consequence of the factor adsorption on amyloid fibrils. If the factor X falls to below 25% of normal, there is a risk of severe bleeding and a requirement that factor X be replaced (reviewed in Ref. [3]).

INFECTIOUS COMPLICATIONS

Incidence and Timing of Infection
Infectious complications remain the major cause of morbidity and mortality in patients with MM [35]. Infectious episodes in MM occur from 0.80 to 2.22 patients per year [3]. This is 7 to 15 times higher than observed in patients who are in the hospital because of other causes. Infection is frequently the cause of death in the context of an advanced phase of the disease. The highest risk of infection is within the first 2 months of initiation of therapy and in patients with relapsed and refractory disease, while patients who have responded to chemotherapy and are in the plateau phase of the disease are at very low risk of infection.

Causes of Infection
The increased susceptibility to infections in MM is multifactorial, with the major cause being the impaired antibody production leading to a decrease in uninvolved immunoglobulins.

> Causes of infection in multiple myeloma
> Decreased synthesis of uninvolved immunoglobulins
> CD4/CD8 imbalances
> Defective opsonization
> Decreased granulocyte adhesiveness
> Impaired leukocyte migration
> Renal function impairment
> Chemotherapy-induced granulocytopenia
> Glucocorticoid treatment (particularly high-dose dexamethasone)

When chemotherapy results in severe granulocytopenia, this is an additional risk factor, particularly in older patients in advanced phases of the disease. Treatment with glucocorticoids, particularly with high-dose dexamethasone, is a risk factor for infection. Renal insufficiency is associated with a higher incidence of infectious complications [3].

Microbiology and Sites of Infection
Streptococcus pneumoniae, *Staphylococcus aureus*, and *Haemophilus influenza* are the more common agents causing respiratory tract infections, while *Escherichia coli*, *Pseudomona* sp, *Proteus* sp, *Enterobacter*, and *Klebsiella* are the usual cause of urinary tract infections. In about 15% of patients with MM, the presenting feature is a bacterial infection. In these untreated patients, *S pneumoniae* is the more common agent. This population is at particular risk of recurrent infections within the first months from initiation of therapy. A temporal biphasic microbial pattern was described a quarter century ago [36–38]. Thus, most infections in newly diagnosed patients and during the first cycles of chemotherapy are caused by *S pneumoniae*, while in patients with renal failure as well as in those with advanced disease receiving salvage chemotherapy, more than 90% of

the infectious episodes are caused by gram-negative bacilli or *S aureus*. Bacteremia is found in more than 50% of patients with MM and severe infections. Contrasting with what happens in patients with acute leukemia, bacteremia in myeloma usually occurs in the absence of granulocytopenia [35]. Active disease is a critical factor for infection [36,39–41].

Treatment and Prophylaxis of Infection

In patients with MM, an infectious episode should be considered as a potentially serious complication requiring immediate therapy. Fever from myeloma mimicking an active infection is extremely rare. Before the causal microorganism is identified, treatment against both encapsulated bacteria and gram-negative microorganisms should be started. The antibiotic choice will be determined by the local flora and by the pattern of antiobiotic resistance at each institution.

The infection prophylaxis in patients with MM is a matter of controversy (reviewed in Ref. [3]). Antibiotic prophylaxis is likely of benefit within the first 2 months of therapy, particularly in patients at high risk of infection (initiation of therapy in patients with history of serious infections, such as recurrent pneumonia, or renal failure) [42,43]. High dose intrevanous immunoglobulins are not recommended [44]. There are patients who develop recurrent pneumococcal infections. The use of prophylactic penicillin is of uncertain efficacy because of the increasing emergency of resistant strains. In selected patients at a very high risk, antibiotic prophylaxis with new macrolides (such as telitromicine) or new fluoquinolones (such as levofloxacin), until a response to chemotherapy is achieved, should be considered. Pneumococcal vaccination is recommended, particularly in patients with IgG myeloma with high-serum M-protein levels (Box 3) [3].

BONE COMPLICATIONS

Frequency and Pathogenesis

The major clinical complication of patients with multiple myeloma is related to the skeletal involvement. Thus 70% of patients with MM have lytic bone

---

Box 3: Infection prophylaxis in multiple myeloma

Immunoglobulin: not recommended

Pneumococcal vaccination

- Recommended, particularly in IgG myeloma with high serum M-protein levels

Antibiotic

- Possible benefit: first two months of therapy
- Recommended in patients at high risk (initiation of therapy in patients with previous serious infections, particularly recurrent pneumonie, renal insufficiency)

Data from Bladé J. Management of renal, hematologic, and infectious complications. In: Malpas JS, Bergsagel DE, Kyle RA, et al, editors. Myeloma: biology and management. 3rd edition. Philadelphia: Saunders, Elsevier Inc.; 2004. p. 251–67.

lesions with or without osteoporosis, while an additional 20% have severe osteopenia with no lytic lesions [24]. The skeletal involvement results in bone pain and may lead to compression fractures, as well as to pathologic fractures of long bones. The most frequent sites of skeletal involvement with potential risk of serious complications include vertebrae, sternum, ribs, pelvis, and proximal humeri and femura. The bone involvement is the result of an imbalance between the increased resorption and a decreased bone formation. The increased osteoclastic activity is mediated through the release of osteoclast-stimulating factors by the bone marrow microenvironment [45]. In this regard, malignant plasma cells as well as bone marrow stromal cells produce cytokines, such as interleukin-1 beta, interleukin-6, and tumor necrosis factor-alpha, which increase the osteoblastic activity [46–48]. Recent studies have shown that the interaction of receptor activator for nuclear factor κB (RANK) and RANK ligand plays an important role in cancer-associated bone disease [49].

In summary, myeloma bone involvement is determined by the alteration of the cytokine network of bone marrow microenvironment. This mechanism may be responsible for uniformity of skeletal involvement in a given patient. Thus, in the authors' experience it is uncommon for patients with no initial lytic lesions to develop significant lytic lesions later in the course of the disease. In these patients, increasing osteopenia can lead to compression fractures. On the other hand, there is a population of patients with large lytic lesions, in general asymetric, with a high-risk of pathologic fracture. Similarly, a number of patients present with multiple small lytic lesions, usually symetric, particularly in femora and humera, with no risk of fracture.

Complications of Bone Disease

Pathologic fractures

Some patients develop long bone fractures requiring orthopedic intervention followed by radiation therapy, in the case of extensive lesions. On the other hand, in patients with large lytic lesions with risk of fracture, a prophylactic orthopedic intervention must be considered. Finally, in patients with vertebral compression fractures and severe bone pain, vertebroplasty or kyphoplasty can be most useful.

Spinal cord compression

Spinal cord compression caused by a vertebral fracture is exceedingly rare in multiple myeloma. The spinal cord compression is usually caused by an extraoseous plasmacytoma arising from a vertebral body (see "neurologic complications" in this article).

Hypercalcemia

Hypercalcemia is observed in 15% to 20% of patients with MM at the time of diagnosis [24,25]. It is associated with polydipsia, polyuria, dehydration, constipation, and neurologic manifestations, including confusion and coma. Renal function impairment caused by interstitial nephritis is a common complication of hypercalcemia. Treatment of hypercalcemia with hydration and bisphosphonates is a medical emergency. Zoledronic acid is the bisphosphonate of choice [50].

Treatment of Bone Disease

There is evidence to support the use of bisphosphonates to treat and prevent bone disease in patients with MM. Both oral clodronate [51,52] and the intravenous compounds pamidronate and zoledronic acid [53,54] have been shown to be of clinical benefit. Oral clodronate is not available in the United States and, even in Europe, has not been extensively used in clinical practice. Pamidronate is administered in a monthly 2-hour infusion. Zoledronic acid is at least as effective as pamidronate, but carries the logistic advantage that it is administered in a monthly 15-minutes infusion. In 2002 an American Society of Clinical Oncology panel recommended the use of a monthly administration of intravenous bisphosphonates, either pamidronate or zoledronic acid, in patients with MM and bone lytic lesions or osteopenia [55]. The panel suggested that once initiated, the treatment should be given indefinitely [55]. However, the recognition of new long-term complications, particularly osteonecrosis of the jaw related to the time of bisphosphonate exposure, has led to a reconsideration of this recommendation [56]. The osteonecrosis of the jaw, observed in up to 10% of patients with MM receiving intravenous bisphosphonates, is related to the time of bisphosphonates exposure, type of bisphosphonate (ie, higher with zoledronic acid than with pamidronate), and to a history of recent dental procedures [57–60]. This has resulted in a Mayo Clinic consensus statement for the use of bisphosphonates in MM [56] consisting of:

Use of pamidronate over zoledronic acid

Discontinuation of bisphosphonate therapy after 2 years of treatment in patients in response

Restart the treatment in patients with active disease while requiring chemotherapy

No treatment with bisphosphonates in patients with asymptomatic monoclonal gammopathies (smoldering myeloma, monoclonal gammopathy of undetermined significance)

Dental evaluation and follow-up in patients receiving bisphophonate therapy.

NEUROLOGIC COMPLICATIONS

The more common neurologic complications in patients with MM are spinal cord compression, nerve root compression, intracraneal plasmacytomas, eptomeningeal involvement, peripheral neuropathy, associated to an IgM protein (in IgM- monoclonal gammopathy of undetermined significance and in Waldenström's macroglobulemia), associated to an IgG or IgA M-protein, amyloid deposititon, associated to neurotoxic drugs, such as vincristine, thalidomide, and bortezomib (reviewed in Ref. [61]).

Spinal Cord Compression

Spinal cord compression from a plasmacytoma arising from a vertebral body is the most frequent and serious neurologic complication in MM, occurring in 10% to 20% of patients [62]. The dorsal spine is the most commonly involved site, followed by the lumbar and sacral regions. The clinical picture of spinal cord compression usually consists of back pain and paraparesis that may evolve over days or weeks, although the onset can be abrupt, leading to severe paraparesis within a few hours. There is usually also a sensitivity level. Lumbar vertebral involvement can lead to a cauda equina syndrome, with low back and radicular pain and weakness of the legs [61]. Spinal cord compression is a medical emergency, and when suspected, an urgent MRI should be done. If confirmed, treatment with dexamethasone (loading dose of 100 mg, followed by 25 mg every 6 hours and then a progressive tapering) [63] plus radiation therapy must be initiated immediately. In case spinal cord compression is caused by vertebral collapse or spinal instability, rather than from extradural extension of a plasmacytoma (which is exceedingly rare), urgent surgical decompression followed by the insertion of a protheses of bone graft of methacrylate is required [61].

Nerve Root Compression

A number of patients develop radicular pain with no evidence of spinal cord compression. These patients complain of back pain with radicular metameric radiation. They may also have radicular sensory involvement. Treatment with dexamethasone plus radiation therapy is helpful before systemic chemotherapy acts.

Intracranial Plasmacytomas

Although the skull is very frequently involved in MM, intracranial myeloma involving the brain is extremely uncommon. However, myeloma involvement of the skull base may extend into the orbits causing orbital pain, exophthalmos, and diplopia [61,64]. Diplopia can result from the direct effect of an orbital plasmacytoma or from ophthalmoplegia caused by cranial nerve involvement within the orbits. When orbital involvement is suspected, the image test, particularly CT, must carefully explore all the regions in order not to miss lesions in this area. Exceptionally, myeloma skull expansion can result in subdural plasmacytoma, direct leptomeningeal infiltration, or even in brain plasmacytoma. Primary intracerebral plasmacytomas are very rare and can be associated with intratumor bleeding [62]. The direct or hematogenous leptomeningeal involvement can result in spastic paraparesis, with MRI imaging suggesting a parasagital meningioma [61,65].

Leptomeningeal Involvement

Involvement of the central nervous system (CNS), with detection of plasma cells in the cerebroespinal fluid (CSF), is very unusual. Fassas and colleagues [66] have reported a series of 25 cases seen at the University of Arkansas, and reviewed the features of 71 reported cases. A summary of their findings is as follows:

Leptomeningeal involvement in multiple myeloma
    Frequency: 1%
    Associated features:
        Unfavorable cytogenetic abnormalities
        Plasmablastic morphology
        Other extramedullary locations (65%)
        Plasma cell leukemia (25%)
        Increased lactate dehydrogenase (40%)
    MRI: diffuse leptomeningeal enhancement plus or minus masses
    Median survival: 3 months

The frequency of leptomeningeal involvement is about 1% and the more relevant presenting features are paraparesis, symptoms from increased intracranial pressure, cranial nerve palsies (particularly nerves V and IV) and confusion. CSF exam usually shows plasma cells with plasmablastic morphology, as well as increased protein levels and a positive immunofixation for the M-protein. The MRI usually shows a diffuse leptomeningeal enhancement, with or without additional findings, such as prominent masses. The more relevant associated features are poor prognosis cytogenetic abnormalities (deletion of chromosome 13, abnormalities of chromosome 11), extramedullary disease in other sites (65% of cases), and a coincidental picture of plasma cell leukemia in one-fourth of the patients. Despite active treatment with intrathecal therapy (methotrexate, hydrocortisone, cytarabine), cranial or cranio-spinal radiation in almost half of the patients, along with systemic treatment, the prognosis is very poor, with a median survival of only 3 months from the diagnoses of the CNS involvement [66].

Peripheral Neuropathy

Clinically relevant peripheral neuropathy at the time of diagnosis is uncommon in patients with MM. Comparatively, peripheral neuropathy is more frequent in WM and in monoclonal gammopathy of undetermined significance (MGUS) (reviewed in Ref. [61]). In some instances the M-protein plays a definite pathogenetic role, such as in the neuropathy associated with IgM antimyelin-associated glycoprotein (anti-MAG) and in patients with WM and IgM-MGUS, while in others it is unclear whether or not the M-protein is involved in the pathogenesis. In patients with IgM peripheral neuropathies, anti-MAG antibodies are found in 50% to 65% of cases [67]. Patients with IgM associated neuropathies are characterized by sensory impairment and tend to have a relatively mild course, with the main disability caused by hand tremor and gait ataxia [68]. Treatment should be reserved for patients with severe disability [68]. Improvement in the anti-MAG associated neuropathy has been reported with plasma exchange, chlorambucil, fludarabine, and rituximab [61,69,70]. In patients with IgG or IgA M-protein, the incidence of peripheral neuropathy is lower than in those with the IgM type. Peripheral neuropathy related to IgG and IgA M-protein resembles chronic inflammatory demyelinating peripheral neuropathy and may be either demyelinating or axonal. Patients with IgG or IgA associated peripheral neuropathies are better responders than those with the IgM type [61].

Peripheral neuropathies in patients with monoclonal gammopathies may be caused by axonal degeneration caused by amyloid deposition. Autonomic nervous system involvement by amyloids may result in severe orthostatic hypotension.

Neuropathies Associated with Neurotoxic Drugs

In the past decades, the most frequently used neurotoxic drug in patients with MM was vincristine. Although not extensively studied, vincristine results in occasional pain, numbness, and paresthesias leading to dose-reduction or treatment discontinuation in a significant number of patients. It can also cause constipation and even paralytic ileus. In the last ten years two other neurotoxic drugs, thalidomide and bortezomib, have been incorporated in the treatment of patients with MM. Thalidomide produces a mainly sensory dose-related peripheral neuropathy in virtually all patients if they have a long-exposure to the drug. It is usually nonreversible. In clinical practice, when a patient starts to complain of numbness and parethesia, the dose must be reduced and the neurologic status carefully followed. In the authors' experience, even with dose reduction the symptoms of peripheral neuropathy usually worsen and the drug must be discontinued [71]. Other neurologic side effects of thalidomide include distal tremor, instability, and ataxia, which are reversible with reduction or drug discontinuation. Bortezomib causes peripheral neuropathy and neuropathic pain in about 35% of patients. In contrast to thalidomide, the bortezomib-associated neuropathy is reversible in more than 70% of the cases with the recommended dose reductions or drug discontinuation. In patients with grade three and four neuropathy, the median time to reversal is 3 months [72]. Bortezomib causes orthostatic hypotension in about 10% of the cases. It can be severe and can last from a few days to 2 months after drug discontinuation. It is dose related and, when resolved, treatment can be resumed at a lower dose level of bortezomib.

References

[1] Alexanian R, Barlogie B, Dixon D. Renal failure in multiple myeloma. Pathogenesis and prognostic implications. Arch Intern Med 1990;150:1693–5.

[2] Bladé J, Fernández-Lama P, Bosch F, et al. Renal failure in multiple myeloma. Presenting features and predictors of outcome in a series of 94 patients. Arch Intern Med 1998;158: 1889–93.

[3] Bladé J. Management of renal, hematologic, and infectious complications. In: Malpas JS, Bergsagel DE, Kyle RA, et al, editors. Myeloma: biology and management. 3rd edition. Philadelphia: Saunders, Elsevier Inc.; 2004. p. 251–67.

[4] Hill GS, Morel-Maroger L, Méry JP, et al. Renal lesions in multiple myeloma: their relationship to associated protein abnormalities. Am J Kidney Dis 1983;4:423–38.

[5] Sanders PW. Pathogenesis and treatment of myeloma kidney. J Lab Clin Med 1994;124: 484–8.

[6] Johnson WJ, Kyle RA, Pineda AA, et al. Treatment of renal failure associated to multiple myeloma. Arch Intern Med 1990;150:863–9.

[7] Kyle RA, Greipp PR. "Idiopathic" Bence Jones proteinuria: long-term follow-up in seven patients. N Engl J Med 1982;306:564–7.

[8] Torra R, Bladé J, Cases A, et al. Patients with multiple myeloma and renal failure requiring long-term dialysis: presenting features, response to therapy, and outcome in a series of 20 cases. Br J Haematol 1995;91:854–9.

[9] Bladé J, Lust JA, Kyle RA. Immunoglobulin D multiple myeloma: presenting features, response to therapy, and survival in a series of 83 patients. J Clin Oncol 1994;12:2398–404.

[10] Randall RE, Williamson WC, Mullinax F, et al. Manifestations of systemic light chain deposition. Am J Med 1976;60:293–9.

[11] Dhodapkar MV, Merlini G, Solomon A. Biology and therapy of immunoglobulin deposition diseases. Hematol Oncol Clin North Am 1997;11:89–110.

[12] Ma CX, Lacy MQ, Rompala JF, et al. Acquired Fanconi syndrome is an indolent disorder in the absence of overt multiple myeloma. Blood 2004;104:40–2.

[13] Bernstein SP, Humes DH. Reversible renal insufficiency in multiple myeloma. Arch Intern Med 1982;142:2083–6.

[14] Cavo M, Baccarani M, Galieni P, et al. Renal failure in multiple myeloma: a study of the presenting findings, response to treatment, and prognosis in 26 patients. Nouv Rev Fr Hematol 1986;28:147–52.

[15] Cohen DJ, Sherman W, Osserman EF. Acute renal failure in patients with multiple myeloma. Am J Med 1984;76:247–56.

[16] Iggo N, Palmer AB, Severn A, et al. Chronic dialysis in patients with multiple myeloma and renal failure: a worthwhile treatment. Q J Med 1989;270:903–10.

[17] Korzets A, Tam F, Russell G, et al. The role of continuous ambulatory peritoneal dialysis in end-stage renal failure due to multiple myeloma. Am J Kidney Dis 1990;6:216–23.

[18] Chanan-Khan AA, Kaufman JL, Metha J, et al. Activity and safety of bortezomib in multiple myeloma patients with advanced renal failure: a multicenter retrospective study. Blood 2007;109:2604–6.

[19] Badros A, Barlogie B, Siegel E, et al. Results of autologous stem cell transplantation in multiple myeloma patients with renal failure. Br J Haematol 2001;114:822–9.

[20] Pasquali S, Casanova S, Zuchelli A, et al. Long-term survival in patients with acute and severe renal failure due to multiple myeloma. Clin Nephrol 1990;34:247–54.

[21] Misiani R, Tiraboschi G, Mingardi G, et al. Management of myeloma kidney: an anti-light-chain approach. Am J Kidney Dis 1987;10:28–33.

[22] Pozzi C, Pasqualli S, Donini U, et al. Prognostic factors and effectiveness of treatment in acute renal failure due to multiple myeloma: review of 50 cases. Clin Nephrol 1987;28:1–9.

[23] Clark WF, Stewart AK, Rock GA, et al. Plasma exchange when myeloma presents as acute renal failure. A randomized, controlled trial. Ann Intern Med 2005;143:777–84.

[24] Kyle RA, Gertz MA, Witzig TE, et al. Review of 1027 patients with newly diagnosed multiple myeloma. Mayo Clin Proc 2003;78:21–33.

[25] Bladé J, San Miguel JF, Fontanillas M, et al. Initial treatment of multiple myeloma: long-term results in 914 patients. Hematol J 2001;2:272–8.

[26] Mecharchand J. Management of haematological complications of myeloma. In: Malpas JS, Bergsagel DE, Kyle RA, et al, editors. Myeloma: biology and management. 2nd edition. Oxford: Oxford University Press. p. 332–57.

[27] Berguin Y, Yerna M, Loo M, et al. Erythropoiesis in multiple myeloma: defective red cell production due to inappropriate erythropoietin production. Br J Haematol 1992;82:648–53.

[28] Rizzo JD, Lichtin AE, Woolf SH, et al. Use of epoietin in patients with cancer: evidence-based clinical pactice guidelines of the American Society of Clinical Oncology and the American Society of Hematology. Blood 2002;100:2303–20.

[29] Rizzo JD, Lichtin AE, Woolf SH, et al. Use of epoietin in patients with cancer: evidence-based clinical practice guidelines of the American Society of Clinical Oncology and the American Society of Hematology. J Clin Oncol 2002;2:40–83.

[30] Bergsagel DE, Bailey AJ, Langley GR, et al. The chemotherapy of plasma cell myeloma and the incidence of acute leukemia. N Engl J Med 1979;301:743–8.

[31] Bergsagel DE. Plasma cell neoplasms and acute leukemia. Clin Haematol 1982;11: 221–34.

[32] Finnish Leukemia Group. Acute leukemia and other secondary neoplasms in patients treated with conventional chemotherapy for multiple myeloma: a Finnish Leukemia Group study. Eur J Haematol 2000;65:123–7.

[33] Cuzick J, Erskine S, Edelman D, et al. A comparison of the incidence of myelodysplastic syndrome and acute leukemia following melphalan and cyclophosphamide treatment for multiple myeloma. Br J Cancer 1987;55:523–9.

[34] Govindarajan R, Jagannath S, Flick JT, et al. Preceding standard therapy is the likely cause of MDS after autotransplants in multiple myeloma. Br J Haematol 1996;95:349–53.

[35] Kelleher P, Chapel H. Infections: principle of prevention and therapy. In: Metha J, Singhal S, editors. Myeloma. London: Martin Dunitz Ldt; 2002. p. 223–39.

[36] Savage DG, Lindenbaum J, Garret TJ. Biphasic pattern of bacterial infection in multiple myeloma. Ann Intern Med 1982;96:47–50.

[37] Meyers BR, Hirschman SZ, Axelrod JA. Current pattern of infection in multiple myeloma. Am J Med 1972;52:87–92.

[38] Shaikh BS, Lombard RM, Appelbaum PC, et al. Changing pattern of infection in patients with multiple myeloma. Oncology 1982;39:78–82.

[39] Hargreaves RM, Lea JR, Griffiths H, et al. Immunological factors and risk of infection in plateau phase myeloma. J Clin Pathol 1995;48:260–6.

[40] Perri RT, Hebbel RP, Oken MM. Influence of treatment and response status on infection in multiple myeloma. Am J Med 1981;71:935–40.

[41] Snowden L, Gibson J, Joshua DE. Frequency of infection in plateau-phase multiple myeloma. Lancet 1994;344:262 [Letter to the Editor].

[42] Oken MM, Pomeroy C, Weisdorf D. Prophylactic antibiotics for the prevention of early infection in multiple myeloma. Am J Med 1996;100:624–8.

[43] Hoen B, Kessler M, Hestin D, et al. Risk factors for bacterial infections in chronic haemodialysis adult patients: a multicenter prospective survey. Nephrol Dial Transplant 1995;10: 377–81.

[44] Salmon SE, Samal BA, Hayes DM, et al. Role of gammaglobulin for immunoprophylaxis in multiple myeloma. N Engl J Med 1967;277:1336–40.

[45] Stashenko P, Dewhirts FE, Peros WJ, et al. Synergistic interactions between interleukin 1, tumor necrosis factor, and lymphotoxin in bone resorption. J Immunol 1987;138:1464–8.

[46] Lacy MQ, Donovan KA, Heimbach JK, et al. Comparison of interleukin-1 beta expression by in situ hybridization in monoclonal gammopathy of undetermined significance and multiple myeloma. Blood 1999;93:300–5.

[47] Lust JA, Donovan KA. The role of interleukin-1 beta in the pathogenesis of multiple myeloma. Hematol Oncol Clin North Am 1999;13:1117–25.

[48] Klein B, Zhang XG, Lu ZY, et al. Interleukin-6 in human multiple myeloma. Blood 1995;85: 863–72.

[49] Li J, Sarosi I, Yan X-Q, et al. RANK is the intrinsic hematopoietic cell surface receptor that controls osteoclastogenesis and regulation of bone mass and calcium metabolism. Proc Natl Acad Sci USA 2000;1566–71.

[50] Major P, Lortholary A, Hon J, et al. Zoledronic acid is superior to pamidronate in the treatment of hypercalcemia of malignancy: a pooled analysis of two randomized, controlled clinical trials. J Clin Oncol 2001;19:558–67.

[51] Lahtinen R, Laakso M, Palva I, et al. Randomized, placebo-controlled multicentre trial of clodronate in multiple myeloma. Lancet 1992;340:1049–52.

[52] McCloskey EV, MacLennan IC, Drayson MT, et al. A randomized trial of the effect of clodronate on skeletal morbidity in multiple myeloma. Br J Haematol 1998;100:317–25.

[53] Berenson JR, Lichtenstein A, Porter L, et al. Efficacy of pamidronate in reducing skeletal events in patients with advanced multiple myeloma. N Engl J Med 1996;334:488–93.

[54] Rosen LS, Gordon D, Kaminski M, et al. Zoledronic acid versus pamidronate in the treatment of skeletal metastases in patients with breast cancer or osteolytic lesions of multiple myeloma: a phase III, double blinded, comparative trial. Cancer J 2001;7:377–87.

[55] Berenson JR, Hillner BE, Kyle RA, et al. American Society of Clinical Oncology practice guidelines: the role of bisphosphonates in multiple myeloma. J Clin Oncol 2002;20: 3719–36.

[56] Lacy MQ, Dispenzieri A, Gertz MA, et al. Mayo Clinic consensus statement for the use of bisphosphonates in multiple myeloma. Mayo Clin Proc 2006;81:1047–53.

[57] Durie BGM, Katz M, Crowley J. Osteonecrosis of the jaw and bisphosphonates [letter]. N Engl J Med 2005;353:99–100.

[58] Badros A, Weikel D, Salama A, et al. Osteonecrosis of the jaw in multiple myeloma patients: clinical features and risk factors. J Clin Oncol 2006;24:945–52.

[59] Bamias A, Kastritis E, Bamia C, et al. Osteonecrosis of the jaw in cancer after treatment with bisphosphonates: incidence and risk factors. J Clin Oncol 2005;23:8580–7.

[60] Woo SB, Hellstein JW, Kalmar JR. Systematic review: bisphosphonates and osteonecrosis of the jaws. Ann Intern Med 2006;144:753–61.

[61] Gawler J. Neurological manifestations of myeloma and their management. In: Malpas JS, Bergsagel DE, Kyle RA, et al, editors. Myeloma: biology and management. 3rd edition. Philadelphia: Saunders, Elsevier Inc.; 2004. p. 269–93.

[62] Henson RA, Urich H. Cancer and nervous system. The neurological manifestations of systemic malignant disease. Oxford: Blackwell Scientific Publications; 1982.

[63] Posner JB. Back pain and epidural spinal cord compression. Med Clin North Am 1987;71: 185–205.

[64] Woodruff RK, Ireton HJC. Multiple nerve palsies as the presenting feature of meningeal myelomatosis. Cancer 1982;49:1710–2.

[65] Spaar FW. Paraproteinemias and multiple myeloma. In: Bryn V, editor. Handbook of clinical neurology. Amsterdan: Elsevier North Holland Biomedical Press; 1980. p. 131–79.

[66] Fassas A, Ward S, Muwalla F, et al. Myeloma of the central nervous system: strong association with unfavorable chromosomal abnormalities and other high-risk disease features. Leuk Lymphoma 2004;45:291–300.

[67] Latov N, Hays AP, Sherman WH. Peripheral neuropathy associated to antiMAG antibodies. Crit Rev Neurobiol 1988;3:301–32.

[68] Nobile-Orazio E, Meucci N, Baldini L, et al. Long term prognosis of neuropathy associated with antiMAG IgM M-proteins and its relationship to immune therapies. Brain 2000;123: 710–7.

[69] Latov N, Sherman WH. Therapy of neuropathy associated with antiMAG IgM monoclonal gammopathy with Rituxan. Neurology 1999;52(Suppl 2):a551.

[70] Levine TD, Pestronk A. IgM antibody related polyneuropathies: B-cell depletion chemotherapy using rituximab. Neurology 1999;52:1701–4.

[71] Cibeira MT, Rosiñol L, Ramiro L, et al. Long-term results of thalidomide in refractory and relapsed multiple myeloma with emphasis on response duration. Eur J Haematol 2006;77: 486–92.

[72] Richardson PG, Briemberg H, Jagannath S, et al. Frequency, characteristics and reversibility of peripheral neuropathy during treatment of advanced multiple myeloma with bortezomib. J Clin Oncol 2006;24:3113–20.

Hematol Oncol Clin N Am 21 (2007) 1247–1273

HEMATOLOGY/ONCOLOGY CLINICS
OF NORTH AMERICA

Complications of Myeloma Therapy

Angela Dispenzieri, MD

Division of Hematology, Mayo Clinic, 200 First Street, Rochester, MN 55905, USA

Appreciating the complications of myeloma therapy is paramount in the twenty-first century. Before the era of novel agents, such as thalidomide, bortezomib, and lenalidomide, median survival for myeloma patients was 3 to 4 years and options were few. Patients received alkylators and corticosteroids fully knowing the risks of these drugs. For the former, one watched predominantly for myelosuppression and in a minority of cases secondary myelodysplasia or leukemia. For the latter, one thought about infection, hyperglycemia, mood swings, insomnia, gastrointestinal bleeding, myopathy, and cataracts. The situation has become far more complicated with the advent of novel agents. Not only are there more complications to consider but patients are also living longer and the risk for delayed complications is becoming more relevant. Patients and physicians must deal with long-term complications. The perfect example of this problem is the issue of bisphosphonate-induced osteonecrosis of the jaw, which is described later.

Our successes for the treatment of multiple myeloma (MM) provide us with additional challenges. Our mission is not only for our patients who have myeloma to live as long as possible but also for them to have the best possible quality of life (ie, as few treatment-related complications as possible). Herein, treatment-related complications are split into two major categories: supportive care therapies and chemotherapy.

SUPPORTIVE CARE

Supportive care is an important adjunct to cancer therapy. Recommendations for conservative measures, such as adequate hydration, a balanced diet, and moderate amounts of low-impact exercise, are universal and noncontroversial. Pharmacologic supportive care measures have also become a mainstay of multiple therapy, but the current use of some of these agents—specifically the bisphosphonates and erythropoietin-stimulating agents—has recently been brought into question because of safety concerns.

Angela Dispenzieri is supported in part by grants CA125614, CA062242, CA107476, CA15083, and CA11345 from the National Cancer Institute.

Support for clinical trials was received from Celgene, Cytogen, and Neurochem.

E-mail address: dispenzieri.angela@mayo.edu

0889-8588/07/$ – see front matter
doi:10.1016/j.hoc.2007.08.002

Bisphosphonates

The knowledge that myeloma bone disease is a significant contributor to morbidity prompted the study of the use of bisphosphonates in these patients. Bisphosphonates, agents that inhibit dissolution of the hydroxyapatite crystals and down-regulate the major osteoclast functions, seemed to be an obvious therapeutic class to study. Indeed, monthly intravenous administration of pamidronate was shown to reduce the likelihood of a skeletal event by almost 50% in patients who had MM [1,2]. In the randomized, blinded controlled study of 392 patients who had Durie-Salmon stage III myeloma and at least one lytic lesion that prompted U.S. Food and Drug Administration (FDA) approval for this indication, there were fewer skeletal-related events in the pamidronate group than in placebo-treated patients (28% versus 44%; $P<.001$) at 12 months. With longer follow-up of 21 months, the difference between groups persisted but narrowed slightly to 28% in the pamidronate group versus 51% in the placebo group ($P<.015$) [3]. Equivalency of pamidronate and zoledronic acid has been demonstrated in two randomized clinical trials, a randomized phase 2 [3] and a randomized phase 3 [4]. In February 2002, the FDA approved an expanded indication for zoledronic acid for the treatment of patients who have bone metastases that included its use in MM.

Indefinite monthly use of bisphosphonate became the standard of care, based on these clinical data [5]. The clinical data were further bolstered by in vitro and in vivo (murine) data that bisphosphonates exert antitumor activity [6] and by the expanding information about the relationships between bone turnover and plasma cell growth and survival [6–10].

In the short term, the drugs were well tolerated—occasional episodes of mild pyrexia, renal function impairment, myalgias, and hypocalcemia were reported. By 2003, however, avascular osteonecrosis of jaw (ONJ) was described as a new complication associated with their use [11–22]. Bisphosphonate-associated ONJ has been described in various malignancies, including MM, breast cancer, and prostate cancer. A management algorithm for ONJ has recently been published [23]. It has been seen in the mandible and the maxilla, but is more frequent in the former. The cause of ONJ is unclear, but is likely multifactorial in origin. Although most patients who develop ONJ have had recent dental or oral surgical procedures (70%), the remainder develop spontaneous ONJ [16]. The leading hypothesis as to mechanism is that bisphosphonate-induced inhibition of osteoclast activity reduces bone turnover and remodeling in addition to suppressing release of bone-specific factors that promote bone formation [24]. In addition, bisphosphonates, particularly zoledronic acid, may have antiangiogenic effects, and impaired blood supply has been implicated in the development of ONJ. Finally, healing of an open bony oral wound is challenged by bacterial insult from oral microflora.

The true incidence of this complication is hard to estimate. Durie and colleagues [19] performed a Web-based survey in 1203 patients who had myeloma and breast cancer and found an incidence of 6.8% in patients who had MM and 4.4% in patients who had breast cancer. The data also suggested the incidence was higher in patients treated with zoledronic acid than with pamidronate [19].

In another study, Bamias and colleagues [18] estimated incidence rates in myeloma patients of 9.9% and found that the time of exposure was strongly associated with development of ONJ and that rates were higher in zoledronic acid–treated patients. Patients who developed ONJ received a median number of 35 infusions (range, 13–68) compared with 15 infusions (range, 6–74) for patients who had no ONJ. Median time of exposure to bisphosphonates was 39.3 months for patients who had ONJ (range, 11–86 months) compared with 19 months (range 4–84.7) for patients who had no osteonecrosis. The likelihood of developing ONJ was 1% during the first year of treatment increasing to 21% at 3 years of treatment for zoledronic acid–treated patients, whereas in the non-zoledronic acid–treated patients the rates were 0% in the first 2 years and 7% after 4 years of treatment.

These observations prompted the Mayo Clinic Myeloma Group to proffer a Consensus Guideline Statement (Table 1) [24], which has been endorsed by the ASCO guidelines [25]. The recommendation is of 2 years of monthly therapy for patients who have myelomatous bone disease, followed by either cessation of therapy in patients who are off active treatment of their myeloma or continuation of therapy every 3 months for those who are receiving myeloma treatment. These recommendations are bolstered by two recent observations. The first is the natural history of myeloma bone disease in the days before bisphosphonate use: the period with the highest rates of bone disease is the first 2 years [26]. The second is a report by the IFM group that pamidronate use after tandem transplant for low-risk patients does not provide any significant reduction in skeletal events [27].

The other major complication of intravenous bisphosphonate use is renal impairment. In a randomized comparison of zoledronic acid versus pamidronate, the incidence of renal deterioration was similar in the two groups; however, in the placebo-controlled trials, the risk for renal deterioration was higher in patients receiving zoledronic acid, especially if the infusion rate was only 5 minutes (16.4% versus 5.6%) [28]. Once the infusion rate had been increased to 15 minutes, the renal toxicity decreased markedly, but there was still a trend toward more renal events with the zoledronic acid group as compared with the placebo group (10.9 versus 6.7%) [28]. In one small long-term study of 57 patients who had cancer treated with either pamidronate or pamidronate plus zoledronic acid, 12% of patients had an increase in serum creatinine [29]. In another smaller study of 22 patients treated with long-term bisphosphonate, 18% had an increase in serum creatinine. Finally in a retrospective observational study of 415 patients who had MM [30], rates of reduction of glomerular filtration rates of 25% or more for patients treated for 18 months with zoledronic acid, pamidronate, or no bisphosphonate were 53.8%, 50.0%, and 33.7%, respectively. Multiple-event analysis found a 2.6-fold risk for renal impairment for zoledronic acid than for pamidronate ($P < .0001$).

Zoledronic acid seems to be more frequently associated with increases in serum creatinine, whereas there are more documented cases of proteinuria in patients treated with pamidronate. There are limited histologic descriptions of bisphosphonate renal toxicity [31,32]. Focal segmental collapsing

Table 1
Mayo Clinic consensus statement for bisphosphonate use in patients who have multiple myeloma

Clinical scenario	Guideline
MM and lytic disease evident on plain radiographs	Intravenous bisphosphonates should be administered monthly
No lytic disease on plain radiographs, but osteopenia or osteoporosis on bone mineral density studies	It is reasonable to start intravenous bisphosphonates in these patients
Smoldering MM	Not recommended outside context of a clinical trial
Duration of bisphosphonate	Patients should receive infusions of bisphosphonates monthly for 2 y
	After 2 y, if the patient has achieved remission and is in stable plateau phase off treatment, the bisphosphonates can be discontinued; if the MM still requires active treatment, the frequency of bisphosphonate infusions can be decreased to every 3 mo
Choice of bisphosphonate	In patients who have newly diagnosed MM, we favor use of pamidronate over zoledronic acid
Dental evaluation and follow-up of patients taking bisphosphonates	Encourage patients to have comprehensive dental evaluation before receiving any bisphosphonate treatment; undergo invasive dental procedures before starting bisphosphonate treatment; see a dentist at least annually and maximize preventive care; report oral/dental symptoms promptly; manage new dental problems conservatively and avoid dental extractions unless absolutely necessary; see an oral and maxillofacial surgeon if surgery is required; practice good dental hygiene
	Encourage physicians to withhold bisphosphonate treatment for at least 1 mo before the procedure and do not resume until the patient has fully recovered and healing of the surgery is complete

From Lacy MQ, Dispenzieri A, Gertz MA, et al. Mayo clinic consensus statement for the use of bisphosphonates in multiple myeloma. Mayo Clin Proc 2006;81:1047–53; with permission.

glomerulosclerosis has been described after high-dose or long-term pamidronate use [31,33–36]. Toxic acute tubular necrosis has been described with zoledronic acid [32]. This same type of injury has also been described with high-dose pamidronate use [37].

Erythropoiesis-Stimulating Agents

The most common clinical feature of MM is anemia. A hemoglobin concentration of less than 12 g/dL occurs in 40% to 73% of patients at presentation [38–40] and contributes to the weakness and fatigue observed in as many as 82% of patients [38–40]. Anemia is often a multifactorial problem, related to direct infiltration and replacement of the bone marrow, renal insufficiency, and chemotherapy.

Anemia is a common complication of cancer or anticancer therapy, with a significant negative impact on the functional status of patients and their quality of life [41]. Recombinant human erythropoietin was developed in the 1980s and was initially developed for the treatment of anemia associated with chronic renal failure. Two placebo-controlled trials in patients who had myeloma demonstrate significantly improved hemoglobin levels and a reduced number of red cell transfusions in patients receiving erythropoietin [42,43]. In these patients, as in any patient who has renal insufficiency, modest doses of recombinant erythropoietin are effective. For patients who have chemotherapy-induced anemia, recombinant erythropoietin may be effective at higher doses. An inappropriately low endogenous erythropoietin concentration is the most important factor predicting response [44].

In general, it was believed that the various erythropoiesis-stimulating agents (ESAs), which are genetically engineered forms of erythropoietin, were safe and increased the quality of life for patients. Their biggest failing was believed to be their cost, but these impressions must now be revised based on several recent FDA alerts (http://www.fda.gov/cder/drug/InfoSheets/HCP/RHE2007HCP.htm) and two publications in the *New England Journal of Medicine* [45,46]. The FDA warning applies specifically to darbepoetin alfa (Aranesp, Amgen Inc.) and epoetin alfa (Epogen, Amgen Inc; and Procrit, Johnson & Johnson). As a point of clarification, all marketed erythropoietins (erythropoietin-alfa, -beta, -gamma, and -omega and darbepoetin alfa) are recombinant erythropoietin with the same 165 amino acid sequence but a slightly different glycosylation pattern (Box 1).

Before discussing the warnings for other patient populations treated with ESAs, the specific risks associated with ESAs in patients who have myeloma is discussed. The major concern about ESA use and thrombosis arose in the context of the immune modulatory drugs (IMiDs), thalidomide and lenalidomide. It is well recognized that with combination chemotherapy and high-dose corticosteroids, the IMiDs are associated with increased risk for thrombosis (Table 2) [47–51]. It was not until comparisons between the North American (MM-009) and the European/Australian (MM-010) relapsed myeloma trials were made that the ESA problem was noted, however [52]. The results of these two large randomized trials showed that patients who had relapsed myeloma randomized to high-dose dexamethasone plus placebo or lenalidomide were identical with regard to efficacy and toxicity, except that the former trial was associated with a much higher thrombosis rate. In an unplanned analysis, the observation was made that the major difference between these trials was the ESA usage; thrombosis rates in patients receiving lenalidomide-dexamethasone versus those not receiving ESA were 23% and 5%, respectively. These findings, although stunning, are not inconsistent with old and emerging data about ESA usage.

As summarized from the FDA web page, in patients who have cancer the use of ESAs to achieve a target hemoglobin of 12 g/dL or greater (1) shortens the

Box 1: FDA recommendations for safe use of erythropoiesis stimulating agents

For all patients

Use the lowest dose possible to gradually increase the hemoglobin (Hgb) concentration to avoid the need for transfusion.

Measure Hgb twice a week for 2 to 6 weeks after any dosage adjustment to ensure that Hgb has stabilized in response to the dose change.

Withhold the dose of the ESA if the Hgb increase exceeds 12 g/dL or increases by 1 g/dL in any 2-week period.

For patients who have cancer

Use of an ESA in anemic patients who have cancer who are not on chemotherapy offered no benefit and may shorten the time to death.

ESAs are not FDA approved to treat anemia in patients who have cancer not receiving chemotherapy

There is a potential risk for shortening the time to tumor progression or disease-free survival

ESAs are administered only to avoid red blood cell transfusions in patients who have cancer. ESAs do not improve the outcome of cancer treatment and do not alleviate fatigue or increase energy.

From United States Food and Drug Administration. Information for healthcare professionals: erythropoiesis stimulating agents (ESA). Available at: http://www.fda.gov/cder/drug/InfoSheets/HCP/RHE2007HCP.htm.

time to tumor progression in patients who have advanced head and neck cancer receiving radiation therapy; (2) increases the risk for death in patients who have active malignant disease not under treatment with chemotherapy or radiation therapy; and (3) shortens overall survival and increased deaths attributed to disease progression in patients who have metastatic breast cancer receiving chemotherapy. In patients who do not have cancer, perioperative venous thrombosis rates are doubled in patients undergoing elective spinal surgery who were randomized to receiving epoetin alfa (Procrit, Ortho Biotech) for pretreatment hemoglobin values between 10 and 13 g/dL. Finally, in patients who had renal failure, targeting normal hemoglobin levels was associated with higher mortality and cardiovascular endpoints [45,46,53].

The data reported to the FDA to prompt these warnings are summarized below. The first admonition arose from results presented to the FDA in 2006 by Amgen. The Danish Head and Neck Cancer Study Group trial is an open-label, randomized trial comparing radiation therapy alone to radiation therapy plus Aranesp (hemoglobin goal of 14.0 to 15.5 g/dL) in the treatment of advanced head and neck cancer (http://conman.au.dk/dahanca). The endpoint was locoregional control rates. The data monitoring committee found that the 3-year locoregional control rate and the overall survival rates were inferior in the Aranesp-treated group (respective P-values of $P = .01$ and .08). In

Table 2
Risk for thrombosis using combination therapy with immune modulatory agents

Reference	N	Regimen	Prophylaxis	TE, n	TE%
Zangari et al	134	TT2	No	19	14
2004 [49]	87	TT2 + Thal	No	30	34
	35	TT2 + Thal	LD warfarin	11	31
	62	TT2	Enox	9	15
	68	TT2 + Thal	Enox	10	15
Baz et al	19	DVd-T	No	11	58
2005 [50]	26	DVd-T	Late ASA	4	15
	58	DVd-T	ASA	11	19
Rajkumar et al	34	Len-Dex	ASA	0	0
2005 [48]					
Palumbo et al	65	MPT	No	11	17
2006 [86]	64	MPT	Enox	2	3
Palumbo et al	50	MPR	ASA	1	2
2006 [87]					
Rajkumar et al	102	Thal-Dex	No	17	17
2006 [47]	102	Dex	No	3	3
Rajkumar and	132	Len-Dex	No	24	18
Blood 2006 [51]	134	Len-LD-Dex	No	5	4
Knight et al	87	Len-Dex + Epo	No	20	23
2006 [52]	83	Len-Dex	No	4	5
	67	Dex + Epo	No	5	7
	103	Dex	No	1	1
Jimenez et al [88]	30	Thal-Dex	No	7	17
	30	Thal-Dex	ASA	1	5

Abbreviations: ASA, aspirin; Dex, dexamethasone; Enox, enoxaparin 40 mg/d; Epo, erythropoietin; LD, low dose; TE, thromboembolism; Thal, thalidomide; TT2, total therapy 2, a complex anthracycline containing multiagent chemotherapy regimen.

hindsight, a similar risk of using erythropoietin beta in head and neck patients was reported at the meeting of the Oncologic Drugs Advisory Committee on May 4, 2004 (http://www.fda.gov/ohrms/dockets/ac/cder04.html#Oncologic).

The new warning not to use ESAs in patients not receiving chemotherapy is from two unpublished studies presented to the FDA in January 2007. The first information was from a 989-patient, multicenter, double-blind, randomized, placebo-controlled study of darbepoetin alfa (Aranesp) in anemic patients who had cancer who were not receiving chemotherapy. The target hemoglobin was 12 g/dL. Aranesp did not reduce the need for red blood cell transfusion and the hazard ratio of death for patients receiving Aranesp was 1.25 (95%CI 1.04, 1.51). The second study prompting the FDA alert not to use ESA in patients who had cancer not receiving chemotherapy was a quality-of-life study in patients who had non–small cell lung cancer not on chemotherapy. The epoetin alpha dose was titrated to maintain a hemoglobin of 12 to 14 g/dL. After enrolling 70 of the 300 planned patients, the data monitoring committee found higher mortality in those treated with epoetin alpha. Median time to death in epoetin alpha arm was 68 days versus the 131 days for those treated with placebo ($P = .04$). The major cause of death reported was disease progression. In this small sample size, there was no evidence that epoetin alpha reduced the need for red cell transfusion or increased the quality of life.

Finally, another randomized, double-blind, placebo-controlled study designed to investigate the effect of erythropoietin treatment to maintain normal hemoglobin concentrations on survival in patients who had metastatic breast cancer suggested inferiority in the erythropoietin arm [54]. A total of 939 patients who had metastatic breast cancer undergoing first-line chemotherapy either received 12 months of erythropoietin (Eprex) as an adjunct to chemotherapy to prevent anemia (goal hemoglobin of >12 g/dL and <14 g/dL) or they did not. The independent data-monitoring committee terminated the study early because of an observed higher mortality at 12 months in the group treated with Eprex (30% versus 24%, $P = .0117$). Much of this difference occurred within the first 4 months of the study and was mainly attributable to an increase in incidence of disease progression (6% versus 3%) and of thrombotic and vascular events (1% versus 0.2%) in the Eprex group as compared with placebo.

Two clinical studies and an editorial published in the *New England Journal of Medicine* in November 2006 addressed safety concerns about the use of ESAs in the treatment of anemia of chronic renal failure [45,46,53]. The 1400-subject CHOIR study demonstrated increases in serious and potentially life-threatening cardiovascular events when epoetin alfa (Procrit) is administered to reach higher target hemoglobin levels (13.5 g/dL) than lower target hemoglobin levels (11.3 g/dL) [45]. The 600-subject CREATE study [46], which used epoetin beta, trended toward more cardiovascular events in a pattern similar to the CHOIR study, strengthening the findings of the CHOIR study. For the former study, the primary endpoint of composite of death and cardiovascular events were statistically significantly worse in the higher-target hemoglobin group ($P = .03$ by log rank test) with a hazard ratio of 1.3 (95% CI 1.03, 1.74).

CHEMOTHERAPY

As early as the late 1960s and early 1970s it was recognized that novel agents for the treatment of MM–the alkylators–put patients at increased risk for secondary myelodysplastic syndrome and acute leukemia [55–58]. Long-term use of corticosteroids causes cataracts, osteoporosis, and atypical infections, among other things. As the list of drugs in the myeloma armamentarium grew, so did the list of possible side effects. The toxicities of drugs may be exaggerated when used in combination with other drugs.

To best try to dissect these complications, we discuss the most serious known adverse effects associated with the most commonly used antimyeloma agents. Specific combinations are discussed as appropriate. Any description of adverse events across studies is fraught with difficulty because of differential ascertainment and reporting. The adverse events observed in newly diagnosed trials are given more weight because it is slightly easier to discern drug toxicity from disease toxicity.

Alkylators

Standard low-dose oral cyclophosphamide or melphalan is well tolerated. Both drugs are most commonly administered with prednisone, and therefore complications are reported in the context of prednisone-containing regimens. Most patients do not experience significant side effects other than myelosuppression. Fewer than 20% of patients receiving MP will have grade 3 to 4 hematologic toxicity [59], which is easily managed by dose reduction in the next cycle. Severe pyogenic infections occur in about 10% of patients, but hemorrhage, psychiatric complications, thrombotic episodes, or severe diabetes is seen in fewer than 5% of patients [59].

The most dreaded treatment-related complication among myeloma patients receiving standard dose alkylator therapy is secondary myelodysplastic syndrome or acute leukemia. After secondary leukemia is diagnosed, median survival tends to be short—about 2 months [60].

For patients receiving melphalan, the risk for myelodysplastic syndrome is approximately 3% at 5 years and 10% at 8 to 9 years [60,61], with estimates as high as 25% at 10 years [62] and multiple other estimates somewhere in between [63–65]. Some authors have suggested that higher cumulative doses of melphalan are associated with a higher risk for acute leukemia [61]. Others have shown no difference in incidence based on the number of courses of chemotherapy or the cumulative melphalan dose between the patients who did and did not develop acute leukemia [60]. In one study, the mean number of chemotherapy cycles was 19.7 and 18.5 in patients who did and did not have secondary leukemia, respectively; mean cumulative melphalan doses were 1440 and 1400 mg, respectively [60]. Although cyclophosphamide has been shown to be leukemogenic, it may be less so than melphalan [61,66,67]. From a practical standpoint, it is much less toxic to platelets.

After stem cell transplantation for myeloma, the risk for myelodysplastic syndrome seems to be related to prior chemotherapy rather than to the transplant itself [68]. The 10-year estimate of secondary myelodysplastic syndrome in patients undergoing high-dose chemotherapy and hematopoietic stem cell transplantation is 7% [69].

Novel Agents

The novel agent category includes bortezomib and the IMiDs (thalidomide, lenalidomide, and CC-4047). For the purpose of discussion, only the three FDA-approved drugs are discussed. Tables 3 and 4 include the more common adverse events associated with these drugs. Although the adverse events for these drugs are listed in one table for ease of viewing, one should not make direct comparisons between the studies because of differences among them in toxicity ascertainment and reporting. Other important adverse events specific to a given drug may be omitted if uncommon for the other drugs.

Thalidomide

Thalidomide is the first in the class of the IMiDs. Its mechanism of action is not completely understood, but it has been shown to reduce angiogenesis,

Table 3
Hematologic adverse events associated with novel agents

Drug	Thal[a]	Thal[b]	Bor[b]	Bor[c]	Len[c]	Len[d]	Dex[b]
Reference	Rajkumar et al [77]	Singhal et al [72]	Richardson et al [90]	Jagannath et al [91]	Rajkumar et al [48]	Richardson et al [85]	Richardson et al [90]
N	31	83	331	32	34	67	332
Anemia							
Grade 1–2	NS	NS	16	NS	6	NS	11
Grade 3–4	NS	<1	10	NS	6	16	11
Neutropenia							
Grade 1–2	NS	<5	5	3 (grade 2)	32	NS	6
Grade 3–4	NS	NS	14	13	12	61	0
Thrombocytopenia							
Grade 1–2	NS	NS	5	3 (grade 2)	27	NS	5
Grade 3–4	NS	<1	30	3	NS	16	6

NS, not stated.
[a]Single agent, newly diagnosed.
[b]Single agent, relapsed diagnosed.
[c]With dexamethasone, newly diagnosed.
[d]With dexamethasone, relapsed disease.

modulate adhesion molecules of myeloma cells and their surrounding stroma, modulate cytokines, and affect natural killer cells [70].

The complication rate, and possibly the response rate [71], of the drug is partially dose-dependent. In the earliest studies, patients were started on 200 mg daily and the dose was pushed to 800 mg daily [72]. Most patients were unable to tolerate these doses, and there was a move to treating patients on daily doses as low as 50 to 100 mg [73–76]. Using lower doses of drug, even in association with dexamethasone, adverse events occurred in 5% to 15% of patients, with only 10% of patients discontinuing therapy because of toxicity [75].

The adverse event most feared is that of fetal malformation in babies born to mothers taking the drug. Because of the System for Thalidomide Education and Prescribing Safety program, which emphasizes the danger of the drug to unborn children, this adverse event has not been seen this decade. The most common side effects reported by patients taking the drug are constipation, fatigue, sedation, and tingling and numbness. In the first report, the frequency of these adverse events differed depending on whether a patient was receiving 200 mg/d or 800 mg/d. The respective rates were as follows: 35% to 59%, 29% to 48%, 34% to 43%, and 12% to 28%, respectively, of patients [72]. Myelosuppression is rare. Other significant side effects are rash (16%–55%), tremor (10%–35%), depression (16%–22%), dizziness (17%–28%), bradycardia (26%), ataxia (16%–22%), and edema (3%–16%) [72,77]. Life-threatening complications have included Stevens-Johnson syndrome and hepatitis [78,79]. Thrombosis is rare in patients receiving single-agent thalidomide, but it is an important risk occurring in as many as 28% of patients receiving concurrent corticosteroids or anthracyclines [80–82] (see Table 2).

The peripheral neuropathy induced by thalidomide deserves special mention because it is common and seemingly irreversible. In one study, the time course of occurrence, possible predictive factors, and the use of serial nerve electrophysiologic studies for detecting onset of neuropathy was studied in 75 patients who had relapsed/refractory myeloma who were participating in a multicenter trial of dose-escalating thalidomide, with or without interferon [83]. Thirty-nine percent had some nerve electrophysiologic studies abnormalities at baseline. Patients received thalidomide at a median dose intensity of 373 mg/d. Forty-one percent of patients developed neuropathy during thalidomide treatment, and 11 patients (15%) discontinued treatment with thalidomide because of neuropathy. The actuarial incidence of neuropathy increased from 38% at 6 months to 73% at 12 months, with 81% of responding patients developing this complication. The only predictor of developing neuropathy was time on therapy: median of 268 versus 89 days ($P = .0001$) for those who did and did not develop PN.

Lenalidomide (CC-5013; Revlimid)
Lenalidomide is a small molecule derivative of thalidomide and a member of the IMiD class that is more potent than thalidomide in mediating direct cytokine-related and immunomodulatory effects against human MM cell lines and patient-derived cells in vitro. It induces apoptosis of myeloma cells,

Table 4
Nonhematologic adverse events associated with novel agents

Drug	Thal[a]	Thal[b]	Bor[b]	Bor[c]	Len[c]	Len[d]	Dex[b]
Reference	Rajkumar et al [77]	Singhal et al [72]	Richardson et al [90]	Jagannath et al [91]	Rajkumar et al [48]	Richardson et al [85]	Richardson et al [90]
N	31	83	331	32	34	67	332
Fatigue							
Grade 1–2	65	29–48	36	19 (grade 2)	41	NS	28
Grade 3–4	3	NS	6	6	15	NS	4
PN							
Grade 1–2	87	12–28	28[e]	16 (grade 2)	21	NS	1[e]
Grade 3–4	3	NS	8[e]	16	0	10	0
Rash							
Grade 1–2	55	16–26	17	6 (grade 2)	6	NS	6
Grade 3–4	0	NS	1	0	6	NS	0
Constipation							
Grade 1–2	87	35–59	40	25 (grade 2)	15	NS	14
Grade 3–4	0	NS	2	3	0	25	1
Diarrhea							
Grade 1–2	NS	NS	50	6 (grade 2)	6	NS	19
Grade 3–4	NS	NS	7	9	0	NS	2
Nausea							
Grade 1–2	NS	12–23	55	16 (grade 2)	3	NS	14
Grade 3–4	NS	NS	2	0	3	NS	0

Emesis					
Grade 1–2	NS	NS	32	NS	5
Grade 3–4	NS	NS	3	NS	1
Edema					
Grade 1–2	16	6–22	NS	6 (grade 2)	NS
Grade 3–4	3	NS	NS	0	NS
Fever					
Grade 1–2	NS	NS	33	NS	15
Grade 3–4	NS	NS	2	NS	1

Abbreviations: Bor, bortezomib; Dex, dexamethasone; Len, lenalidomide; NS, not stated; PN, peripheral neuropathy; Thal, thalidomide.

[a]Single agent, newly diagnosed.
[b]Single agent, relapsed diagnosed.
[c]With dexamethasone, newly diagnosed.
[d]With dexamethasone, relapsed disease.
[e]Unclear what total number is because in manuscript, paresthesias and peripheral neuropathy are counted as separate categories. For thalidomide, 19% and 2% had grade 1–2 and 3–4 paresthesias, respectively; for dexamethasone-treated patients; 1% had grade 1–2 paresthesias.

overcomes cytokine and bone marrow stromal cell-mediated drug resistance, has antiangiogenic effects, and stimulates host antimyeloma T and natural killer cell immunity [84,85].

Lenalidomide has never been studied as a single agent in newly diagnosed myeloma, but adverse event information is available from limited single-agent trials in relapsed/refractory patients and from newly diagnosed patient trials in combination with dexamethasone.

In the original phase 1 and phase 2 trials, there is limited toxicity information available. In the phase 1 trial that included 25 patients treated with 5 to 50 mg of drug per day, the most common adverse events for treated patients included grade 3 neutropenia in 76% and grade 3 thrombocytopenia in 20%. Other adverse events included grade 1 lightheadedness (~18%), leg cramps (~44%), and fatigue (~35%). Grade 1 to 2 rash was observed in about 40% of patients [84]. For those patients receiving 30 mg of lenalidomide in the phase 2 setting, there was grade 3 to 4 neutropenia (61%), thrombocytopenia (31%), and anemia (17%) [85]. Treatment-emergent neuropathy occurred in 10% of patients (Tables 3 and 4).

These rates differ slightly from those reported in the up-front setting using lenalidomide and dexamethasone (Tables 3 and 4) [48]. Only 9% of patients treated with standard-dose lenalidomide and high-dose dexamethasone had grade 3 to 4 neutropenia, and none had grade 3 to 4 thrombocytopenia. Also seen were dizziness (9%), infection (~9%), elevated alkaline phosphatase (6%), thrombosis (3%), and nausea (3%). Grade 1 to 2 depression was reported, but it is unclear whether that side effect was dexamethasone or lenalidomide related. No peripheral neuropathy was observed.

Risk for thrombosis when using immune modulatory drugs as combination therapy
Thrombosis is an important complication in patients undergoing treatment with ImiDs (thalidomide or lenalidomide). As a single agents, there does not seem to be any heightened risk; however, concomitant chemotherapy [86]—especially anthracyclines [49,50], high-dose corticosteroids [47,51], and erythropoietin [52]—seems to increase the risk for thrombosis to as high as 58% (Table 2). Prophylactic low molecular heparin (eg, enoxaparin 40 mg daily) [49,86] abrogates that risk. Daily aspirin also seems to be protective in the lower-risk setting [47,48,52,87,88]. At the 2006 American Society of Hematology Meeting, Jimenez and colleagues [88] presented their data of a small trial in which 60 patients who had myeloma being treated with thalidomide-dexamethasone were randomized to aspirin prophylaxis or no prophylaxis. The thrombosis rates were 17% versus 5%, in favor of aspirin prophylaxis.

Low-dose warfarin is not protective. Although full anticoagulation with full-dose warfarin is commonly recommended, there are no trial data substantiating this recommendation; the concern with warfarin anticoagulation is the difficulty of maintaining a therapeutic INR while cycling the IMiDs, corticosteroids, and other chemotherapeutic agents. It is for this reason that the current recommendation for thromboembolism protection in intermediate-risk patients is either aspirin or warfarin. The risk for bleeding when using any of the thromboembolism-protective agents must be weighed against the risk for bleeding in any given patient.

Bortezomib

Bortezomib is the first drug in its class of proteasome inhibitors. It is a boronic acid dipeptide that reversibly and selectively inhibits the proteasome, an intracellular complex that degrades primarily ubiquitinated proteins. The proteasome has a key role in protein degradation, cell-cycle regulation, and gene expression. Tumor cells, including MM, are heavily dependent on proteasome-regulated proteins for their growth and interaction with stromal cells. Inhibition of the proteasome has emerged as an important antitumor target, and bortezomib has been shown in vitro and in vivo to cause growth arrest, to induce apoptosis, and to inhibit angiogenesis [89].

The most common adverse events (Tables 3 and 4) associated with standard schedule bortezomib (1.3 mg/m^2 days 1, 4, 8, 11, every 21 days) are: diarrhea (57%), nausea (16%–55%), vomiting (35%), constipation (28%–42%), fatigue (25%–42%), peripheral neuropathy (~32%), thrombocytopenia (6%–35%), and neutropenia (16%–24%) [90,91]. In the large phase 3, randomized APEX study, 75% of patients treated with bortezomib had serious (grade 3–4) adverse events [90]. Herpes zoster was seen in 13% of patients treated with bortezomib. Fever occurred in 35% of patients, but it is unclear whether this fever was related to infection or febrile reaction. Because infection is not listed as an adverse event, one could assume that these reported fevers were in the context of an infection.

Peripheral neuropathy deserves special mention, because it is a common adverse event. In one study reported by Richardson and colleagues [92], peripheral neuropathy was assessed in 256 relapsed or refractory myeloma patients participating in two phase 2 studies using bortezomib 1.0 or 1.3 mg/m^2 according to the standard schedule, for up to eight cycles. Peripheral neuropathy was evaluated at baseline, during the study, and after the study by patient-reported symptoms using the Functional Assessment of Cancer Therapy Scale/Gynecologic Oncology Group–Neurotoxicity (FACT/GOG-Ntx) questionnaire and neurologic examination. Of interest, before treatment approximately 80% of patients had peripheral neuropathy. Treatment-emergent neuropathy was reported in 35% of patients, including 37% (84 of 228 patients) receiving bortezomib 1.3 mg/m^2 and 21% (6 of 28 patients) receiving bortezomib 1.0 mg/m^2, and grade 3 to 4 neuropathy was more likely to occur in patients who had baseline neuropathy (14% versus 4%, respectively). Grade 1 or 2, 3, and 4 neuropathy occurred in 22%, 13%, and 0.4% of patients, respectively. Neuropathy led to dose reduction in 12% and discontinuation in 5% of patients. Of 35 patients who had neuropathy greater than or equal to grade 3 or requiring discontinuation, resolution to baseline or improvement occurred in 71%.

An unusual toxicity, seemly more common in people of Japanese ancestry, is severe pulmonary toxicity. In a report of 13 Japanese patients who had MM treated with bortezomib, 4 developed severe pulmonary complications, and 2 died of respiratory failure without progression of underlying disease [93].

Low-dose bortezomib (1.0 mg/m^2) is better tolerated—but slightly less effective—than standard dose (1.3 mg/m^2) bortezomib [94]. Although no direct comparisons were made in a randomized phase 2 study, in the low-dose group there seemed to be a lower rate of dose reductions (11% versus 35%) and adverse events. For low-dose and standard-dose patients, the respective grade 3 to 4 adverse events were: peripheral neuropathy (8% versus 15%), weakness (4% versus 12%), neutropenia (11% versus 23%), and pneumonia (0 versus 15%) [94]. Although the original studies using bortezomib included only eight cycles of therapy, 63 patients were treated on an extension study without significantly more serious adverse events than were seen on the parent studies of eight cycles alone [95].

Corticosteroids

Corticosteroid-based therapy has been used since 1950 when Thorn and colleagues [96] reported the first observations on the beneficial effects of adrenocorticotropic hormone in myeloma. The mechanism of action of this drug class is complex. Corticosteroids suppress the production of cytokines important in myeloma growth, such as IL-6 and IL-1β, and reduce nuclear factor κB activity, resulting in enhanced apoptosis [97–100].

As a class, corticosteroids have been an important therapy for myeloma patients, used for tumor burden reduction, treatment of hypercalcemia, and as an adjunct for patients who have spinal cord compression. Alone or in combination, they have been used in patients who have newly diagnosed, relapsed, and refractory disease [101–103]. Although they clearly induce hematologic responses and increase response rates when used as an adjunct with other drugs [85,91,104,105], they have not been shown to produce a survival advantage [106,107]. There are emerging data in the newly diagnosed setting that dose-intensive dexamethasone may be associated with more morbidity and a worse overall survival [59,108].

Some of the most common side effects seen with high-dose corticosteroids are shown in Table 3. Common grade 3 to 4 toxicities include hyperglycemia (15%), dyspnea (10%), fatigue (10%), insomnia (5%), hypertension (3%), and anxiety (3%) [47].

Anthracyclines

For the treatment of myeloma, doxorubicin is the most commonly used anthracycline, but its activity as a single agent in relapsed or refractory disease is modest, with response rates of about 10% [109,110]. Doxorubicin is one of the original anthracyclines isolated from the bacterium *Streptomyces peucetius*. Its mechanism of action is multifaceted. It intercalates into DNA, thus interfering with macromolecule synthesis. It contributes to generation of reactive oxygen species, binds to and alkylates DNA contributing to cross-linking, and inhibits topoisomerase II.

The most common side effects associated with doxorubicin are listed in the context of myeloma regimens. One of the more important toxicities of this drug is its acute and chronic effects on the cardiovascular system. The acute effects, which include arrhythmias, hypotension, and various electrocardiographic changes, occur in approximately 11% of patients during or soon after (within a couple of days) administration and are generally reversible and clinically manageable. Less commonly, acute left ventricular failure, pericarditis, and myocarditis may be seen in the acute setting [111].

The chronic effects of doxorubicin, however, are dose-dependent, irreversible cardiomyopathic changes leading to congestive heart failure with a poor prognosis. The incidence of doxorubicin-induced cardiomyopathy is 1.7%, and the mortality rate is more than 50%. The cardiotoxicity is clearly related to the total cumulative dose administered, and to acute peak levels, age at exposure, and the concurrent administration of other cardiotoxic antineoplastic agents. Studies from the 1970s illustrated that cardiomyopathy and congestive heart failure developed in more than 4% of patients who received a cumulative dose of 500 to 550 mg/m^2, in more than 18% of those who received 551 to 600 mg/m^2, and in about 36% of those receiving more than 601 mg/m^2 [112]. Cardiomyopathy occurred an average of 34 days after the last administration, but among long survivors after doxorubicin chemotherapy, many developed heart failure 6 to 10 years after therapy. In one study with a median follow-up of 11 years, the incidence of a clinical cardiac event among 191 patients who had Hodgkin lymphoma treated with doxorubicin, bleomycin, vinblastine, and dacarbazine was 9% [113].

The best long-term toxicity data are available from patients treated as children. These data may have limited generalizability because toxicity could be greater in a growing heart than in a full-grown adult heart; however, pediatric follow-up data are often more complete because of better follow-up and better overall long-term survival rates. Most of the studies have described cardiac abnormalities 5 to10 years after anthracycline therapy at an incidence of 5% to 10% of long-term survivors; however, the incidence dramatically increases after 10 years of follow-up [114].

Antioxidants have been explored as agents to protect against cardiac toxicity. Vitamin E seemed protective against acute cardiotoxic effects of doxorubicin, but ineffective against the development of chronic cardiomyopathy. Other antioxidants have been used with limited success. Carvedilol, which acts as a β-adrenergic receptor blocker and an antioxidant, also seems to reduce doxorubicin cardiotoxicity. The iron-chelating agent dexrazoxane has a cardioprotective effect, but it aggravates myelosuppression and may even interfere with cancer therapy. Cytokines, such as erythropoietin, granulocyte colony-stimulating factor, and thrombopoietin, may have some cardioprotective effects also [111].

In principle, the use of liposomes to target doxorubicin delivery should reduce its cardiotoxicity. Liposome-encapsulated or liposomal anthracyclines have reduced cardiotoxicity in clinical trials [111]. The use of anthracyclines has increased in patients who have MM since the introduction of liposomal doxorubicin (Doxil, Caelyx), partially based on the perceived improved safety profile, but partially based on the synergy seen with novel agents, especially bortezomib [115].

When liposomal doxorubicin is used with vincristine and dexamethasone, the most common side effects include: nausea (~50%), asthenia (~50%), constipation (44%), anemia (~40%), fever (25%–30%), stomatitis (20%–30%), neutropenia (20%–30%), pneumonia (5%–10%), deep venous thrombosis (7%–10%), and syncope (4%–7%) [116]. Alopecia, injection-site reactions, and grade 3 or 4 neutropenia were less common in the group receiving liposomal doxorubicin, whereas hand-foot syndrome was significantly more common. Two patients receiving infusional doxorubicin developed grade 3 to 4 congestive heart failure in comparison to none in the liposomal doxorubicin group.

In patients receiving bortezomib and liposomal doxorubicin [117], the most common grade 3 to 4 adverse advents observed were: fatigue (14%), thrombocytopenia (43%), neutropenia (17%), pneumonia (14%), diarrhea (10%), febrile neutropenia (10%), syncope (7%), sinusitis (5%), bowel obstruction (7%), fever (7%), dyspnea (5%), hypotension (5%), and gastrointestinal bleeding (5%). Other common, but less severe, toxicities included: nausea (64%), constipation (60%), peripheral neuropathy (55%), anemia (52%), anorexia (43%), rash (40%), mucositis (33%), headache (24%), cough (24%), weight loss (21%), plantar-palmar erythrodysesthesia (21%), and bruising (21%).

Other Drugs: Vincristine and Arsenic Trioxide
Vincristine
Vincristine is one of the least-effective agents against MM that is currently in use. Although never evaluated as a single agent in newly diagnosed myeloma, vincristine has little activity as a single agent in refractory disease. In the one single-agent study, of the 21 patients treated, 2 patients had transient responses (1.2 and 2.2 months) [118]. Although there was initial theoretic benefit to its use in myeloma [119–121], randomized trials do not support its use [122–125]. The toxicity profile of vincristine is well understood with the most common side effects being constipation, nausea, vomiting, peripheral neuropathy, diplopia, alopecia, and myelosuppression.

Arsenic trioxide
In vitro, arsenic trioxide (ATO) induces growth inhibition and apoptosis [126]. Generation of reactive oxygen species with subsequent accumulation of hydrogen peroxide enhances ATO-induced apoptosis. Because glutathione is believed to salvage free radicals, methods to reduce glutathione have been explored, the most popular of which is coadministration of ascorbic acid. In vitro, this approach has seemed to be more effective against myeloma cells of patients

who had refractory disease than those who had newly diagnosed disease [127]. As a single agent in refractory disease, however, the overall partial response rate is 7.1% [128] with a total of one third achieving a 25% reduction in M-protein in one study [129]. Using the daily 60-day schedule commonly used in acute promyelocytic leukemia, the most common side effects were neutropenia (79%), infection (36%), thrombosis (21%), and extreme fatigue (14%) [128]. Using a less-frequent infusion schedule is more tolerable. In one study in which arsenic trioxide was combined with dexamethasone and ascorbic acid, grade 3 neutropenia, fatigue, hyponatremia, dehydration, burning at the intravenous site, and syncope each occurred in 5% of patients treated. Grade 3 to 4 hyperglycemia occurring in 15% of patients [130].

SUMMARY

Cognizance of the complications of myeloma therapy and supportive care is essential. All physicians should know about the risks of osteonecrosis of the jaw and renal insufficiency with prolonged, intensive dosing of intravenous bisphosphonates. They should be aware of the risks of overzealous use of erythropoiesis-stimulating agents in general (more cardiovascular events, shortened overall survival, and possibly poorer control of carcinoma) and more specifically in conjunction with the immunomodulatory drugs, such as thalidomide and lenalidomide (higher rates of thrombotic events). Moreover, awareness of the shifting spectrum of toxicities induced by myeloma therapies is important. With older therapies myelosuppression, alopecia, mucositis, nausea, vomiting, and diarrhea were the rule; however, with bortezomib, peripheral neuropathy (Table 5) is a major recurring toxicity. In addition, a heightened thrombotic risk when using thalidomide or lenalidomide in combination with other agents should be foremost in the physician's mind.

With the exception of alkylators, anthracyclines, and bisphosphonates, we have focused on short-term adverse effects of the newer agents. Short-term effects are obviously important from the standpoint of quality of life and early mortality. How these short-term effects will play into long-term survival and quality of life can only be speculated on, however. What is the implication of introducing irreversible neuropathy by thalidomide and (less commonly) by bortezomib

Table 5 Antitumor agents that cause neurotoxicity			
Agent	Likelihood	Peripheral	Central
Cisplatin	High	x	
Interferon	High		x
Vinca alkaloids	High	x	
Thalidomide	High	x	x
Lenalidomide	Low	x	
Bortezomib	High	x	

Table 6
Initial therapy and early mortality

Regimen	RR	Deaths%
Dex (E1A00) (Rajkuma et al [47])	41%	11%
Dex ± IFN (IFM 95-01) (Facon et al [59])	41%	10.5%
MP (IFM 99-06) (Facon et al [139])	40%	8%
Thal/Dex (E1A00) (Rajkuma et al [47])	63%	7%
Rev/Dex (E4A03) (Rajkumar et al [108])	?	4.9%
MPT (IFM 99-06) (Facon et al [139])	81%	3%
Rev/low-dose Dex (E4A03) (Rajkumar et al [108])	?	0.5%
Bortezomib (Jagannath et al [91])	40%	0%
Bortezomib + dexamethasone (Harousseau et al [140])	66%	0%
MRC trials 1980–2002 (Augustson et al [141])	Mixed	10%

Abbreviations: Dex, dexamethasone; IFN, interferon; MP, melphalan and prednisone; MRC, Medical Research Council; Thal, thalidomide; Rev, lenalidomide.

Data from Dispenzieri A, Rajkumar SV, Gertz MA, et al. Treatment of newly diagnosed multiple myeloma based on Mayo stratification of myeloma and risk-adapted therapy (mSMART): consensus statement. Mayo Clin Proc 2007;82:323–41.

to a patient's long-term picture? What about combining neurotoxic agents, such as vincristine and thalidomide, as in the thalidomide, vincristine, doxorubicin, dexamethasone regimen [131,132]? Or combining thalidomide with bortezomib as is done in the highly active bortezomib, thalidomide, dexamethasone regimen [133–135]? What is the implication of combining bortezomib with anthracyclines as is done in the bortezomib, doxorubicin, dexamethasone regimen [136] or in the liposomal doxorubicin and bortezomib regimens? [117,137,138] Although there is no increase in early cardiac toxicity, might there be delayed cardiac toxicity? Will the long-term benefits of more morbid induction combination therapies be worthwhile by reducing early mortality because of more rapid control of disease? As shown in Table 6 [139–142], early mortality of newly diagnosed myeloma patients participating in clinical trials ranges from 0 to 11%. It is unclear what portion of early mortality is patient condition versus lack of disease control versus toxicity of therapy. There seems to be a trend toward regimens with higher response rates being associated with higher survival rates. Will it be that higher up-front morbidity will be the price to pay for lower mortality? In the context of dexamethasone dose intensity, the converse seems to be true [108].

As always, there are more questions than answers; however, it is encouraging that there are new drugs available for our myeloma patients. With that perk comes the challenge of deciphering new complications, risks, and benefits. What a small price to pay!

References

[1] Berenson JR, Lichtenstein A, Porter L, et al. Efficacy of pamidronate in reducing skeletal events in patients with advanced multiple myeloma. Myeloma Aredia Study Group. N Engl J Med 1996;334:488–93.

[2] Berenson JR, Lichtenstein A, Porter L, et al. Long-term pamidronate treatment of advanced multiple myeloma patients reduces skeletal events. Myeloma Aredia Study Group. J Clin Oncol 1998;16:593–602.

[3] Berenson JR, Rosen LS, Howell A, et al. Zoledronic acid reduces skeletal-related events in patients with osteolytic metastases. Cancer 2001;91:1191–200.

[4] Rosen LS, Gordon D, Antonio BS, et al. Zoledronic acid versus pamidronate in the treatment of skeletal metastases in patients with breast cancer or osteolytic lesions of multiple myeloma: a phase III, double-blind, comparative trial. Cancer J 2001;7:377–87.

[5] Berenson JR, Hillner BE, Kyle RA, et al. American Society of Clinical Oncology clinical practice guidelines: the role of bisphosphonates in multiple myeloma. J Clin Oncol 2002;20:3719–36.

[6] Abe M, Hiura K, Wilde J, et al. Osteoclasts enhance myeloma cell growth and survival via cell-cell contact: a vicious cycle between bone destruction and myeloma expansion. Blood 2004;104:2484–91.

[7] Yaccoby S, Wezeman MJ, Zangari M, et al. Inhibitory effects of osteoblasts and increased bone formation on myeloma in novel culture systems and a myelomatous mouse model. Haematologica 2006;91:192–9.

[8] Stewart JP, Shaughnessy JD Jr. Role of osteoblast suppression in multiple myeloma. J Cell Biochem 2006;98:1–13.

[9] Terpos E, Politou M, Szydlo R, et al. Serum levels of macrophage inflammatory protein-1 alpha (MIP-1alpha) correlate with the extent of bone disease and survival in patients with multiple myeloma. Br J Haematol 2003;123:106–9.

[10] Silvestris F, Lombardi L, De Matteo M, et al. Myeloma bone disease: pathogenetic mechanisms and clinical assessment. Leuk Res 2007;31:129–38.

[11] Marx RE. Pamidronate (Aredia) and zoledronate (Zometa) induced avascular necrosis of the jaws: a growing epidemic. J Oral Maxillofac Surg 2003;61:1115–7.

[12] Carter GD, Goss AN. Bisphosphonates and avascular necrosis of the jaws. Aust Dent J 2003;48:268.

[13] Lugassy G, Shaham R, Nemets A, et al. Severe osteomyelitis of the jaw in long-term survivors of multiple myeloma: a new clinical entity. Am J Med 2004;117:440–1.

[14] Migliorati CA. Bisphosphanates and oral cavity avascular bone necrosis. J Clin Oncol 2003;21:4253–4.

[15] Tarassoff P, Csermak K. Avascular necrosis of the jaws: risk factors in metastatic cancer patients. J Oral Maxillofac Surg 2003;61:1238–9.

[16] Ruggiero SL, Mehrotra B, Rosenberg TJ, et al. Osteonecrosis of the jaws associated with the use of bisphosphonates: a review of 63 cases. J Oral Maxillofac Surg 2004;62:527–34.

[17] Bagan JV, Murillo J, Jimenez Y, et al. Avascular jaw osteonecrosis in association with cancer chemotherapy: series of 10 cases. J Oral Pathol Med 2005;34:120–3.

[18] Bamias A, Kastritis E, Bamia C, et al. Osteonecrosis of the jaw in cancer after treatment with bisphosphonates: incidence and risk factors. J Clin Oncol 2005;23:8580–7.

[19] Durie BG, Katz M, Crowley J. Osteonecrosis of the jaw and bisphosphonates. N Engl J Med 2005;353:99–102 [discussion: 199–102].

[20] Marx RE, Sawatari Y, Fortin M, et al. Bisphosphonate-induced exposed bone (osteonecrosis/osteopetrosis) of the jaws: risk factors, recognition, prevention, and treatment. J Oral Maxillofac Surg 2005;63:1567–75.

[21] Badros A, Weikel D, Salama A, et al. Osteonecrosis of the jaw in multiple myeloma patients: clinical features and risk factors. J Clin Oncol 2006;24:945–52.

[22] Kanat O, Ozet A, Arpaci F, et al. Bisphosphonate-associated osteonecrosis of the jaws: case reports and analysis of 184 cases. J Clin Oncol [Meeting abstracts] 2006;24:18595.

[23] Migliorati CA, Casiglia J, Epstein J, et al. Managing the care of patients with bisphosphonate-associated osteonecrosis: an American Academy of Oral Medicine position paper. J Am Dent Assoc 2005;136:1658–68.

[24] Lacy MQ, Dispenzieri A, Gertz MA, et al. Mayo clinic consensus statement for the use of bisphosphonates in multiple myeloma. Mayo Clin Proc 2006;81(8):1047–53.

[25] Kyle RA, Yee GC, Somerfield MR, et al. American Society of Clinical Oncology 2007 clinical practice guideline update on the role of bisphosphonates in multiple myeloma. J Clin Oncol 2007;27:2464–72.

[26] Melton LJ 3rd, Kyle RA, Achenbach SJ, et al. Fracture risk with multiple myeloma: a population-based study. J Bone Miner Res 2005;20:487–93.

[27] Attal M, Harousseau JL, Leyvraz S, et al. Maintenance therapy with thalidomide improves survival in patients with multiple myeloma. Blood 2006;108:3289–94.

[28] Rosen LS, Gordon D, Tchekmedyian S, et al. Zoledronic acid versus placebo in the treatment of skeletal metastases in patients with lung cancer and other solid tumors: a phase III, double-blind, randomized trial—the Zoledronic Acid Lung Cancer and Other Solid Tumors Study Group. J Clin Oncol 2003;21:3150–7.

[29] Guarneri V, Donati S, Nicolini M, et al. Renal safety and efficacy of i.v. bisphosphonates in patients with skeletal metastases treated for up to 10 Years. Oncologist 2005;10:842–8.

[30] Nickolas TL, Chen L, Markowitz G, et al. Renal toxicity associated with zoledronic acid and pamidronate in multiple myeloma patients: a retrospective study. J Clin Oncol [Meeting abstracts] 2006;24:17515.

[31] Markowitz GS, Appel GB, Fine PL, et al. Collapsing focal segmental glomerulosclerosis following treatment with high-dose pamidronate. J Am Soc Nephrol 2001;12:1164–72.

[32] Markowitz GS, Fine PL, Stack JI, et al. Toxic acute tubular necrosis following treatment with zoledronate (Zometa). Kidney Int 2003;64:281–9.

[33] Dijkman HB, Weening JJ, Smeets B, et al. Proliferating cells in HIV and pamidronate-associated collapsing focal segmental glomerulosclerosis are parietal epithelial cells. Kidney Int 2006;70:338–44.

[34] Sauter M, Julg B, Porubsky S, et al. Nephrotic-range proteinuria following pamidronate therapy in a patient with metastatic breast cancer: mitochondrial toxicity as a pathogenetic concept? Am J Kidney Dis 2006;47:1075–80.

[35] Kunin M, Kopolovic J, Avigdor A, et al. Collapsing glomerulopathy induced by long-term treatment with standard-dose pamidronate in a myeloma patient. Nephrol Dial Transplant 2004;19:723–6.

[36] Barri YM, Munshi NC, Sukumalchantra S, et al. Podocyte injury associated glomerulopathies induced by pamidronate. Kidney Int 2004;65:634–41.

[37] Banerjee D, Asif A, Striker L, et al. Short-term, high-dose pamidronate-induced acute tubular necrosis: the postulated mechanisms of bisphosphonate nephrotoxicity. Am J Kidney Dis 2003;41:E18.

[38] Kyle RA. Multiple myeloma: review of 869 cases. Mayo Clin Proc 1975;50:29–40.

[39] Riccardi A, Gobbi PG, Ucci G, et al. Changing clinical presentation of multiple myeloma. Eur J Cancer 1991;27:1401–5.

[40] Kyle RA, Gertz MA, Witzig TE, et al. Review of 1027 patients with newly diagnosed multiple myeloma. Mayo Clin Proc 2003;78:21–33.

[41] Desai J, Demetri GD. Recombinant human erythropoietin in cancer-related anemia: an evidence-based review. Best Pract Res Clin Haematol 2005;18:389–406.

[42] Garton JP, Gertz MA, Witzig TE, et al. Epoetin alfa for the treatment of the anemia of multiple myeloma. A prospective, randomized, placebo-controlled, double-blind trial. Arch Intern Med 1995;155:2069–74.

[43] Dammacco F, Castoldi G, Rodjer S. Efficacy of epoetin alfa in the treatment of anaemia of multiple myeloma. Br J Haematol 2001;113:172–9.

[44] Osterborg A, Boogaerts MA, Cimino R, et al. Recombinant human erythropoietin in transfusion-dependent anemic patients with multiple myeloma and non-Hodgkin's lymphoma—a randomized multicenter study. The European Study Group of Erythropoietin (Epoetin Beta) Treatment in Multiple Myeloma and Non-Hodgkin's Lymphoma. Blood 1996;87:2675–82.

[45] Singh AK, Szczech L, Tang KL, et al. Correction of anemia with epoetin alfa in chronic kidney disease. N Engl J Med 2006;355:2085–98.

[46] Drueke TB, Locatelli F, Clyne N, et al. Normalization of hemoglobin level in patients with chronic kidney disease and anemia. N Engl J Med 2006;355:2071–84.

[47] Rajkumar SV, Blood E, Vesole D, et al. Phase III clinical trial of thalidomide plus dexamethasone compared with dexamethasone alone in newly diagnosed multiple myeloma: a clinical trial coordinated by the Eastern Cooperative Oncology Group. J Clin Oncol 2006;24:431–6.

[48] Rajkumar SV, Hayman SR, Lacy MQ, et al. Combination therapy with lenalidomide plus dexamethasone (Rev/Dex) for newly diagnosed myeloma. Blood 2005;106:4050–3.

[49] Zangari M, Barlogie B, Anaissie E, et al. Deep vein thrombosis in patients with multiple myeloma treated with thalidomide and chemotherapy: effects of prophylactic and therapeutic anticoagulation. Br J Haematol 2004;126:715–21.

[50] Baz R, Li L, Kottke-Marchant K, et al. The role of aspirin in the prevention of thrombotic complications of thalidomide and anthracycline-based chemotherapy for multiple myeloma. Mayo Clin Proc 2005;80:1568–74.

[51] Rajkumar SV, Blood E. Lenalidomide and venous thrombosis in multiple myeloma. N Engl J Med 2006;354:2079–80.

[52] Knight R, DeLap RJ, Zeldis JB. Lenalidomide and venous thrombosis in multiple myeloma. N Engl J Med 2006;354:2079–80.

[53] Remuzzi G, Ingelfinger JR. Correction of anemia—payoffs and problems. N Engl J Med 2006;355:2144–6.

[54] Leyland-Jones B. Breast cancer trial with erythropoietin terminated unexpectedly. Lancet Oncol 2003;4:459–60.

[55] Nordenson N. Myelomatosis: a clinical review of 310 cases. Acta Med Scand 1966;445(Suppl):178–86.

[56] Osserman EF, Takatsuki K, Talal N. The pathogenesis of "amyloidosis". Semin Hematol 1964;1:3–85.

[57] Edwards GA, Zawadzki ZA. Extraosseous lesions in plasma cell myeloma: a report of six cases. Am J Med 1967;43:194–205.

[58] Kyle RA, Pierre RV, Bayrd ED. Multiple myeloma and acute myelomonocytic leukemia. N Engl J Med 1970;283:1121–5.

[59] Facon T, Mary JY, Pegourie B, et al. Dexamethasone-based regimens versus melphalan-prednisone for elderly multiple myeloma patients ineligible for high-dose therapy. Blood 2006;107:1292–8.

[60] Acute leukaemia and other secondary neoplasms in patients treated with conventional chemotherapy for multiple myeloma: a Finnish Leukaemia Group study. Eur J Haematol 2000;65:123–7.

[61] Cuzick J, Erskine S, Edelman D, et al. A comparison of the incidence of the myelodysplastic syndrome and acute myeloid leukaemia following melphalan and cyclophosphamide treatment for myelomatosis. A report to the Medical Research Council's working party on leukaemia in adults. Br J Cancer 1987;55:523–9.

[62] Bergsagel DE. Chemotherapy of myeloma: drug combinations versus single agents, an overview, and comments on acute leukemia in myeloma. Hematol Oncol 1988;6:159–66.

[63] Oken MM, Harrington DP, Abramson N, et al. Comparison of melphalan and prednisone with vincristine, carmustine, melphalan, cyclophosphamide, and prednisone in the treatment of multiple myeloma: results of Eastern Cooperative Oncology Group Study E2479. Cancer 1997;79:1561–7.

[64] Gonzalez F, Trujillo JM, Alexanian R. Acute leukemia in multiple myeloma. Ann Intern Med 1977;86:440–3.

[65] Bergsagel DE, Bailey AJ, Langley GR, et al. The chemotherapy on plasma-cell myeloma and the incidence of acute leukemia. N Engl J Med 1979;301:743–8.

[66] West WO. Acute erythroid leukemia after cyclophosphamide therapy for multiple myeloma: report of two cases. South Med J 1976;69:1331–2.

[67] Greene MH, Harris EL, Gershenson DM, et al. Melphalan may be a more potent leukemogen than cyclophosphamide. Ann Intern Med 1986;105:360–7.

[68] Govindarajan R, Jagannath S, Flick JT, et al. Preceding standard therapy is the likely cause of MDS after autotransplants for multiple myeloma. Br J Haematol 1996;95:349–53.

[69] Tricot G, Reiner M, Sawyer J, et al. Low frequency of treatment-related myelodysplastic syndromes (t-MDS) after autotransplants (AT) for multiple myeloma (MM), especially if at is applied early during treatment. Blood 2005;106:706.

[70] Rajkumar SV. Current status of thalidomide in the treatment of cancer. Oncology 2001;867–74.

[71] Yakoub-Agha I, Doyen C, Hulin C, et al. A multicenter prospective randomized study testing non-inferiority of thalidomide 100 mg/day as compared with 400 mg/day in patients with refractory/relapsed multiple myeloma: Results of the final analysis of the IFM 01-02 study. J Clin Oncol [Meeting abstracts] 2006;24:7520.

[72] Singhal S, Mehta J, Desikan R, et al. Antitumor activity of thalidomide in refractory multiple myeloma. N Engl J Med 1999;341:1565–71.

[73] Durie BGM, Stephan DE. Efficacy of low dose thalidomide in multiple myeloma [abstract]. Blood 1999;96:168a.

[74] Pini M, Baraldi A, Pietrasanta D, et al. Low-dose of thalidomide in the treatment of refractory myeloma. Haematologica 2000;85:1111–2.

[75] Palumbo A, Giaccone L, Bertola A, et al. Low-dose thalidomide plus dexamethasone is an effective salvage therapy for advanced myeloma. Haematologica 2001;86:399–403.

[76] Coleman M, Leonard J, Lyons L, et al. BLT-D (clarithromycin [Biaxin], low-dose thalidomide, and dexamethasone) for the treatment of myeloma and Waldenstrom's macroglobulinemia. Leuk Lymphoma 2002;43:1777–82.

[77] Rajkumar SV, Gertz MA, Lacy MQ, et al. Thalidomide as initial therapy for early-stage myeloma. Leukemia 2003;17:775–9.

[78] Rajkumar SV, Gertz MA, Witzig TE. Life-threatening toxic epidermal necrolysis with thalidomide therapy for myeloma. N Engl J Med 2000;343:972–3.

[79] Fowler R, Imrie K. Thalidomide-associated hepatitis: a case report. Am J Hematol 2001;66:300–2.

[80] Zangari M, Anaissie E, Barlogie B, et al. Increased risk of deep-vein thrombosis in patients with multiple myeloma receiving thalidomide and chemotherapy. Blood 2001;98:1614–5.

[81] Osman K, Comenzo R, Rajkumar SV. Deep venous thrombosis and thalidomide therapy for multiple myeloma. N Engl J Med 2001;344:1951–2.

[82] Camba L, Peccatori J, Pescarollo A, et al. Thalidomide and thrombosis in patients with multiple myeloma. Haematologica 2001;86:1108–9.

[83] Mileshkin LR, Stark R, Day B, et al. Development of neuropathy in patients (pts) with multiple myeloma (MM) treated with thalidomide (thal)—patterns of occurrence and the role of electrophysiologic monitoring. J Clin Oncol [Meeting abstracts] 2006;24:7618.

[84] Richardson PG, Schlossman RL, Weller E, et al. Immunomodulatory drug CC-5013 overcomes drug resistance and is well tolerated in patients with relapsed multiple myeloma. Blood 2002;100:3063–7.

[85] Richardson PG, Blood E, Mitsiades CS, et al. A randomized phase 2 study of lenalidomide therapy for patients with relapsed or relapsed and refractory multiple myeloma. Blood 2006;108:3458–64.

[86] Palumbo A, Bringhen S, Caravita T, et al. Oral melphalan and prednisone chemotherapy plus thalidomide compared with melphalan and prednisone alone in elderly patients with multiple myeloma: randomised controlled trial. Lancet 2006;367:825–31.

[87] Palumbo A, Falco P, Benevolo G, et al. Oral lenalidomide plus melphalan and prednisone (R-MP) for newly diagnosed multiple myeloma. J Clin Oncol [Meeting abstracts] 2006;24:7518.

[88] Jimenez VH, Dominguez V, Reynoso E, et al. Thromboprophylaxis with aspirin for newly diagnosed multiple myeloma treated with thalidomide plus dexamethasone: a preliminary report. Blood 2006;108(11):5091.

[89] Hideshima T, Mitsiades C, Akiyama M, et al. Molecular mechanisms mediating antimyeloma activity of proteasome inhibitor PS-341. Blood 2003;101:1530–4.

[90] Richardson PG, Sonneveld P, Schuster MW, et al. Bortezomib or high-dose dexamethasone for relapsed multiple myeloma. N Engl J Med 2005;352:2487–98.

[91] Jagannath S, Durie BG, Wolf J, et al. Bortezomib therapy alone and in combination with dexamethasone for previously untreated symptomatic multiple myeloma. Br J Haematol 2005;129:776–83.

[92] Richardson PG, Briemberg H, Jagannath S, et al. Frequency, characteristics, and reversibility of peripheral neuropathy during treatment of advanced multiple myeloma with bortezomib. J Clin Oncol 2006;24:3113–20.

[93] Miyakoshi S, Kami M, Yuji K, et al. Severe pulmonary complications in Japanese patients after bortezomib treatment for refractory multiple myeloma. Blood 2006;107:3492–4.

[94] Jagannath S, Barlogie B, Berenson J, et al. A phase 2 study of two doses of bortezomib in relapsed or refractory myeloma. Br J Haematol 2004;127:165–72.

[95] Berenson JR, Jagannath S, Barlogie B, et al. Safety of prolonged therapy with bortezomib in relapsed or refractory multiple myeloma. Cancer 2005;104:2141–8.

[96] Thorn GW, Forsham PH, Frawley RF, et al. The clinical usefulness of ACTH and cortisone. N Engl J Med 1950;242:824.

[97] Feinman R, Koury J, Thames M, et al. Role of NF-kappaB in the rescue of multiple myeloma cells from glucocorticoid-induced apoptosis by bcl-2. Blood 1999;93:3044–52.

[98] Karadag A, Oyajobi BO, Apperley JF, et al. Human myeloma cells promote the production of interleukin 6 by primary human osteoblasts. Br J Haematol 2000;108:383–90.

[99] De Bosscher K, Vanden Berghe W, Vermeulen L, et al. Glucocorticoids repress NF-kappaB-driven genes by disturbing the interaction of p65 with the basal transcription machinery, irrespective of coactivator levels in the cell. Proc Natl Acad Sci U S A 2000;97:3919–24.

[100] Kawano M, Tanaka H, Ishikawa H, et al. Interleukin-1 accelerates autocrine growth of myeloma cells through interleukin-6 in human myeloma. Blood 1989;73:2145–8.

[101] Alexanian R, Yap BS, Bodey GP. Prednisone pulse therapy for refractory myeloma. Blood 1983;62:572–7.

[102] Alexanian R, Barlogie B, Dixon D. High-dose glucocorticoid treatment of resistant myeloma. Ann Intern Med 1986;105:8–11.

[103] Gertz MA, Garton JP, Greipp PR, et al. A phase II study of high-dose methylprednisolone in refractory or relapsed multiple myeloma. Leukemia 1995;9:2115–8.

[104] Weber D, Rankin K, Gavino M, et al. Thalidomide alone or with dexamethasone for previously untreated multiple myeloma. J Clin Oncol 2003;21:16–9.

[105] Jagannath S, Richardson PG, Barlogie B, et al. Bortezomib in combination with dexamethasone for the treatment of patients with relapsed and/or refractory multiple myeloma with less than optimal response to bortezomib alone. Haematologica 2006;91:929–34.

[106] Mass RE. A comparison of the effect of prednisone and a placebo in the treatment of multiple myeloma. Cancer Chemother Rep 1962;16:257–9.

[107] Palva IP, Ala-Harja K, Almqvist A, et al. Corticosteroid is not beneficial in multiple-drug combination chemotherapy for multiple myeloma. Finnish Leukaemia Group. Eur J Haematol 1993;51:98–101.

[108] Rajkumar SV, Jacobus S, Callander N, et al. A randomized phase III trial of lenalidomide plus high-dose dexamethasone versus lenalidomide plus low-dose dexamethasone in newly diagnosed multiple myeloma (e4a03): a Trial Coordinated by the Eastern Cooperative Oncology Group [abstract]. Blood 2006;108:799.

[109] Bennett JM, Silber R, Ezdinli E, et al. Phase II study of Adriamycin and bleomycin in patients with multiple myeloma. Cancer Treat Rep 1978;62:1367–9.

[110] Alberts DS, Salmon SE. Adriamycin (NSC-123127) in the treatment of alkylator-resistant multiple myeloma: a pilot study. Cancer Chemother Rep 1975;59:345–50.

[111] Takemura G, Fujiwara H. Doxorubicin-induced cardiomyopathy from the cardiotoxic mechanisms to management. Prog Cardiovasc Dis 2007;49:330–52.

[112] Lefrak EA, Pitha J, Rosenheim S, et al. A clinicopathologic analysis of Adriamycin cardiotoxicity. Cancer 1973;32:302–14.

[113] Aviles A, Neri N, Nambo JM, et al. Late cardiac toxicity secondary to treatment in Hodgkin's disease. A study comparing doxorubicin, epirubicin and mitoxantrone in combined therapy. Leuk Lymphoma 2005;46:1023–8.

[114] Elbl L, Hrstkova H, Tomaskova I, et al. Late anthracycline cardiotoxicity protection by dexraxane (ICRF-187) in pediatric patients: echocardiographic follow-up. Support Care Cancer 2006;14:128–36.

[115] Ma MH, Yang HH, Parker K, et al. The proteasome inhibitor PS-341 markedly enhances sensitivity of multiple myeloma tumor cells to chemotherapeutic agents. Clin Cancer Res 2003;9:1136–44.

[116] Rifkin RM, Gregory SA, Mohrbacher A, et al. Pegylated liposomal doxorubicin, vincristine, and dexamethasone provide significant reduction in toxicity compared with doxorubicin, vincristine, and dexamethasone in patients with newly diagnosed multiple myeloma: a Phase III multicenter randomized trial. Cancer 2006;106:848–58.

[117] Orlowski RZ, Voorhees PM, Garcia RA, et al. Phase 1 trial of the proteasome inhibitor bortezomib and pegylated liposomal doxorubicin in patients with advanced hematologic malignancies. Blood 2005;105:3058–65.

[118] Jackson DV, Case LD, Pope EK, et al. Single agent vincristine by infusion in refractory multiple myeloma. J Clin Oncol 1985;3:1508–12.

[119] Salmon SE. Immunoglobulin synthesis and tumor kinetics of multiple myeloma. Semin Hematol 1973;10:135–44.

[120] Alexanian R, Salmon S, Bonnet J, et al. Combination therapy for multiple myeloma. Cancer 1977;40:2765–71.

[121] Alexanian R, Dreicer R. Chemotherapy for multiple myeloma. Cancer 1984;53:583–8.

[122] Cornwell GG 3rd, Pajak TF, Kochwa S, et al. Comparison of oral melphalan, CCNU, and BCNU with and without vincristine and prednisone in the treatment of multiple myeloma. Cancer and Leukemia Group B experience. Cancer 1982;50:1669–75.

[123] Hansen OP, Clausen NA, Drivsholm A, et al. Phase III study of intermittent 5-drug regimen (VBCMP) versus intermittent 3-drug regimen (VMP) versus intermittent melphalan and prednisone (MP) in myelomatosis. Scand J Haematol 1985;35:518–24.

[124] MacLennan IC, Cusick J. Objective evaluation of the role of vincristine in induction and maintenance therapy for myelomatosis. Medical Research Council Working Party on Leukaemia in Adults. Br J Cancer 1985;52:153–8.

[125] Tribalto M, Amadori S, Cantonetti M, et al. Treatment of multiple myeloma: a randomized study of three different regimens. Leuk Res 1985;9:1043–9.

[126] Rousselot P, Labaume S, Marolleau JP, et al. Arsenic trioxide and melarsoprol induce apoptosis in plasma cell lines and in plasma cells from myeloma patients. Cancer Res 1999;59:1041–8.

[127] Kalmadi SR, Hussein MA. The emerging role of arsenic trioxide as an immunomodulatory agent in the management of multiple myeloma. Acta Haematol 2006;116:1–7.

[128] Munshi NC, Tricot G, Desikan R, et al. Clinical activity of arsenic trioxide for the treatment of multiple myeloma. Leukemia 2002;16:1835–7.

[129] Hussein MA, Saleh M, Ravandi F, et al. Phase 2 study of arsenic trioxide in patients with relapsed or refractory multiple myeloma. Br J Haematol 2004;125:470–6.

[130] Abou-Jawde RM, Reed J, Kelly M, et al. Efficacy and safety results with the combination therapy of arsenic trioxide, dexamethasone, and ascorbic acid in multiple myeloma patients: a phase 2 trial. Med Oncol 2006;23:263–72.

[131] Zervas K, Dimopoulos MA, Hatzicharissi E, et al. Primary treatment of multiple myeloma with thalidomide, vincristine, liposomal doxorubicin and dexamethasone (T-VAD Doxil): a phase II multicenter study. Ann Oncol 2004;15:134–8.

[132] Hussein MA, Wood L, Hsi E, et al. A Phase II trial of pegylated liposomal doxorubicin, vincristine, and reduced-dose dexamethasone combination therapy in newly diagnosed multiple myeloma patients. Cancer 2002;95:2160–8.

[133] Ciolli S, Leoni F, Gigli F, et al. Low dose Velcade, thalidomide and dexamethasone (LD-VTD): an effective regimen for relapsed and refractory multiple myeloma patients. Leuk Lymphoma 2006;47:171–3.

[134] Zangari M, Barlogi B, Jacobson J, et al. VTD regimen comprising Velcade (V) + thalidomide (T) and added DEX (D) for non-responders to V + T effects a 57% PR Rate among 56 patients with myeloma (M) relapsing after autologous transplant. Blood 2003;102: 830a.

[135] Wang M, Delasalle K, Giralt S, et al. Rapid control of previously untreated multiple myeloma with bortezomib-thalidomide-dexamethasone followed by early intensive therapy. Blood 2005; [784].

[136] Oakervee HE, Popat R, Curry N, et al. PAD combination therapy (PS-341/bortezomib, doxorubicin and dexamethasone) for previously untreated patients with multiple myeloma. Br J Haematol 2005;129:755–62.

[137] Orlowski RZ, Peterson BL, Sanford B, et al. Bortezomib and pegylated liposomal doxorubicin as induction therapy for adult patients with symptomatic multiple myeloma: Cancer and Leukemia Group B Study 10301. Blood 2006;108(11):797.

[138] Orlowski RZ, Zhuang SH, Parekh T, et al, the DOXIL-MMY-3001 Study Investigators. The combination of pegylated liposomal doxorubicin and bortezomib significantly improves time to progression of patients with relapsed/refractory multiple myeloma compared with bortezomib alone: results from a planned interim analysis of a randomized phase III study. Blood 2006;108(11):404.

[139] Facon T, Mary J, Harousseau J, et al. Superiority of melphalan-prednisone (MP) + thalidomide (THAL) over MP and autologous stem cell transplantation in the treatment of newly diagnosed elderly patients with multiple myeloma. J Clin Oncol [Meeting abstracts] 2006;24:1.

[140] Harousseau JL, Attal M, Leleu X, et al. Bortezomib plus dexamethasone as induction treatment prior to autologous stem cell transplantation in patients with newly diagnosed multiple myeloma: results of an IFM phase II study. Haematologica 2006;91:1498–505.

[141] Augustson BM, Begum G, Dunn JA, et al. Early mortality after diagnosis of multiple myeloma: analysis of patients entered onto the United Kingdom medical research council trials between 1980 and 2002—Medical Research Council Adult Leukaemia Working Party. J Clin Oncol 2005;23:9219–26.

[142] Dispenzieri A, Rajkumar SV, Gertz MA, et al. Treatment of newly diagnosed multiple myeloma based on Mayo stratification of myeloma and risk-adapted therapy (mSMART): consensus statement. Mayo Clin Proc 2007;82:323–41.

INDEX

0889-8588/07/$ – see front matter
doi:10.1016/S0889-8588(07)00156-6

Moving?

Make sure your subscription moves with you!

To notify us of your new address, find your **Clinics Account Number** (located on your mailing label above your name), and contact customer service at:

E-mail: elspcs@elsevier.com

800-654-2452 (subscribers in the U.S. & Canada)
407-345-4000 (subscribers outside of the U.S. & Canada)

Fax number: 407-363-9661

Elsevier Periodicals Customer Service
6277 Sea Harbor Drive
Orlando, FL 32887-4800

*To ensure uninterrupted delivery of your subscription, please notify us at least 4 weeks in advance of move.